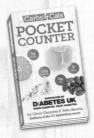

POC

★ Over 7

★ Great a
CARB

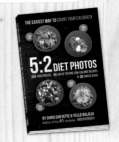

5:2 DIET PHOTOS

★ Delicious inspiration for your fasting days

★ Helps you stick to your 500 calorie budget

★ 600 photos, 60 recipes and 30 snack ideas

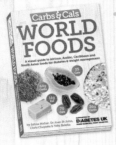

WORLD FOODS

★ 750 photos of food & drinks from African, Arabic, Caribbean & South Asian communities

★ Uses new 'blood glucose icons' to show food's possible effect on blood glucose levels

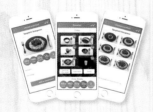

MOBILE APP

Available for iPhone & Android

★ Over 3,500 photos (inc branded foods)

★ The perfect portable calorie counter for weight loss, portion control & diabetes

PLUS...
FREE HEALTH RESOURCES

FREE!

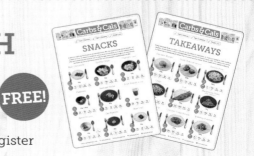

★ Register for FREE access to 50 PDF resources

★ www.carbsandcals.com/register

www.carbsandcals.com

Carbs & Cals

CARB & CALORIE COUNTER

Count your carbs & calories with over 1,700 food photos!

6TH EDITION

First published in Great Britain in 2010
by Chello Publishing Limited
Registered Company Number 7237986

www.chellopublishing.co.uk | info@chellopublishing.co.uk

Copyright © Chello Publishing Limited 2016

In memory of our dear friend Tom Rawlins

With special thanks to: Anita Beckwith, Barry & Joan Cheyette, Dave Charlton, Dougie Twenefour, Eleana Papadopoulou, Emma Jenkins, Fran Turner, George Malache, Jasmine Walton, Justine Rose, Marianne Ouaknin, Maxine Gregory, Pat & Akbar Balolia, Peter Rose, Ravinder Kundi, Sean O'Dell, Simon Callaghan, Stuey McMillan, Victoria Francis, Yoshi Balolia, Zoë Harrison, DSG committee of the BDA, and Diabetes UK.

The information contained in this book is not a substitute for medical or other professional guidance. Please consult your GP before making any alterations to medications or changing medical treatment. Although all reasonable care has been taken in the writing of this book, the authors and publisher are not responsible for any specific health needs; they do not accept any legal responsibility or liability for any personal injury or other consequences, damage or loss arising from any use of information and advice contained within this book.

The authors have asserted their moral rights.

ISBN: 978-1-908261-15-1 Printed in the UK 0919

Authors	Chris Cheyette BSc (Hons) MSc RD
	Yello Balolia BA (Hons)
Photography (food portions)	Yello Balolia BA (Hons)
Design Concept	George F Malache
Graphic Design	Maxine Gregory BA (Hons)
Additional Layout	Yello Balolia BA (Hons)
Introduction Text	Chris Cheyette BSc (Hons) MSc RD
	Eleana Papadopoulou MPH MSc (Oxon) RD
	Victoria Francis BSc (Hons) RD
Editing & Proofreading	Yoshi Balolia BA (Hons) PGCE

For more information, please visit: **www.carbsandcals.com**

 Contents

Foreword by Diabetes UK 4
Introduction 5
  Nutrients in our food 9
  Guide to weight loss 18
  Diabetes 22
  How to use this book 30
Food Photos 32
  Biscuits & Crackers 32
  Bread 38
  Breakfast 49
  Cakes & Bakery 67
  Cheese 77
  Desserts 84
  Drinks 99
  Eggs 114
  Fruit 117
  Gluten Free 136
  Meals 144
  Meal Accompaniments 167
  Meat, Chicken & Fish 170
  Milk & Cream 195
  Nuts & Seeds 201
  Pasta & Noodles 206
  Potatoes & Tubers 221
  Rice & Grains 233
  Sandwiches 244
  Snacks & Confectionery 247
  Soup 257
  Spreads & Sauces 260
  Vegetables & Pulses 278
  Vegetarian Alternatives 306
  Yogurt 308
Eating Out 311
Index 340
About the Authors / Awards 352

Foreword

Carbohydrate counting is an important part of diabetes management, especially for people with Type 1 diabetes.

Carbs & Cals is a great tool for those people with diabetes who count carbohydrates as part of the management of their condition. This easy-to-use visual reference guide allows you to compare what is on your plate with the pictures in the book, to find out the amount of carbohydrate and calories in the food you are eating. Knowing how many calories are in a portion of food is also really helpful information for people who are trying to lose weight, and may let you know that you need to eat a smaller portion or opt for something a little healthier.

Having all of this information at your fingertips, in an easy to understand format, will help to give you greater control over your diabetes and also give you the information you need to help you make healthier choices at meal times. Whatever your goals, we are sure that you will find Carbs & Cals a great help in achieving them.

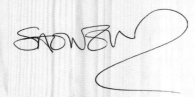

Simon O'Neill
Director of Health Intelligence and Professional Liaison
Diabetes UK

DIABETES UK
KNOW DIABETES. FIGHT DIABETES.

www.diabetes.org.uk

Introduction

Welcome to *Carbs & Cals*. This book contains over 1,700 photos of a wide range of popular food and drink items. The carbohydrate, calorie, protein, fat, saturated fat and fibre values are clearly displayed in colour-coded circles below each photo. This highly visual approach makes it incredibly quick and easy to see the nutrient content of the food and drink you consume. *Carbs & Cals* is the perfect support tool for carbohydrate counting in diabetes, weight management, portion control and general healthy eating.

Healthy Eating Principles

A healthy, balanced diet is important for maintaining good health, as it improves general wellbeing, helps with weight management and reduces the risk of long-term conditions such as heart disease, type 2 diabetes and cancer.

What does 'healthy eating' really mean?

Nutrients such as proteins, fats, vitamins and minerals are the building blocks for good health. Foods within our diet are grouped together according to the main nutrients they provide e.g. meat, fish, eggs and nuts are grouped as high quality proteins whilst milk, cheese and yogurt are grouped as dairy foods and are a rich source of calcium. Healthy eating means eating a wide variety of nutrient dense foods in the right proportions to achieve and maintain a healthy balanced weight and provide a range of nutrients such as:

* Antioxidants, vitamins and minerals from fruit and vegetables
* Calcium from dairy foods such as milk and yogurt
* B vitamins and fibre from wholegrain carbohydrates such as oats, pearl barley and brown rice
* Good quality protein from meat, fish, nuts, eggs and quinoa
* Omega-3 oils from oily fish and nuts

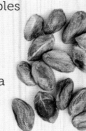

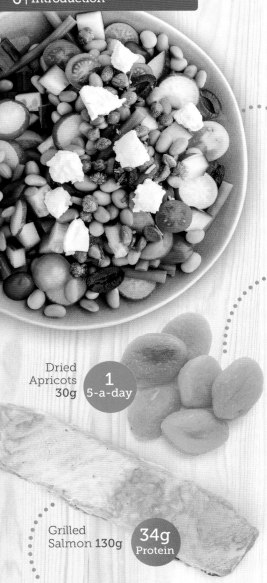

Tips for Healthy Eating

Aim for three meals each day

Avoid skipping meals and spread breakfast, lunch and dinner across the day to keep your energy levels topped up and help you avoid snacking.

Reach your 5-a-day fruit & veg!

The World Health Organisation recommends eating a minimum of 5 portions of fruit and vegetables each day to reduce the risk of long-term conditions such as heart disease and type 2 diabetes. They are packed with vitamins and minerals, are excellent sources of dietary fibre and are low in fat and calories. When choosing fruit & veg, select a rainbow of colours, as this will provide a wider variety of vitamins and minerals.

Dried Apricots 30g

1 5-a-day

Grilled Salmon 130g

34g Protein

Eat more fish!

Fish is a good source of protein. It is recommended to have at least 2 portions of fish per week, including 1 portion of oily fish, such as mackerel, salmon, fresh tuna or trout. Oily fish contains a type of polyunsaturated fat called omega-3, which lowers triglyceride levels and helps protect against heart disease. People with diabetes are advised to have at least 2 portions of oily fish per week.

Eat more plant based proteins such as beans and lentils

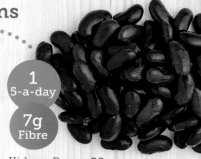

Pulses such as beans, peas and lentils are a cheap source of protein and have many nutritional benefits, including:

★ Count as one of your 5-a-day
★ Low in fat and calories
★ High in soluble fibre (known to improve cholesterol levels)
★ If you have diabetes, pulses have minimal effect on your blood glucose levels

1 5-a-day

7g Fibre

Kidney Beans **80g**

Choose wholegrain carbohydrates

Wholegrain carbohydrates provide energy, are a good source of B vitamins and a great source of fibre. Examples of wholegrain foods include wholegrain breakfast cereals such as porridge, whole wheat pasta, wholegrain bread, and brown rice.

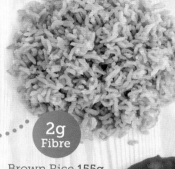

2g Fibre

Brown Rice **155g**

Limit sugar and sugary foods

Latest guidelines are to limit our added sugar ('free sugar') intake to 30g per day, to address the increasing obesity and type 2 diabetes epidemic. You can enjoy a small amount of sugar as part of your healthy diet, but choose sugar free options where possible, for example sugar free or diet fizzy drinks/squash. Cutting down your sugar intake will help with weight maintenance, weight loss and dental health.

Choose lower fat dairy products

Milk, yogurts and cheese are a great source of calcium, which is important for keeping our bones and teeth strong. Aim for 3 portions of dairy per day (one portion is 200ml milk, 125g pot yogurt or matchbox size cheese).

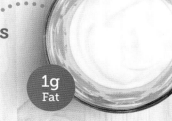

1g Fat

Natural Yogurt (low fat) **125g**

Choose healthy fats

Choose foods high in monounsaturated fats (such as avocado, olive oil and nuts) and polyunsaturated fats (oily fish and seeds). Limit saturated fat, to maintain healthy cholesterol levels and for heart health. Good suggestions include:

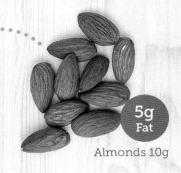

5g Fat

Almonds 10g

★ Choose lean meat cuts and limit the amount of processed meat, such as burgers and sausages
★ Remove the visible fat from meat, and skin from chicken
★ Use olive oil in cooking and salad dressings
★ Nuts are a great nutritious snack compared to chocolate or crisps

Drink alcohol in moderation

New guidelines (currently in consultation) recommend that men and women do not drink more than 14 units of alcohol per week and that it is best spread evenly across the week. Having several alcohol free days a week is a good way to cut down. If weight maintenance or weight loss is your goal, cutting back on alcohol will help, as alcohol is high in calories and these calories have no nutritional value.

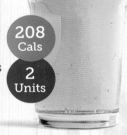

208 Cals

2 Units

Limit salt intake to 6g per day

A diet that is high in salt can raise your blood pressure, increasing the risk of stroke and heart disease. Use herbs and spices, instead of salt, for flavour and where possible aim to cook fresh rather than relying on processed foods. Read labels to choose lower salt options where possible.

Diabetic products

Diabetic foods are of no benefit to people with diabetes. They tend to be more expensive than the conventional products, can be high in fat and calories, often still affect blood glucose levels and may have a laxative effect.

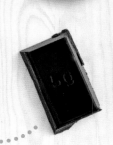

Nutrients in our food

Carbohydrate

The term carbohydrate encompasses a variety of foods, from the sugar we put in our hot drinks to the humble potato. Carbohydrate has become a forbidden word in recent times, in part due to the rise of celebrity fad diets. However, our bodies need it! It is the body's main source of glucose for energy and the brain's preferred source of energy!

The two main types are starchy carbohydrates and sugars. Starchy carbohydrates include bread, pasta, chapatis, potatoes, yam and cereals. Sugars can be categorised as natural sugars and added sugars (or 'free sugars'). Free sugars include those added to food by manufacturers, cooks or consumers (such as granulated sugar) and those naturally present in honey, syrups and unsweetened fruit juice.

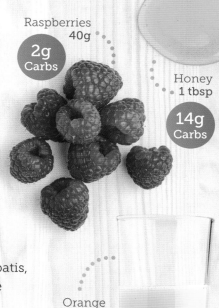

Raspberries
40g

2g
Carbs

Honey
1 tbsp

14g
Carbs

Orange
Juice
150ml

12g
Carbs

Natural Sugars	Free Sugars	
Fruit sugar (known as fructose) is present in all types of whole fruit	Table sugar (sucrose)	Honey
Milk sugar (known as lactose) is present in milk and yogurt	Glucose syrup	Unsweetened fruit juice

How much carbohydrate should I eat each day?

Carbohydrate requirements vary depending on:

★ gender　　★ age　　★ weight　　★ physical activity

Science does not support the popular belief that starchy foods cause more weight gain than other foods. Starchy foods, fruit and vegetables should probably contribute around 50% of your energy needs. Some people may prefer to get more of their calories from other food groups and thus have a lower carbohydrate intake. For people with diabetes, there is a lot of debate in support of a lower carbohydrate intake to improve long-term blood glucose control. However, this may not be appropriate for everyone, and there is no evidence that this approach is better than others in the long term, which is why Diabetes UK guidelines encourage the need for an individualised approach.

Sugar should not play such a significant role in our diets!

In 2015, the Scientific Advisory Committee on Nutrition (SACN) updated its recommendations on the amount of free sugars in our diet, to address the growing obesity and diabetes crisis and reduce the risk of tooth decay.

4-6 year old
19g per day
(5 cubes)

7-10 year old
24g per day
(6 cubes)

What are the new recommendations and what does that mean to your daily diet?

SACN advises that free sugars should account for no more than 5% of a person's daily energy intake.

11 years +
30g per day
(7 cubes)

The NHS Change4Life campaign has introduced 'Sugar Swaps' to help people reduce their sugar intake and reach these new recommendations. Simple practical sugar swap ideas include:

★ Replacing a sugary drink with a diet drink
★ Choosing a plain oatcake or crackers instead of a sweet biscuit
★ Replace sugar coated breakfast cereals with wholegrain plain cereals such as wheat biscuits

change
4 life

Protein

Why do you need protein?

Sources of protein include meat, fish, eggs, pulses, nuts and tofu. Protein has a number of uses in the human body:

* Cell growth
* Maintenance and repair of cells
* Proper functioning of the immune system
* Production of hormones and enzymes

How much do you need?

For most adults, 1g of protein per kg of body weight is enough to meet the daily requirements. If you weigh 70kg, for example, a protein intake of 70g is sufficient. In the UK, protein intake is usually in excess of requirements.

Endurance and strength athletes are likely to require higher amounts of protein in their diet (up to 1.7g per kg of body weight per day). Protein acts as an additional source of fuel and also provides the building blocks for muscle repair and development.

Can I eat more than the recommendations?

Some high protein foods (such as full fat dairy products and meat) are high in saturated fat, which is not good for heart health. Eating larger quantities of protein has not been shown to improve sports performance or increase muscle mass. The body is only able to use a certain amount of protein and eating large amounts offers no additional nutritional benefit. Excess intake of protein is not advisable for people with kidney disease.

9g Protein
Tofu 40g

Cashews 10g

2g Protein

42g Protein
Tuna Steak 130g

3g Protein
Chickpeas 40g

64g Protein
Chicken Breast 200g

Fried Egg
8g Protein

Fat

Why is fat an essential part of our diet?

- ★ It is a major source of energy for the body
- ★ It is essential for the absorption of the fat-soluble vitamins A, D, E and K
- ★ It insulates the body and provides a protective layer around the essential organs
- ★ It is a structural component of all cell membranes

Main types of fat

Type / Source	Effect on body
Saturated fat Animal sources, such as meat fat and processed meat, milk, cheese and butter, and also in vegetable sources, such as coconut oil and palm oil	Raises total cholesterol levels and unhealthy LDL cholesterol levels, increasing the risk of heart disease
	May impair glucose control by increasing insulin resistance
Monounsaturated fat Olive and rapeseed oil, some nuts and seeds, avocados and in some spreads	Lowers unhealthy LDL cholesterol levels, but does not lower healthy HDL levels, thus decreasing the risk of heart disease
Polyunsaturated fat Sunflower oil and spreads, corn oil, oily fish (such as mackerel), nuts and seeds	Lowers unhealthy LDL cholesterol levels, but may also lower healthy HDL cholesterol levels
	Omega-3, found in oily fish, lowers blood triglyceride levels

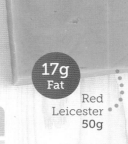

17g Fat

Red Leicester 50g

Pumpkin Seeds 10g

5g Fat

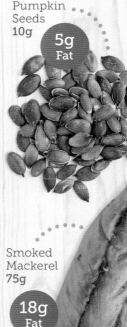

Smoked Mackerel 75g

18g Fat

Information on the fat and saturated fat content of foods and drinks is included in this book to help you to monitor your fat intake and stay within your requirements.

The table below shows the adult reference intake (RI, formerly known as GDA) for fat and saturated fat. The RIs for an adult are based on the requirements for an average female with no special dietary requirements and an assumed energy intake of 2000 calories. Your individual needs may be higher or lower, depending on your calorie requirements and your specific nutritional goals.

Energy or nutrient	Reference Intake
Energy	2000 calories
Total Fat	70g
Saturated Fat	20g

Why should we watch our intake of fat?

Fat contains the most calories per gram when compared to carbohydrate, protein and alcohol. Therefore, eating too much of it can lead to weight gain, which increases the risk of heart disease, type 2 diabetes and some cancers.

A word on processed foods

The term 'processed' applies to any food that has been altered from its natural state in some way, either for safety reasons or convenience. Meats including salami, bacon, sausages, ham and pâté all come under the umbrella of processed meats. When meat is preserved by smoking, curing or salting, or by the addition of preservatives, cancer-causing substances (carcinogens) can be formed.

There is strong evidence linking the consumption of processed meat with bowel cancer. Therefore, the Department of Health has advised that people who eat more than 90g (cooked weight) of red and processed meat a day cut down to 70g (500g per week) and choose unprocessed meat where possible, or turn to a plant source of protein instead e.g. beans, soya, nuts and seeds.

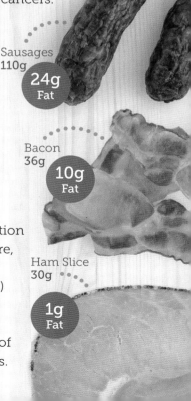

Sausages
110g

24g
Fat

Bacon
36g

10g
Fat

Ham Slice
30g

1g
Fat

Fibre

What is all the fuss about fibre?

Dietary fibre is only found in foods of plant origin, such as fruit, vegetables, cereals and pulses. It has no calories and it passes through the gut largely undigested. There are two types of fibre, soluble and insoluble, and most foods containing fibre have a mixture of the two.

4g Fibre

Apple Rings 30g

Why should we eat it?

Strong evidence shows that increasing total fibre intake, particularly cereal grains and wholegrains, is associated with a lower risk of cardio-metabolic disease and colo-rectal cancer. Increasing fibre intake can help with weight loss, as it slows down the rate at which the stomach is emptying, helping to keep you fuller for longer. The proven benefits of fibre have led to the SACN revising its recommendations and advising people to increase their daily intake of fibre.

3g Fibre

Mango 80g

The new recommendations are:

Age Range	Fibre Intake per day
2 - 5	15g
5 - 11	20g
11 - 16	25g
16 - 18 and older	30g

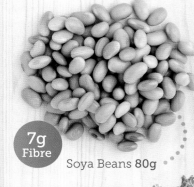

7g Fibre

Soya Beans 80g

How can we reach our 30g fibre per day?

The National Diet and Nutrition Survey in 2011 found that the most commonly consumed food type was bread. This would explain why the average fibre intake is only 19g per day. If we are to meet these new recommendations, we need to change our eating habits. This book can help you work out if you are meeting your daily fibre requirement.

3g Fibre

Muesli 30g

Simple swaps

Corn Flakes v Muesli

Oats and fruit boost the intake of soluble fibre, to help slow down the rate at which glucose enters the bloodstream.

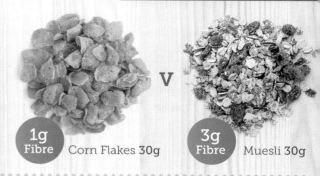

V

1g Fibre — Corn Flakes 30g

3g Fibre — Muesli 30g

Rice v Pearl Barley

Soluble fibre forms a gel-like substance in the stomach, keeping us feeling full for longer.

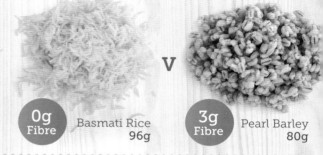

V

0g Fibre — Basmati Rice 96g

3g Fibre — Pearl Barley 80g

Crisps v Nuts

Soluble fibre in nuts can help lower cholesterol, reducing the risk of heart disease and stroke.

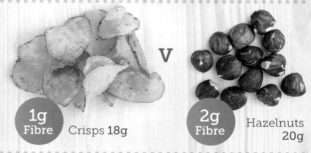

V

1g Fibre — Crisps 18g

2g Fibre — Hazelnuts 20g

White Bread v Granary Bread

Increases the intake of insoluble fibre, which speeds up the time it takes for food to pass through your gut, so aids a healthy, regular digestive system.

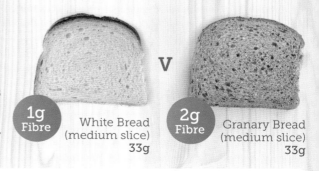

V

1g Fibre — White Bread (medium slice) 33g

2g Fibre — Granary Bread (medium slice) 33g

Important note: Any increase in dietary fibre consumption should be accompanied by an increase in fluid intake.

Alcohol

Although most people can enjoy moderate consumption of alcohol safely, exceeding the recommended limit of 14 units per week and/or binge drinking can contribute to a number of health problems, such as liver disease, cancer, high blood pressure and obesity.

Do you know the limit?

This is what 14 units looks like:

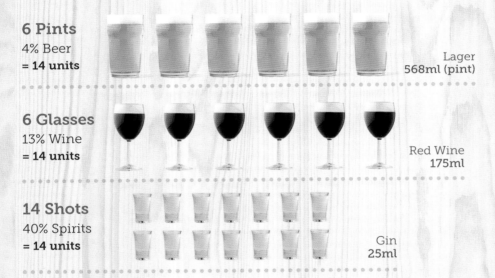

6 Pints
4% Beer
= 14 units

Lager
568ml (pint)

6 Glasses
13% Wine
= 14 units

Red Wine
175ml

14 Shots
40% Spirits
= 14 units

Gin
25ml

Over the years, the alcohol content of most drinks has risen and a drink may therefore contain more units of alcohol than you think. The number of units each alcoholic drink portion contains has been included in this book to make it easier for you to monitor your alcohol intake.

Does alcohol provide any nutritional benefit?

Alcohol contains 7 calories per gram and these are usually 'empty calories', meaning they are of no nutritional value – an important consideration for weight management.

To keep on top of your calorie intake, choose sugar free mixers instead of sugary ones or fruit juice.

Calories

Calories are not nutrients in themselves; they are actually the units used to measure the amount of energy in food and drink. The number of calories varies according to the nutritional composition of each item of food and drink we consume. The calorie content per gram of carbohydrate, protein, fat and alcohol is as follows:

1g carbohydrate = 4 cals

1g protein = 4 cals

1g fat = 9 cals

1g alcohol = 7 cals

Fat has twice the amount of calories per gram compared to carbohydrate and protein, which explains why if you eat foods that are high in fat, you are likely to consume more calories and gain weight.

How many calories should I aim for each day?

Age, gender, physical activity levels and weight goal (maintenance, weight loss or gain) all affect your calorie requirements. A registered dietitian can help give you a more accurate idea. The reference intake for calories is 2,000 for an average adult, who has no special dietary needs.

Why count calories?

Calorie counting helps you understand the number of calories in food and drink you consume. You can then choose appropriate food to avoid excess, select healthier options (usually lower fat options) and maintain a healthy weight. If you are currently gaining weight, this indicates that you are consuming more calories than you burn through physical activity and while doing your everyday activities. This can easily happen:

100 cals per day extra = **36,500 cals** over a year = Weight gain of around **5kg / 11 lb** in one year

This book makes it easier to see where you can reduce portion sizes or make lower fat and calorie choices in order to lose weight. It can also help you to identify where you can make small changes that actually make a big overall difference.

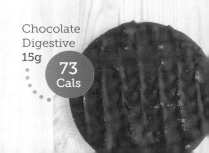

Chocolate Digestive 15g

73 Cals

Guide to weight loss

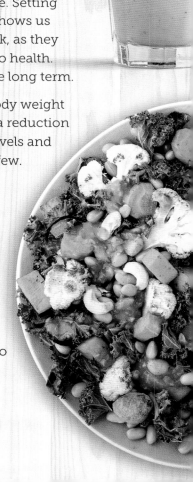

Take a moment to ask yourself:

★ Why do I want to lose weight?
★ What is my weight goal (realistic goal)?
★ What have I tried before that has worked?
★ What hasn't worked before in the past (e.g. diet too strict)?
★ What support do I need? Is it the right time for me?

Losing weight in a healthy way is a big challenge. Setting yourself realistic expectations is key! Evidence shows us that short term 'quick fix' diets don't usually work, as they are unsustainable and may even be dangerous to health. Losing weight gradually is more beneficial in the long term.

Studies have shown that losing 5-10% of your body weight can bring significant health benefits, including a reduction in blood pressure, cholesterol and triglyceride levels and a lowered risk of type 2 diabetes, to name just a few.

Keeping the weight off can be even harder. Some words of support:

★ If you don't achieve your target/re-gain some of the weight you lost, do not despair! Accept the occasional slip up as a learning experience, focus on your aim and always remember your hard work and the progress you have made.
★ Whatever your goals may be, it is important to discuss your diet plan and what you want to get out of it with your healthcare team. Let them know your main aim and they will help you set realistic short-term goals to help you get there.

What is a healthy weight?

Your Body Mass Index (BMI) is a measure of your weight in relation to your height, and tells you whether you are a healthy weight. You can use our online BMI calculator at www.carbsandcals.com/BMI, ask your healthcare team, or work it out yourself using the following equation:

$$BMI = Weight_{(kg)} \div Height_{(m)}^2$$

For example, if your weight is 72kg and your height is 1.68m, then your BMI = 72 ÷ (1.68 x 1.68) = 25.5 kg/m². Once you have your BMI, you can see which range it falls into by comparing it to this table:

BMI (kg/m²)	Category
Under 18.5	Underweight
18.5 - 24.9 Asian: 18.5 - 22.9	Healthy weight
25 - 29.9	Overweight
30 - 35	Obese
Over 35	Morbidly obese

Important note: If you have a large amount of muscle, your BMI may be in the overweight range, even though you have little body fat. People from black, Asian and minority ethnic backgrounds should aim for low BMI cut-offs.

Waist circumference, an indication of body fat distribution, is another way to check your weight. Measure the circumference of your waist at the midway point between the bottom of your ribs and the top of your hips.

The table below shows the waist sizes that increase the risk of a number of health conditions, such as type 2 diabetes, cardiovascular disease, cancer and stroke. Having a BMI of 25 or over increases your risk too.

	At Increased Risk	At High Risk
Men	Over 94cm / 37 inches Asian: Over 90cm / 35.5 inches	Over 102cm / 40 inches
Women	Over 80cm / 31.5 inches	Over 88cm / 34.5 inches

How to lose weight safely

A safe weight loss rate is 0.5-1kg (1-2 lbs) of body weight each week. Losing more weight than this may place you at risk of nutrient deficiencies. Reducing your dietary intake by about 600 calories per day (4,200 calories per week) can help you achieve weight loss at this safe rate. This reduction could be by diet alone or by a combination of diet and increased physical activity.

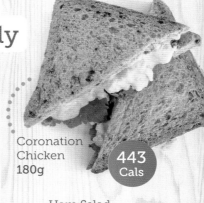

Coronation Chicken 180g

443 Cals

Does 600 calories sound unrealistic? Try breaking it up into smaller 100–200 calorie reductions. For example, eat a smaller portion at a meal, or choose a lower-calorie drink, and you can easily save yourself 100 calories. Small changes like these can make a big difference! A simple sandwich swap could save over 180 calories.

Ham Salad 160g

261 Cals

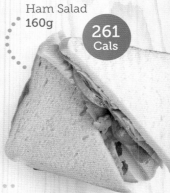

This book makes it easier to see which foods to eat in smaller quantities or avoid altogether if you are trying to cut down on calories or reduce your fat intake.

For example, you could consider swapping deep fried chips with oven chips and thus save 187 calories and 16g fat.

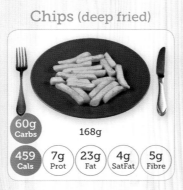

Chips (deep fried)

60g Carbs	168g			
459 Cals	**7g** Prot	**23g** Fat	**4g** SatFat	**5g** Fibre

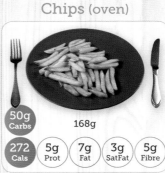

Chips (oven)

50g Carbs	168g			
272 Cals	**5g** Prot	**7g** Fat	**3g** SatFat	**5g** Fibre

Calories matter:

Evidence shows that different diets can work, if you stick to them! For success, find the right diet that suits you and your lifestyle.

Which diet is right for me?

Calorie reduction and weight loss can be achieved in a number of ways, and different types of diet suit different people. Some diets aren't considered to be nutritionally balanced because they don't provide all the nutrients your body requires. They usually involve cutting out whole food groups entirely, for example carbohydrates or dairy foods. It is unnecessary to avoid whole food groups to lose weight and this could even be dangerous. A Registered Dietitian can give you individualised advice about which diets may suit you best.

★ Low Calorie

Low calorie diets are defined as 800 to 1,600 calories per day. This can be achieved through careful selection of foods and controlling portion sizes.

★ Low Fat

Fat contains more calories per gram than any other nutrient, so reducing the fat content of foods is a great way to lower calorie intake.

★ Very Low Calorie

This involves eating under 800 calories per day for up to 12 weeks and often relies on commercial meal-replacement products. Very Low Calorie diets should only be followed under supervision, ideally from a Registered Dietitian, and may require medical monitoring.

★ Low Carbohydrate / High Protein

Foods high in protein help you to feel fuller for longer, so increasing the proportion of protein in the diet and reducing the amount of carbohydrate may help to lower overall calories. Depending on the level of carbohydrate restriction and on careful selection of foods, it should be possible to achieve a healthy balance with this diet.

★ Intermittent Fasting / 5:2 Diet

The 5:2 diet works by fasting on 2 days of the week and eating a healthy balanced diet on the remaining 5 days. This achieves a 25% reduction in calories. Other forms of fasting include alternate day fasting. Check out our 5:2 Diet Photos book at www.carbsandcals.com/5-2

Diabetes

Diabetes is a condition where glucose levels in the blood are too high, because the body cannot use the glucose properly. Diabetes can lead to heart disease, eye and kidney problems, which can be prevented by keeping blood glucose, blood fats and blood pressure levels within the normal range and maintaining a healthy active lifestyle.

Type 1 diabetes

Type 1 diabetes develops when the body's immune system destroys the cells of the pancreas that produce insulin. The pancreas is then unable to produce insulin, leading to increased blood glucose levels. It is treated by daily insulin administration, through injections or a pump.

Type 2 diabetes

Type 2 diabetes is more common than type 1. It develops when the pancreas does not produce enough insulin, or when the body can't use it effectively (known as insulin resistance). Type 2 is often associated with being overweight and usually occurs after the age of 40 (or from 25 for people of South Asian origin). It is also becoming more common in younger people of all ethnicities, due to rising levels of obesity.

Type 2 diabetes is primarily treated with a healthy diet and increased physical activity. However, it is a progressive condition and following a healthy eating plan and being physically active are often not enough to control blood glucose levels. If this is the case, your healthcare team may advise you to take diabetes medication and/or insulin.

Is it possible to prevent type 2 diabetes?

There is strong evidence that lifestyle changes, including weight loss strategies such as calorie restriction, can prevent type 2 diabetes in high-risk individuals. Every 1kg lost can lead to a 16% reduction in the risk of developing type 2 diabetes in overweight people.

Carbohydrate counting

Carbohydrate is the main nutrient that affects the rise in blood glucose levels and therefore carbohydrate counting has a key role in the management of type 1 diabetes. Carbohydrate counting is also being incorporated into the education and management of type 2 diabetes and diabetes in pregnancy.

Carb counting for type 1 diabetes

For people with type 1 diabetes, carbohydrate counting allows them to adjust their insulin dose according to their carbohydrate intake (in meals and snacks) and manage everyday life including:

* alcohol intake   * stress   * illness
* activity levels including sports and hobbies

There is strong evidence that matching insulin doses to carbohydrate intake improves blood glucose levels. Understanding and learning the carbohydrate in food and drink allows insulin doses to be adjusted accurately, to keep blood glucose levels as near normal as possible. Healthy dietary principles already discussed at the beginning of this book and regular physical activity are also important in the management of type 1 diabetes.

Carb counting for type 2 diabetes

In type 2 diabetes, the evidence about the effect of carbohydrate counting, even in those treated with insulin, is still inconclusive. What we do know is the larger the carbohydrate intake, the greater the rise in blood glucose levels after eating. Therefore, carbohydrate counting can help people with type 2 diabetes manage their carbohydrate intake at mealtimes and snacks, and may be an effective strategy in controlling blood glucose levels and weight maintenance/loss.

People with type 2 diabetes on a flexible insulin regimen may find that matching their insulin dose to carbohydrate improves their blood glucose levels. Your healthcare team will be able to provide you with the appropriate advice on which treatment is best for you.

Learning to count carbs

If you are new to carb counting, the following is a good place to start:

1. Learn what carb counting is and how to estimate the amount of carbs in food and drinks you consume in your diet by using this book, along with other methods such as weighing food and checking labels.

2. Understand how food, drink, diabetes medication, alcohol and exercise affects blood glucose levels and learn to manage these factors.

3. If you have diabetes and are on multiple daily injections (basal bolus) or use an insulin pump, this book can help you with insulin dose adjustment, i.e. how to match your quick-acting insulin to carbohydrate using your personal insulin-to-carbohydrate ratio.

The carb content of food and drink can be estimated either in grams or as carb portions (CPs). Use the method that works best for you.

This book shows the carb content in grams. To convert to CPs:

$$\frac{\text{Total carb content (g)}}{10}$$

For example 100g chips contains 30g carbs:

$$\frac{30g}{10} = 3 \text{ CPs}$$

You can use this book to calculate the total carbs in a meal:

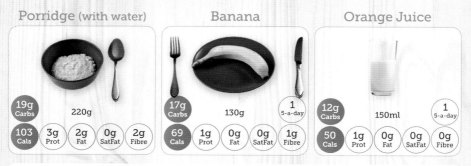

Porridge (with water)

| 19g Carbs | 220g | | | |
| 103 Cals | 3g Prot | 2g Fat | 0g SatFat | 2g Fibre |

Banana

| 17g Carbs | 130g | | | 1 5-a-day |
| 69 Cals | 1g Prot | 0g Fat | 0g SatFat | 1g Fibre |

Orange Juice

| 12g Carbs | 150ml | | | 1 5-a-day |
| 50 Cals | 1g Prot | 0g Fat | 0g SatFat | 0g Fibre |

Porridge: 19g + Banana: 17g + Juice: 12g = 48g Carbs or 5 CPs

Learning to estimate the carbohydrate content of food and drink is a valuable skill that is worth mastering. It will become easier with practice and in time second nature to you. Build your confidence up by calculating the carbohydrate content of foods you eat regularly in your diet, as these will have the greatest impact on your blood glucose levels and overall diabetes control. Calculating the carbohydrate in meals when eating out/with friends or in a takeaway will be difficult and will involve some estimating. By reflecting back upon your experience you can see if your calculations were right or if adjustments need to be made next time.

By focusing on carbohydrate only, it is easy to lose sight of the overall nutrient composition of the diet. For example, focusing on carbohydrate only and forgetting the calorie and fat content of food may lead to undesirable weight gain and increased risk of complications, such as heart disease. Remember the tips for healthy eating already discussed, as these still apply:

Aim for three meals each day.

Reach your 5-a-day!

Eat more fish!

Eat more pulses

Limit sugar and sugary foods

Drink alcohol in moderation

Cut down on fat, particularly saturated fat

Choose lower fat dairy products

Limit salt intake to 6g a day

This book makes carbohydrate counting easier when at home or out and about, and helps you keep an eye on the overall nutrient composition and calorie content of your diet too!

Example: A portion of crème brûlée only contains 19g carbs, but it has 27g fat and 333 cals. A portion of basmati rice contains 51g carbs, 233 cals and only 1g fat.

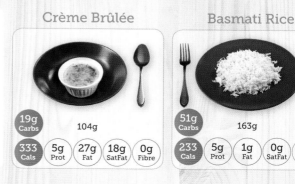

Crème Brûlée — 104g — 19g Carbs, 333 Cals, 5g Prot, 27g Fat, 18g SatFat, 0g Fibre

Basmati Rice — 163g — 51g Carbs, 233 Cals, 5g Prot, 1g Fat, 0g SatFat, 1g Fibre

Carbohydrate counting and insulin dose adjustment

The development of insulin has enabled people with diabetes to effectively adjust insulin doses to the carbohydrate content of their meals. This offers more flexible eating, reduces the risk of hypoglycaemia and improves blood glucose control.

As mentioned earlier, the carbohydrate from the food and drink we consume is digested and broken down into glucose. This glucose enters the blood, from where it is then carried into the cells of the body by the hormone insulin.

★ **Long-acting insulin** (basal) deals with the glucose produced by the liver and influences the blood glucose levels between meals.

★ **Quick-acting insulin** (bolus) deals with the glucose produced from the carbohydrate in the food and drink that is consumed.

The amount of quick-acting insulin needed is directly related to the total amount of carbohydrate consumed. Meals with little or no carbohydrate e.g. omelette and salad generally do not need any quick-acting insulin, as your long-acting insulin will deal with the glucose that is produced by the liver, if the dose is correct for you.

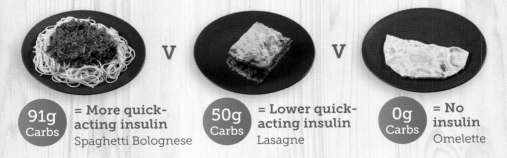

91g Carbs = **More quick-acting insulin** Spaghetti Bolognese

V

50g Carbs = **Lower quick-acting insulin** Lasagne

V

0g Carbs = **No insulin** Omelette

If you are on multiple daily injections of insulin (basal-bolus or MDI regimen) or on an insulin pump, carbohydrate counting can help you decide how much insulin to use. If you are on 2 insulin injections a day, you may also find it useful to count carbohydrate in order to aim for consistent amounts of carbohydrate at meals and minimise big fluctuations in blood glucose.

Calculating how much quick acting insulin to give

The amount of insulin that is required (known as insulin-to-carbohydrate ratio) varies from person to person and can also vary at different times of the day. Typically, most people start with 1 unit of quick-acting insulin for every 10g carbohydrate or 1 CP. Your diabetes team will work with you to help you understand the appropriate insulin-to-carbohydrate ratio for you.

Learning how to adjust insulin doses and how to count carbohydrates can be a complex process. This book is not designed to teach you how to adjust your insulin, but to help you work out how much carbohydrate is in your diet. It is important that you have the support of appropriately trained healthcare professionals, such as a diabetes specialist nurse and diabetes specialist dietitian.

There are many structured education programmes offered in the UK, such as:

Type 1 diabetes	Type 2 diabetes	Type 1 & 2 and those at risk of developing diabetes
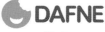	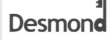	

Alcohol and carbohydrate counting

This book includes a variety of alcoholic drinks and displays their carbohydrate values. People who are carbohydrate counting and adjusting their insulin should use these values as a reference guide only, as it is usually not recommended to take additional insulin for the carbohydrate found in most alcoholic drinks. Extreme caution should be taken when giving additional units of insulin with alcohol, as alcohol is associated with an increased risk of hypoglycaemia. Your diabetes team can advise you on this in greater detail.

Glycaemic Index

The rate at which carbohydrate is broken down depends on the type of carbohydrate consumed; this is known as the Glycaemic Index (GI).

Food or drinks with a high GI are broken down quickly, causing a rapid rise in blood glucose levels.

Foods with a low GI are broken down slowly, giving a more gradual rise in blood glucose levels.

For people with diabetes, having an idea of the GI of food and drink can be helpful in predicting blood glucose fluctuations after eating or drinking. A registered dietitian can help you with more information on this subject.

It is important to bear in mind that GI does not take into account the other nutrients in a meal (protein, fat and fibre, which can slow down the absorption of glucose in the blood) or the amount of carbohydrate in the meal, which is a much better predictor of how high the blood glucose levels will go.

A note of caution: It is important to note that certain foods release glucose at a very slow rate and may not require insulin, or may require a reduced or delayed dose. Examples include foods such as pearl barley, peas, beans and lentils, and some vegetables such as sweetcorn, squash/pumpkin and parsnips. It is advisable to speak to your diabetes team about your insulin requirements for these foods as they may vary from person to person and depend on the portion size consumed.

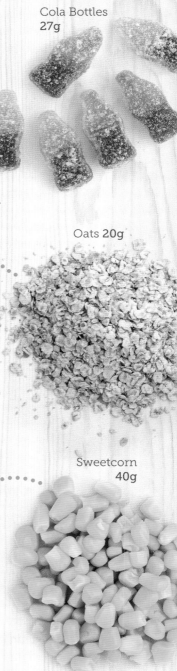

Cola Bottles
27g

Oats **20g**

Sweetcorn
40g

Diabetes & Weight Management

Weight loss is the primary strategy to control blood glucose levels, especially in overweight or obese people with type 2 diabetes. People with type 1 diabetes should also keep to a healthy weight, as being overweight may put them at a higher risk of complications, such as heart disease.

Reducing the total calorie content of the diet and increasing physical activity levels are the best ways of losing weight healthily and keeping it off for good. To date, it is still unclear which is the most effective weight loss plan and which proportion of carbohydrate, protein and fat those with diabetes should consume in order to lose weight. Some people lose weight by following a low fat diet, while others do well on a low carbohydrate diet.

Avocado
70g

Recent evidence has shown that a very low calorie diet of under 800 calories per day for two months could reverse the insulin resistance that is common in type 2 diabetes and slow down the progressive decline of the insulin-producing cells of the pancreas. However, more research is required to show the long-term benefit and it is important to discuss this kind of diet with your healthcare team before considering it as an option for weight loss.

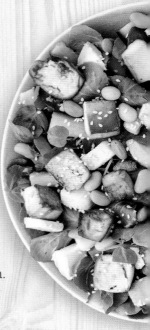

Commercial diet programmes utilise a variety of weight loss methods, such as dietary advice, personalised meal plans, physical activity and group therapy. The evidence about the effect of such programmes on people with diabetes is still unknown. Fad diets, which usually promise quick weight loss by following a restrictive, nutrient-deficient diet of an unusual combination of foods, offer no benefit in the long term and most people put the weight back on.

How to use this book

This book has been written with complete practicality in mind. Simply follow the steps outlined below:

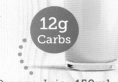

12g Carbs

Orange Juice **150ml**

1. Decide what you want to eat or drink and find the meal, drink or snack in the book.

2. Look at the circles below the photo for the values you are interested in. These show the values for carbs, calories, protein, fat, saturated fat, fibre and 5-a-day.

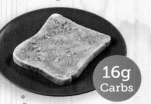

16g Carbs

Toast with Peanut Butter

3. Choose your portion size and assemble your meal.

4. Add up the carbs, cals, protein, fat, sat fat, fibre and 5-a-day values for the different food components, to give the totals for your meal.

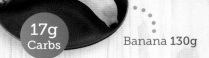

17g Carbs

Banana **130g**

Key points when using this book

★ To help with scale, each food photo displays either a knife and fork, or a dessert spoon. You may find it useful to measure your own dinnerware and compare against the dinnerware in the photos. Alternatively, you may wish to use plates and bowls that are the same size as the ones in the book.

★ The weight of each portion is stated below each photo, just in case you want to double check the weight of your own portion. This is always the cooked/prepared weight.

★ Values for carbohydrate, protein, fat, saturated fat and fibre are given to the nearest gram. Therefore, if a food has 0.4g of fat, the fat value will be listed as 0g. If a food has 0.6g of fat, the fat value will be listed as 1g.

★ If you are eating a meal with more than one component (e.g. steak, chips and salad), you will need to find each component in the book and add them up separately. For example, your steak, chips and salad meal:

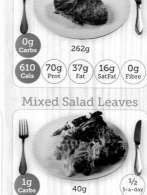

Sirloin Steak (fried)

0g Carbs   262g
610 Cals | 70g Prot | 37g Fat | 16g SatFat | 0g Fibre

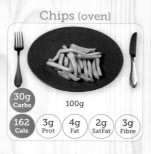

Chips (oven)

30g Carbs   100g
162 Cals | 3g Prot | 4g Fat | 2g SatFat | 3g Fibre

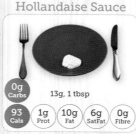

Hollandaise Sauce

0g Carbs   13g, 1 tbsp
93 Cals | 1g Prot | 10g Fat | 6g SatFat | 0g Fibre

Mixed Salad Leaves

1g Carbs   40g   ½ 5-a-day
4 Cals | 0g Prot | 0g Fat | 0g SatFat | 1g Fibre

★ All foods in the book are displayed on either a plate or bowl as shown below (the size is displayed at the top of each page as a reminder):

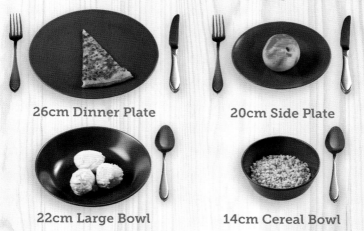

26cm Dinner Plate

20cm Side Plate

22cm Large Bowl

14cm Cereal Bowl

★ Each food in the book has between 1 and 6 portion photos to help you easily judge the nutrient and calorie content of your particular portion, simply by looking at the different photos. For example, a digestive biscuit is always the same size and therefore only 1 photo has been included. However, there are 6 different portion pictures of lasagne included, so that you can choose the portion that is closest to the portion on your plate.

20cm Side Plate

Bourbon Cream

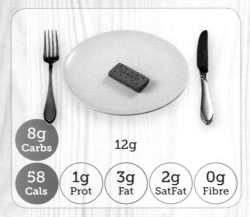

8g Carbs 12g

58 Cals | 1g Prot | 3g Fat | 2g SatFat | 0g Fibre

Chocolate Digestive

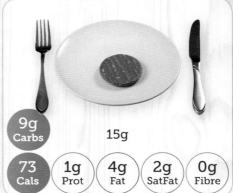

9g Carbs 15g

73 Cals | 1g Prot | 4g Fat | 2g SatFat | 0g Fibre

Chocolate Chip Cookie

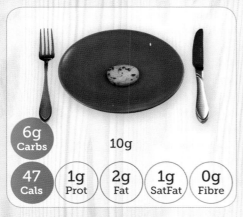

6g Carbs 10g

47 Cals | 1g Prot | 2g Fat | 1g SatFat | 0g Fibre

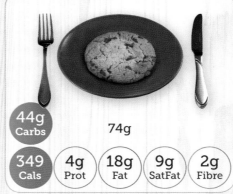

44g Carbs 74g

349 Cals | 4g Prot | 18g Fat | 9g SatFat | 2g Fibre

Chocolate Oat Biscuit

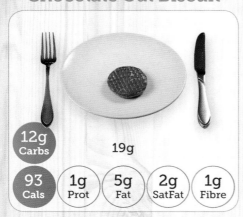

12g Carbs 19g

93 Cals | 1g Prot | 5g Fat | 2g SatFat | 1g Fibre

Chocolate Sandwich Biscuit

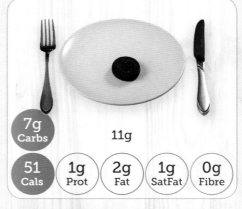

7g Carbs 11g

51 Cals | 1g Prot | 2g Fat | 1g SatFat | 0g Fibre

Custard Cream

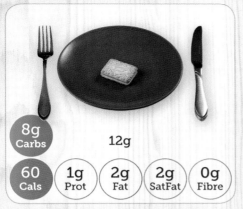

8g Carbs

12g

60 Cals | 1g Prot | 2g Fat | 2g SatFat | 0g Fibre

Digestive

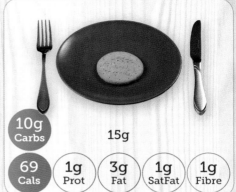

10g Carbs

15g

69 Cals | 1g Prot | 3g Fat | 1g SatFat | 1g Fibre

Fig Roll

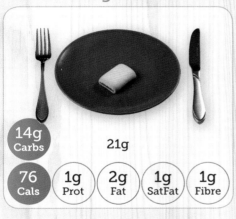

14g Carbs

21g

76 Cals | 1g Prot | 2g Fat | 1g SatFat | 1g Fibre

Ginger Biscuit

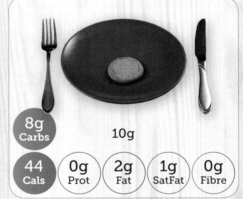

8g Carbs

10g

44 Cals | 0g Prot | 2g Fat | 1g SatFat | 0g Fibre

Gingerbread Man

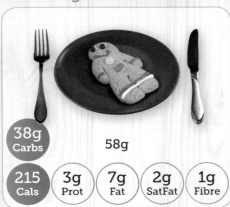

38g Carbs

58g

215 Cals | 3g Prot | 7g Fat | 2g SatFat | 1g Fibre

Iced Ring

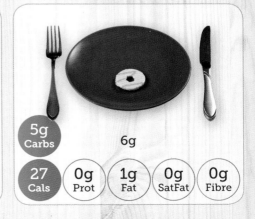

5g Carbs

6g

27 Cals | 0g Prot | 1g Fat | 0g SatFat | 0g Fibre

20cm Side Plate

Jaffa Cake

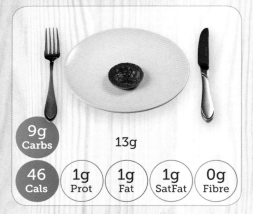

9g Carbs
13g
46 Cals | **1g** Prot | **1g** Fat | **1g** SatFat | **0g** Fibre

Jam Ring

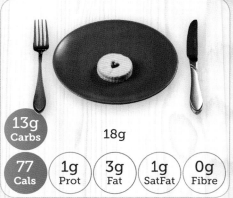

13g Carbs
18g
77 Cals | **1g** Prot | **3g** Fat | **1g** SatFat | **0g** Fibre

Malted Milk

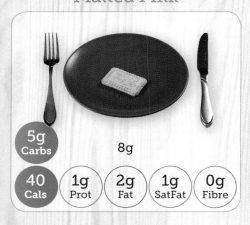

5g Carbs
8g
40 Cals | **1g** Prot | **2g** Fat | **1g** SatFat | **0g** Fibre

Milk Chocolate Biscuit Bar

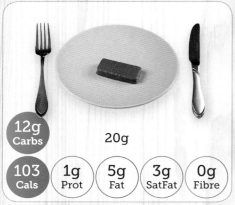

12g Carbs
20g
103 Cals | **1g** Prot | **5g** Fat | **3g** SatFat | **0g** Fibre

Milk Chocolate Finger

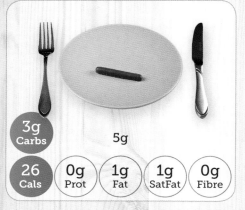

3g Carbs
5g
26 Cals | **0g** Prot | **1g** Fat | **1g** SatFat | **0g** Fibre

Milk Chocolate Wafer

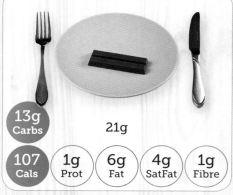

13g Carbs
21g
107 Cals | **1g** Prot | **6g** Fat | **4g** SatFat | **1g** Fibre

Nice Biscuit

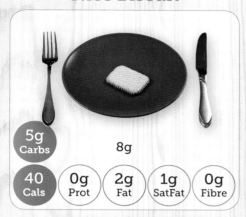

5g Carbs

8g

40 Cals | **0g** Prot | **2g** Fat | **1g** SatFat | **0g** Fibre

Oat Biscuit

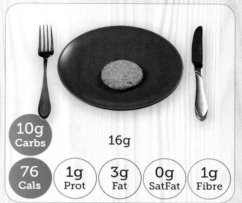

10g Carbs

16g

76 Cals | **1g** Prot | **3g** Fat | **0g** SatFat | **1g** Fibre

Pink Wafer

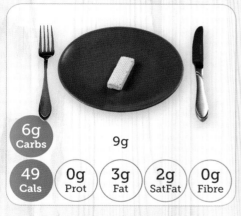

6g Carbs

9g

49 Cals | **0g** Prot | **3g** Fat | **2g** SatFat | **0g** Fibre

Rich Tea

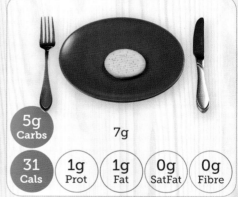

5g Carbs

7g

31 Cals | **1g** Prot | **1g** Fat | **0g** SatFat | **0g** Fibre

Shortbread Finger

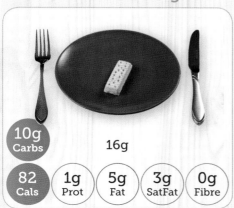

10g Carbs

16g

82 Cals | **1g** Prot | **5g** Fat | **3g** SatFat | **0g** Fibre

Shortcake

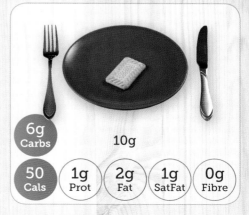

6g Carbs

10g

50 Cals | **1g** Prot | **2g** Fat | **1g** SatFat | **0g** Fibre

20cm Side Plate

Breadstick

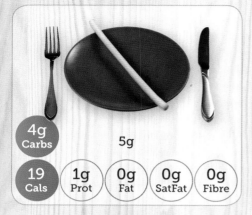

4g Carbs

5g

19 Cals | **1g** Prot | **0g** Fat | **0g** SatFat | **0g** Fibre

Cheddar

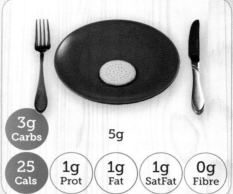

3g Carbs

5g

25 Cals | **1g** Prot | **1g** Fat | **1g** SatFat | **0g** Fibre

Cheese Straw

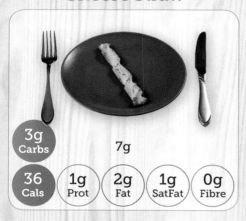

3g Carbs

7g

36 Cals | **1g** Prot | **2g** Fat | **1g** SatFat | **0g** Fibre

Cream Cracker

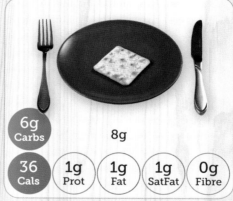

6g Carbs

8g

36 Cals | **1g** Prot | **1g** Fat | **1g** SatFat | **0g** Fibre

Crispbread

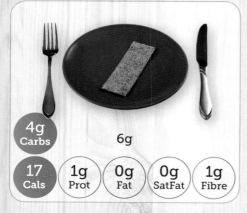

4g Carbs

6g

17 Cals | **1g** Prot | **0g** Fat | **0g** SatFat | **1g** Fibre

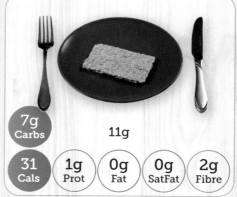

7g Carbs

11g

31 Cals | **1g** Prot | **0g** Fat | **0g** SatFat | **2g** Fibre

Digestive (savoury)

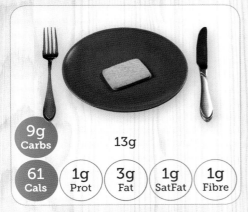

9g Carbs
13g
61 Cals | **1g Prot** | **3g Fat** | **1g SatFat** | **1g Fibre**

Oatcake

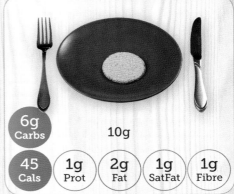

6g Carbs
10g
45 Cals | **1g Prot** | **2g Fat** | **1g SatFat** | **1g Fibre**

Puffed Cracker

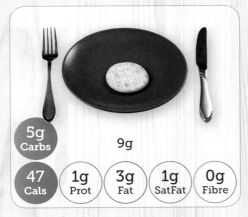

5g Carbs
9g
47 Cals | **1g Prot** | **3g Fat** | **1g SatFat** | **0g Fibre**

Rice Cake

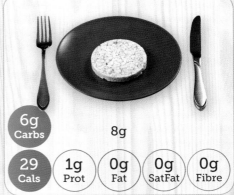

6g Carbs
8g
29 Cals | **1g Prot** | **0g Fat** | **0g SatFat** | **0g Fibre**

Water Biscuit

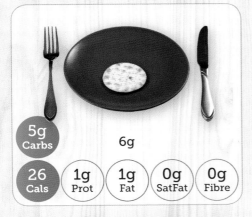

5g Carbs
6g
26 Cals | **1g Prot** | **1g Fat** | **0g SatFat** | **0g Fibre**

Wholegrain Cracker

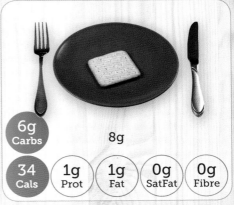

6g Carbs
8g
34 Cals | **1g Prot** | **1g Fat** | **0g SatFat** | **0g Fibre**

20cm Side Plate

Granary Bread

White Bread

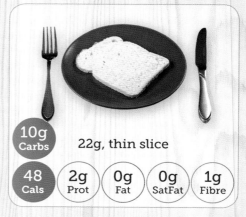

10g Carbs — Granary, 22g, thin slice
52 Cals | **2g** Prot | **1g** Fat | **0g** SatFat | **1g** Fibre

10g Carbs — White, 22g, thin slice
48 Cals | **2g** Prot | **0g** Fat | **0g** SatFat | **1g** Fibre

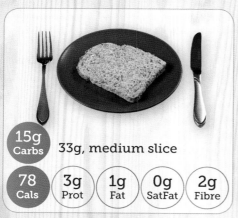
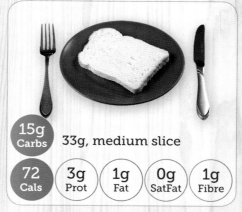

15g Carbs — 33g, medium slice
78 Cals | **3g** Prot | **1g** Fat | **0g** SatFat | **2g** Fibre

15g Carbs — 33g, medium slice
72 Cals | **3g** Prot | **1g** Fat | **0g** SatFat | **1g** Fibre

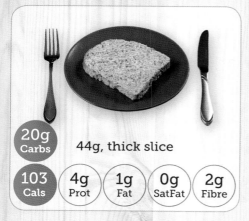
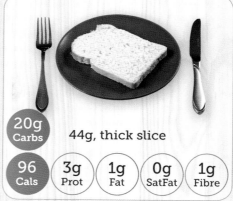

20g Carbs — 44g, thick slice
103 Cals | **4g** Prot | **1g** Fat | **0g** SatFat | **2g** Fibre

20g Carbs — 44g, thick slice
96 Cals | **3g** Prot | **1g** Fat | **0g** SatFat | **1g** Fibre

Wholemeal Bread

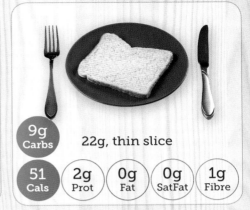

9g Carbs   22g, thin slice

48 Cals | **2g** Prot | **1g** Fat | **0g** SatFat | **2g** Fibre

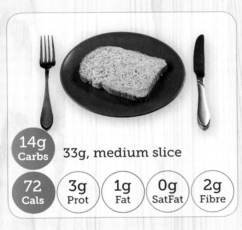

14g Carbs   33g, medium slice

72 Cals | **3g** Prot | **1g** Fat | **0g** SatFat | **2g** Fibre

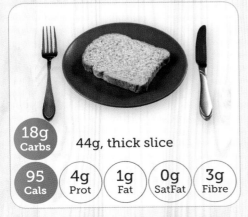

18g Carbs   44g, thick slice

95 Cals | **4g** Prot | **1g** Fat | **0g** SatFat | **3g** Fibre

White Wholemeal Bread

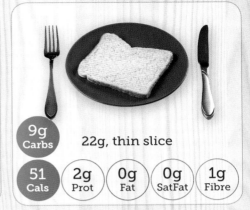

9g Carbs   22g, thin slice

51 Cals | **2g** Prot | **0g** Fat | **0g** SatFat | **1g** Fibre

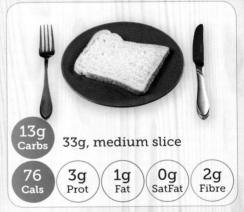

13g Carbs   33g, medium slice

76 Cals | **3g** Prot | **1g** Fat | **0g** SatFat | **2g** Fibre

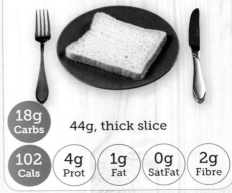

18g Carbs   44g, thick slice

102 Cals | **4g** Prot | **1g** Fat | **0g** SatFat | **2g** Fibre

20cm Side Plate

Bap (white)

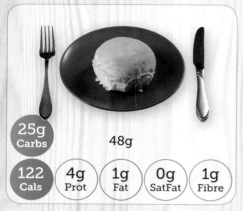

25g Carbs
48g
122 Cals | 4g Prot | 1g Fat | 0g SatFat | 1g Fibre

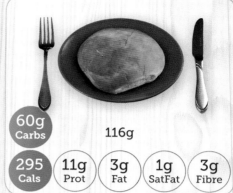

60g Carbs
116g
295 Cals | 11g Prot | 3g Fat | 1g SatFat | 3g Fibre

Bap (wholemeal)

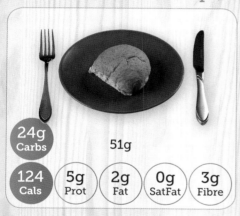

24g Carbs
51g
124 Cals | 5g Prot | 2g Fat | 0g SatFat | 3g Fibre

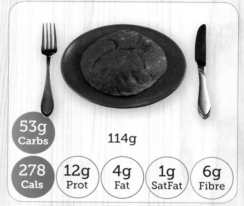

53g Carbs
114g
278 Cals | 12g Prot | 4g Fat | 1g SatFat | 6g Fibre

Crusty Roll (white)

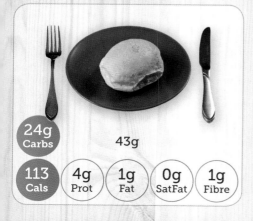

24g Carbs
43g
113 Cals | 4g Prot | 1g Fat | 0g SatFat | 1g Fibre

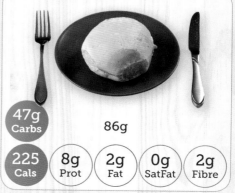

47g Carbs
86g
225 Cals | 8g Prot | 2g Fat | 0g SatFat | 2g Fibre

Bagel

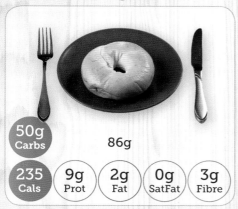

50g Carbs
86g

235 Cals | **9g** Prot | **2g** Fat | **0g** SatFat | **3g** Fibre

English Muffin

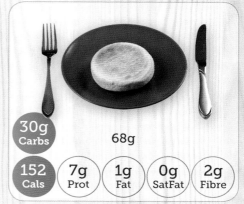

30g Carbs
68g

152 Cals | **7g** Prot | **1g** Fat | **0g** SatFat | **2g** Fibre

Crumpet

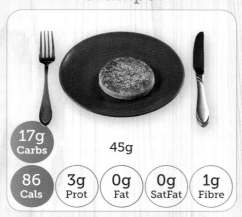

17g Carbs
45g

86 Cals | **3g** Prot | **0g** Fat | **0g** SatFat | **1g** Fibre

Crumpet (square)

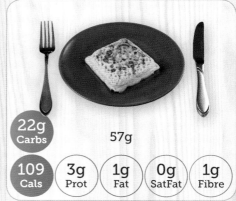

22g Carbs
57g

109 Cals | **3g** Prot | **1g** Fat | **0g** SatFat | **1g** Fibre

Poppy Seeded Roll

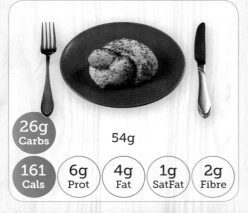

26g Carbs
54g

161 Cals | **6g** Prot | **4g** Fat | **1g** SatFat | **2g** Fibre

Tea Cake

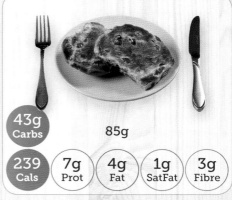

43g Carbs
85g

239 Cals | **7g** Prot | **4g** Fat | **1g** SatFat | **3g** Fibre

20cm Side Plate

Burger Bun

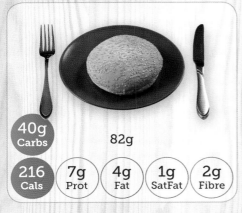

40g Carbs

82g

216 Cals | **7g** Prot | **4g** Fat | **1g** SatFat | **2g** Fibre

Finger Roll

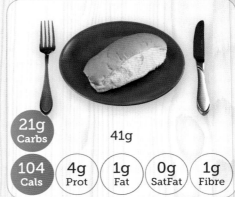

21g Carbs

41g

104 Cals | **4g** Prot | **1g** Fat | **0g** SatFat | **1g** Fibre

Croutons

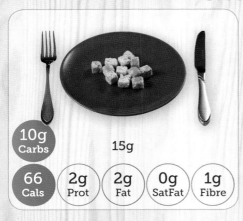

10g Carbs

15g

66 Cals | **2g** Prot | **2g** Fat | **0g** SatFat | **1g** Fibre

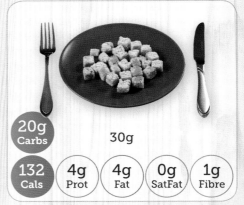

20g Carbs

30g

132 Cals | **4g** Prot | **4g** Fat | **0g** SatFat | **1g** Fibre

Ciabatta

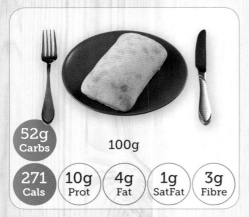

52g Carbs

100g

271 Cals | **10g** Prot | **4g** Fat | **1g** SatFat | **3g** Fibre

Panini

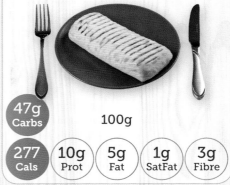

47g Carbs

100g

277 Cals | **10g** Prot | **5g** Fat | **1g** SatFat | **3g** Fibre

Baguette

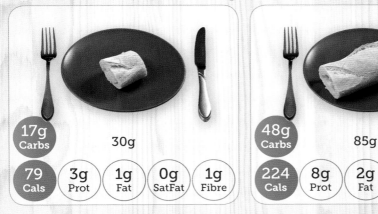

17g Carbs

30g

79 Cals | **3g** Prot | **1g** Fat | **0g** SatFat | **1g** Fibre

48g Carbs

85g

224 Cals | **8g** Prot | **2g** Fat | **0g** SatFat | **3g** Fibre

Banana Bread

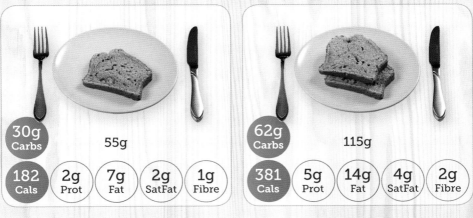

30g Carbs

55g

182 Cals | **2g** Prot | **7g** Fat | **2g** SatFat | **1g** Fibre

62g Carbs

115g

381 Cals | **5g** Prot | **14g** Fat | **4g** SatFat | **2g** Fibre

Focaccia

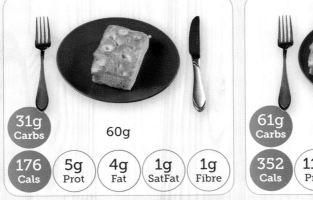

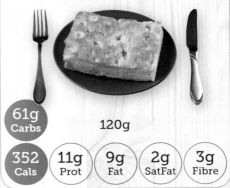

31g Carbs

60g

176 Cals | **5g** Prot | **4g** Fat | **1g** SatFat | **1g** Fibre

61g Carbs

120g

352 Cals | **11g** Prot | **9g** Fat | **2g** SatFat | **3g** Fibre

20cm Side Plate

Garlic Bread

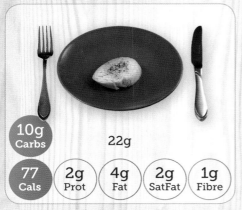

10g Carbs

22g

77 Cals | 2g Prot | 4g Fat | 2g SatFat | 1g Fibre

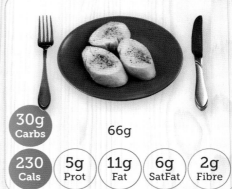

30g Carbs

66g

230 Cals | 5g Prot | 11g Fat | 6g SatFat | 2g Fibre

Pumpernickel

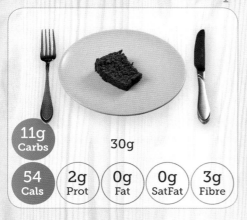

11g Carbs

30g

54 Cals | 2g Prot | 0g Fat | 0g SatFat | 3g Fibre

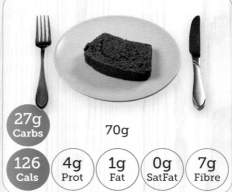

27g Carbs

70g

126 Cals | 4g Prot | 1g Fat | 0g SatFat | 7g Fibre

Raisin Bread

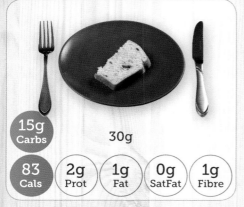

15g Carbs

30g

83 Cals | 2g Prot | 1g Fat | 0g SatFat | 1g Fibre

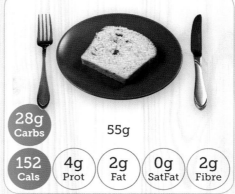

28g Carbs

55g

152 Cals | 4g Prot | 2g Fat | 0g SatFat | 2g Fibre

Rye Bread

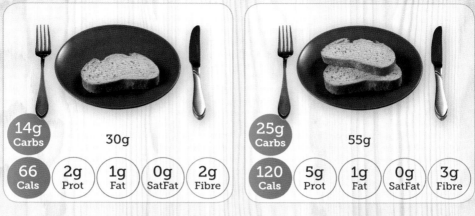

14g Carbs — 30g
66 Cals | **2g** Prot | **1g** Fat | **0g** SatFat | **2g** Fibre

25g Carbs — 55g
120 Cals | **5g** Prot | **1g** Fat | **0g** SatFat | **3g** Fibre

Sourdough

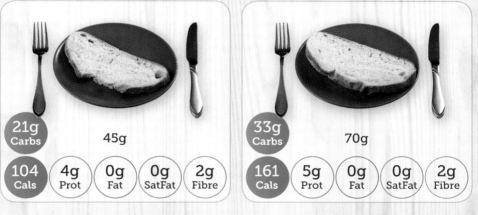

21g Carbs — 45g
104 Cals | **4g** Prot | **0g** Fat | **0g** SatFat | **2g** Fibre

33g Carbs — 70g
161 Cals | **5g** Prot | **0g** Fat | **0g** SatFat | **2g** Fibre

Spelt Bread

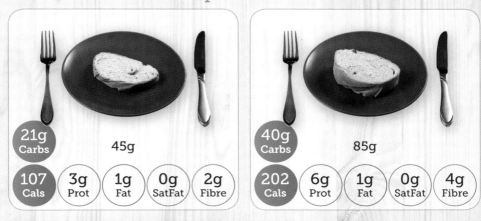

21g Carbs — 45g
107 Cals | **3g** Prot | **1g** Fat | **0g** SatFat | **2g** Fibre

40g Carbs — 85g
202 Cals | **6g** Prot | **1g** Fat | **0g** SatFat | **4g** Fibre

Pitta Bread (white)

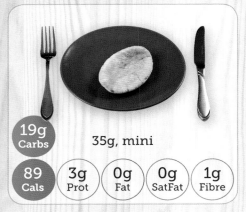

19g Carbs

35g, mini

89 Cals · **3g** Prot · **0g** Fat · **0g** SatFat · **1g** Fibre

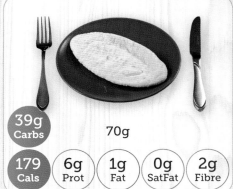

39g Carbs

70g

179 Cals · **6g** Prot · **1g** Fat · **0g** SatFat · **2g** Fibre

Pitta Bread (wholemeal)

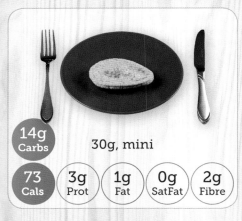

14g Carbs

30g, mini

73 Cals · **3g** Prot · **1g** Fat · **0g** SatFat · **2g** Fibre

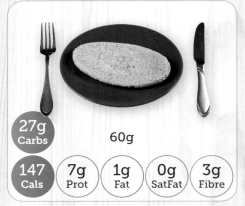

27g Carbs

60g

147 Cals · **7g** Prot · **1g** Fat · **0g** SatFat · **3g** Fibre

Turkish Flatbread

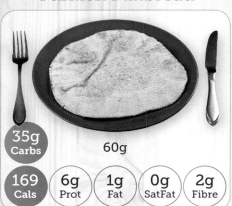

35g Carbs

60g

169 Cals · **6g** Prot · **1g** Fat · **0g** SatFat · **2g** Fibre

Taco Shell

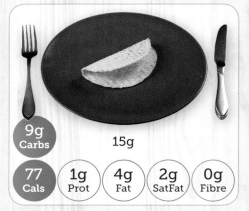

9g Carbs

15g

77 Cals · **1g** Prot · **4g** Fat · **2g** SatFat · **0g** Fibre

Tortilla (flour)

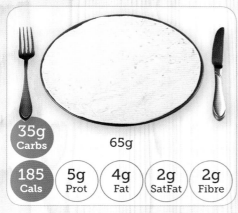

35g Carbs

65g

185 Cals | **5g** Prot | **4g** Fat | **2g** SatFat | **2g** Fibre

Tortilla (wholemeal)

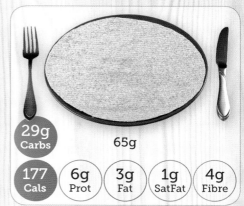

29g Carbs

65g

177 Cals | **6g** Prot | **3g** Fat | **1g** SatFat | **4g** Fibre

Naan Bread

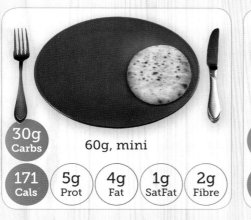

30g Carbs

60g, mini

171 Cals | **5g** Prot | **4g** Fat | **1g** SatFat | **2g** Fibre

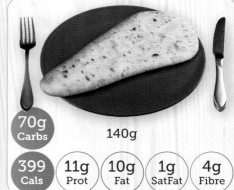

70g Carbs

140g

399 Cals | **11g** Prot | **10g** Fat | **1g** SatFat | **4g** Fibre

Poppadom

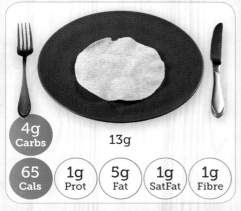

4g Carbs

13g

65 Cals | **1g** Prot | **5g** Fat | **1g** SatFat | **1g** Fibre

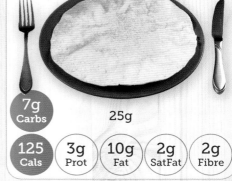

7g Carbs

25g

125 Cals | **3g** Prot | **10g** Fat | **2g** SatFat | **2g** Fibre

Chapati (without fat)

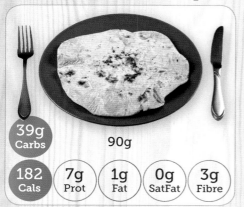

39g Carbs — 90g

182 Cals | **7g** Prot | **1g** Fat | **0g** SatFat | **3g** Fibre

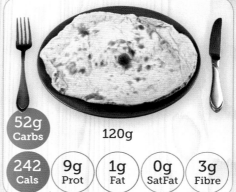

52g Carbs — 120g

242 Cals | **9g** Prot | **1g** Fat | **0g** SatFat | **3g** Fibre

Chapati (with butter)

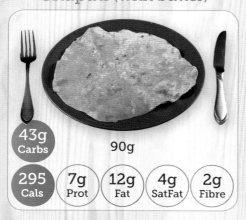

43g Carbs — 90g

295 Cals | **7g** Prot | **12g** Fat | **4g** SatFat | **2g** Fibre

Paratha

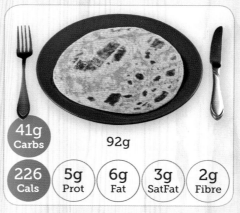

41g Carbs — 92g

226 Cals | **5g** Prot | **6g** Fat | **3g** SatFat | **2g** Fibre

Puri

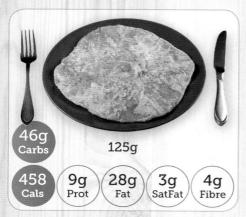

46g Carbs — 125g

458 Cals | **9g** Prot | **28g** Fat | **3g** SatFat | **4g** Fibre

Roti

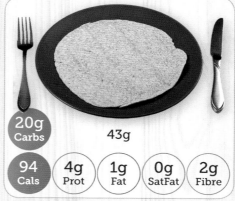

20g Carbs — 43g

94 Cals | **4g** Prot | **1g** Fat | **0g** SatFat | **2g** Fibre

Brioche

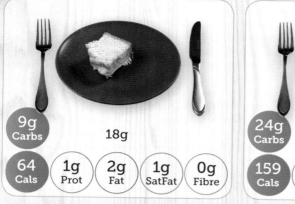

9g Carbs

18g

64 Cals — **1g** Prot — **2g** Fat — **1g** SatFat — **0g** Fibre

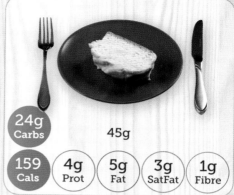

24g Carbs

45g

159 Cals — **4g** Prot — **5g** Fat — **3g** SatFat — **1g** Fibre

Croissant

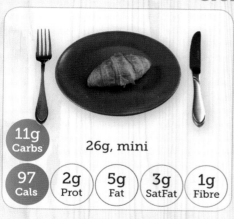

11g Carbs

26g, mini

97 Cals — **2g** Prot — **5g** Fat — **3g** SatFat — **1g** Fibre

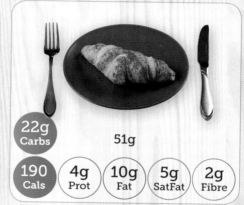

22g Carbs

51g

190 Cals — **4g** Prot — **10g** Fat — **5g** SatFat — **2g** Fibre

Pain au Chocolat

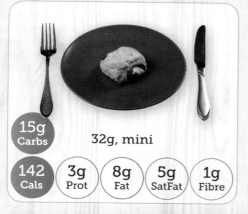

15g Carbs

32g, mini

142 Cals — **3g** Prot — **8g** Fat — **5g** SatFat — **1g** Fibre

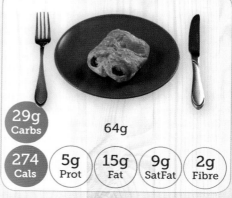

29g Carbs

64g

274 Cals — **5g** Prot — **15g** Fat — **9g** SatFat — **2g** Fibre

All Bran

Bran Flakes

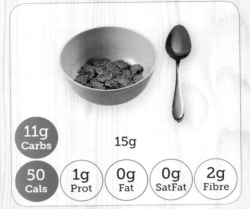

All Bran — 20g

10g Carbs

67 Cals | **3g** Prot | **1g** Fat | **0g** SatFat | **5g** Fibre

Bran Flakes — 15g

11g Carbs

50 Cals | **1g** Prot | **0g** Fat | **0g** SatFat | **2g** Fibre

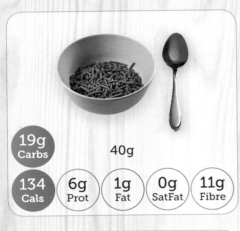

All Bran — 40g

19g Carbs

134 Cals | **6g** Prot | **1g** Fat | **0g** SatFat | **11g** Fibre

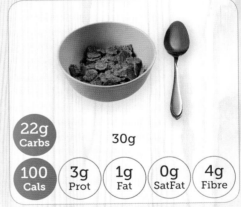

Bran Flakes — 30g

22g Carbs

100 Cals | **3g** Prot | **1g** Fat | **0g** SatFat | **4g** Fibre

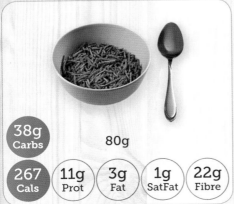

All Bran — 80g

38g Carbs

267 Cals | **11g** Prot | **3g** Fat | **1g** SatFat | **22g** Fibre

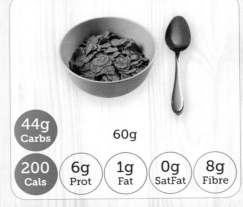

Bran Flakes — 60g

44g Carbs

200 Cals | **6g** Prot | **1g** Fat | **0g** SatFat | **8g** Fibre

Chocolate Snaps

Corn Flakes

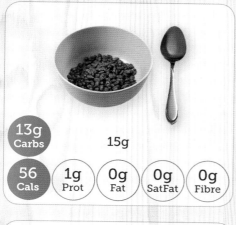

13g Carbs

15g

56 Cals | **1g** Prot | **0g** Fat | **0g** SatFat | **0g** Fibre

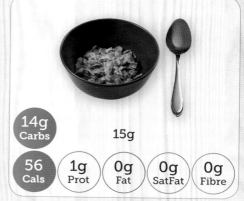

14g Carbs

15g

56 Cals | **1g** Prot | **0g** Fat | **0g** SatFat | **0g** Fibre

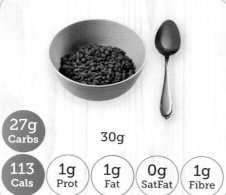

27g Carbs

30g

113 Cals | **1g** Prot | **1g** Fat | **0g** SatFat | **1g** Fibre

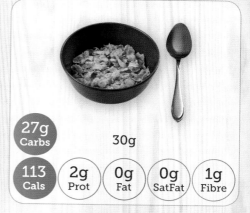

27g Carbs

30g

113 Cals | **2g** Prot | **0g** Fat | **0g** SatFat | **1g** Fibre

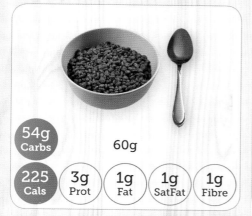

54g Carbs

60g

225 Cals | **3g** Prot | **1g** Fat | **1g** SatFat | **1g** Fibre

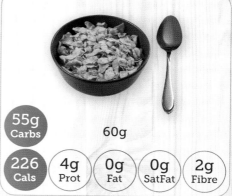

55g Carbs

60g

226 Cals | **4g** Prot | **0g** Fat | **0g** SatFat | **2g** Fibre

Frosted Flakes

Fruit & Fibre

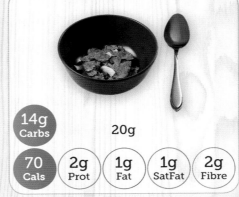

13g Carbs — 15g

53 Cals | **1g** Prot | **0g** Fat | **0g** SatFat | **0g** Fibre

14g Carbs — 20g

70 Cals | **2g** Prot | **1g** Fat | **1g** SatFat | **2g** Fibre

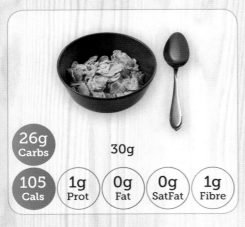
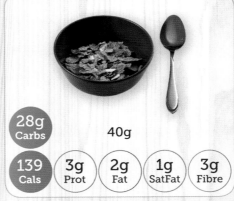

26g Carbs — 30g

105 Cals | **1g** Prot | **0g** Fat | **0g** SatFat | **1g** Fibre

28g Carbs — 40g

139 Cals | **3g** Prot | **2g** Fat | **1g** SatFat | **3g** Fibre

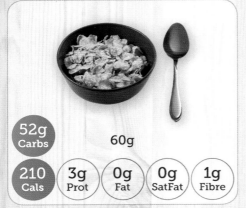
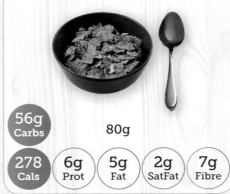

52g Carbs — 60g

210 Cals | **3g** Prot | **0g** Fat | **0g** SatFat | **1g** Fibre

56g Carbs — 80g

278 Cals | **6g** Prot | **5g** Fat | **2g** SatFat | **7g** Fibre

Granola

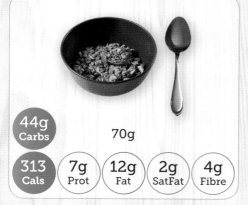

22g Carbs
35g
157 Cals | **3g** Prot | **6g** Fat | **1g** SatFat | **2g** Fibre

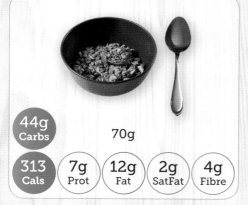

44g Carbs
70g
313 Cals | **7g** Prot | **12g** Fat | **2g** SatFat | **4g** Fibre

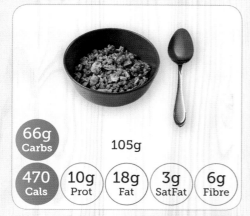

66g Carbs
105g
470 Cals | **10g** Prot | **18g** Fat | **3g** SatFat | **6g** Fibre

Honey Nut Flakes

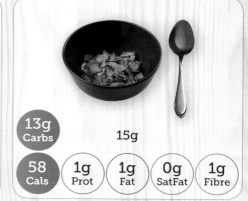

13g Carbs
15g
58 Cals | **1g** Prot | **1g** Fat | **0g** SatFat | **1g** Fibre

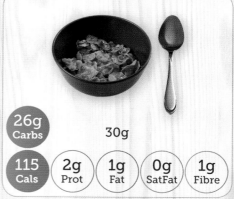

26g Carbs
30g
115 Cals | **2g** Prot | **1g** Fat | **0g** SatFat | **1g** Fibre

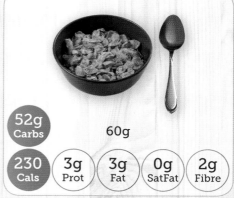

52g Carbs
60g
230 Cals | **3g** Prot | **3g** Fat | **0g** SatFat | **2g** Fibre

Honey Puffed Wheat

Malted Wheats

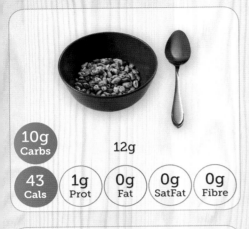

10g Carbs
12g
43 Cals | **1g** Prot | **0g** Fat | **0g** SatFat | **0g** Fibre

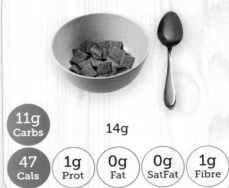

11g Carbs
14g
47 Cals | **1g** Prot | **0g** Fat | **0g** SatFat | **1g** Fibre

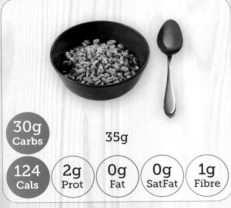

30g Carbs
35g
124 Cals | **2g** Prot | **0g** Fat | **0g** SatFat | **1g** Fibre

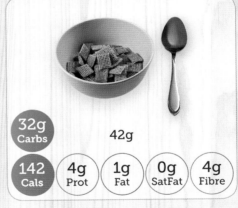

32g Carbs
42g
142 Cals | **4g** Prot | **1g** Fat | **0g** SatFat | **4g** Fibre

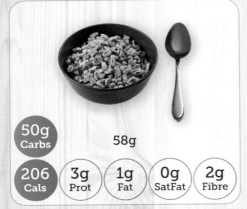

50g Carbs
58g
206 Cals | **3g** Prot | **1g** Fat | **0g** SatFat | **2g** Fibre

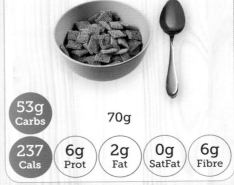

53g Carbs
70g
237 Cals | **6g** Prot | **2g** Fat | **0g** SatFat | **6g** Fibre

Muesli

Muesli (no added sugar)

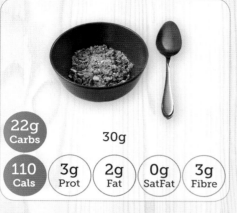

22g Carbs

30g

110 Cals | **3g** Prot | **2g** Fat | **0g** SatFat | **3g** Fibre

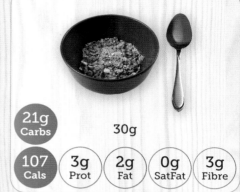

21g Carbs

30g

107 Cals | **3g** Prot | **2g** Fat | **0g** SatFat | **3g** Fibre

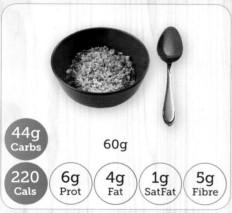

44g Carbs

60g

220 Cals | **6g** Prot | **4g** Fat | **1g** SatFat | **5g** Fibre

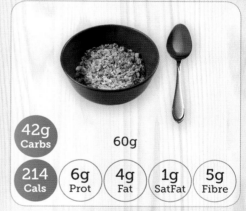

42g Carbs

60g

214 Cals | **6g** Prot | **4g** Fat | **1g** SatFat | **5g** Fibre

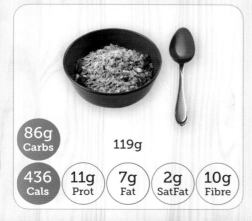

86g Carbs

119g

436 Cals | **11g** Prot | **7g** Fat | **2g** SatFat | **10g** Fibre

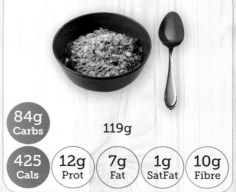

84g Carbs

119g

425 Cals | **12g** Prot | **7g** Fat | **1g** SatFat | **10g** Fibre

Multigrain Hoops

Raisin Bites

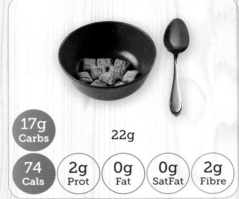

Multigrain Hoops — 15g

12g Carbs				
55 Cals	1g Prot	1g Fat	0g SatFat	1g Fibre

Raisin Bites — 22g

17g Carbs				
74 Cals	2g Prot	0g Fat	0g SatFat	2g Fibre

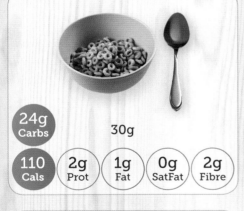

Multigrain Hoops — 30g

24g Carbs				
110 Cals	2g Prot	1g Fat	0g SatFat	2g Fibre

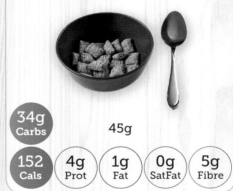

Raisin Bites — 45g

34g Carbs				
152 Cals	4g Prot	1g Fat	0g SatFat	5g Fibre

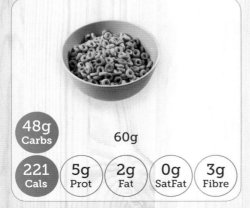

Multigrain Hoops — 60g

48g Carbs				
221 Cals	5g Prot	2g Fat	0g SatFat	3g Fibre

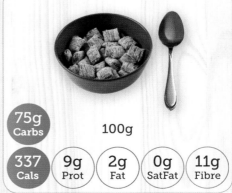

Raisin Bites — 100g

75g Carbs				
337 Cals	9g Prot	2g Fat	0g SatFat	11g Fibre

14cm Cereal Bowl

Rice Snaps

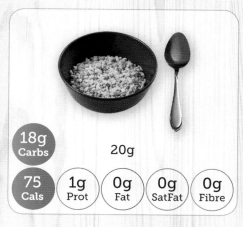

9g Carbs

10g

37 Cals

1g Prot

0g Fat

0g SatFat

0g Fibre

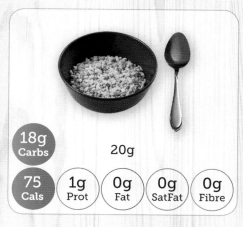

18g Carbs

20g

75 Cals

1g Prot

0g Fat

0g SatFat

0g Fibre

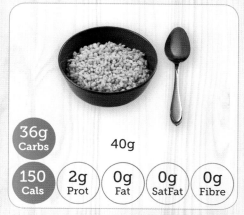

36g Carbs

40g

150 Cals

2g Prot

0g Fat

0g SatFat

0g Fibre

Special Flakes with Berries

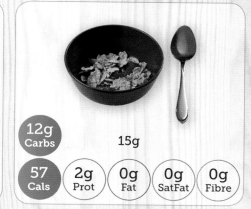

12g Carbs

15g

57 Cals

2g Prot

0g Fat

0g SatFat

0g Fibre

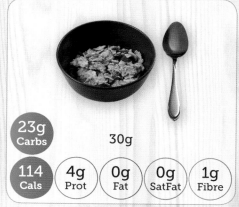

23g Carbs

30g

114 Cals

4g Prot

0g Fat

0g SatFat

1g Fibre

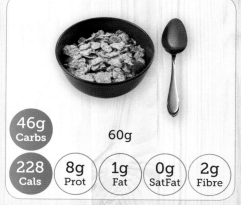

46g Carbs

60g

228 Cals

8g Prot

1g Fat

0g SatFat

2g Fibre

14cm Cereal Bowl

Oat Biscuit

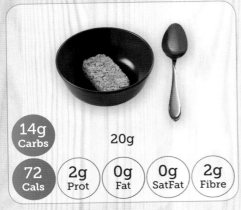

14g Carbs

20g

72 Cals | **2g** Prot | **0g** Fat | **0g** SatFat | **2g** Fibre

Milk (whole)

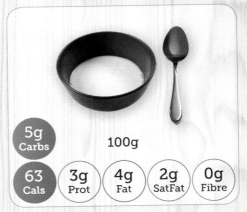

5g Carbs

100g

63 Cals | **3g** Prot | **4g** Fat | **2g** SatFat | **0g** Fibre

Wheat Biscuit

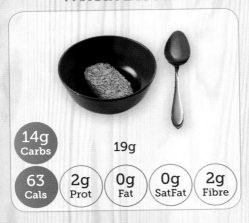

14g Carbs

19g

63 Cals | **2g** Prot | **0g** Fat | **0g** SatFat | **2g** Fibre

Milk (semi-skimmed)

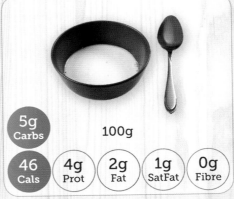

5g Carbs

100g

46 Cals | **4g** Prot | **2g** Fat | **1g** SatFat | **0g** Fibre

Wheat Pillow

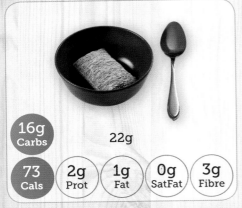

16g Carbs

22g

73 Cals | **2g** Prot | **1g** Fat | **0g** SatFat | **3g** Fibre

Milk (skimmed)

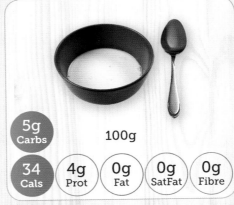

5g Carbs

100g

34 Cals | **4g** Prot | **0g** Fat | **0g** SatFat | **0g** Fibre

Cornmeal Porridge
(with condensed milk & sugar)

Cornmeal Porridge
(with water)

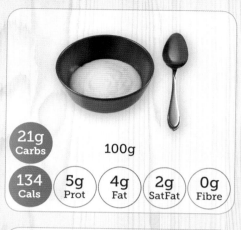

21g Carbs

100g

134 Cals | 5g Prot | 4g Fat | 2g SatFat | 0g Fibre

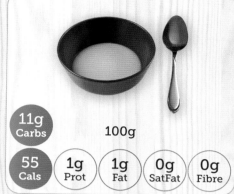

11g Carbs

100g

55 Cals | 1g Prot | 1g Fat | 0g SatFat | 0g Fibre

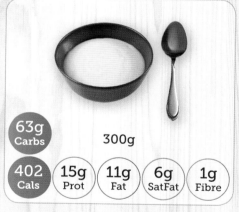

63g Carbs

300g

402 Cals | 15g Prot | 11g Fat | 6g SatFat | 1g Fibre

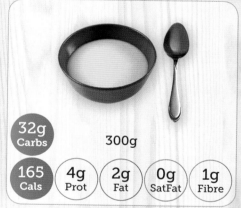

32g Carbs

300g

165 Cals | 4g Prot | 2g Fat | 0g SatFat | 1g Fibre

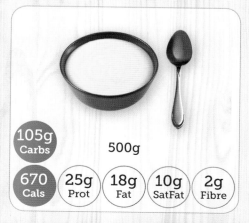

105g Carbs

500g

670 Cals | 25g Prot | 18g Fat | 10g SatFat | 2g Fibre

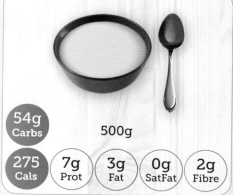

54g Carbs

500g

275 Cals | 7g Prot | 3g Fat | 0g SatFat | 2g Fibre

14cm Cereal Bowl

Porridge
(with semi-skimmed milk)

Porridge
(with water)

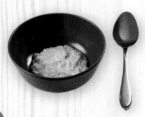

9g Carbs · 75g (9g oats)
63 Cals · **3g** Prot · **2g** Fat · **1g** SatFat · **1g** Fibre

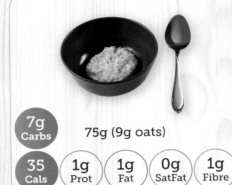

7g Carbs · 75g (9g oats)
35 Cals · **1g** Prot · **1g** Fat · **0g** SatFat · **1g** Fibre

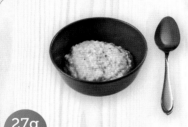

27g Carbs · 220g (27g oats)
185 Cals · **10g** Prot · **5g** Fat · **2g** SatFat · **2g** Fibre

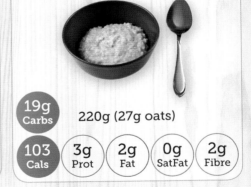

19g Carbs · 220g (27g oats)
103 Cals · **3g** Prot · **2g** Fat · **0g** SatFat · **2g** Fibre

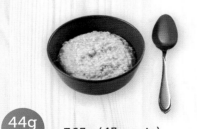

44g Carbs · 365g (45g oats)
307 Cals · **17g** Prot · **8g** Fat · **4g** SatFat · **4g** Fibre

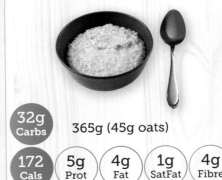

32g Carbs · 365g (45g oats)
172 Cals · **5g** Prot · **4g** Fat · **1g** SatFat · **4g** Fibre

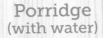

Cereals (per 100g weight)

	Carbs	Cals	Prot	Fat	SatFat	Fibre
All Bran	48g	334	14g	4g	1g	27g
All Bran Golden Crunch	62g	405	8g	11g	2g	13g
Bran Flakes	73g	333	10g	2g	0g	13g
Chocolate Snaps	90g	375	5g	2g	1g	2g
Corn Flakes	91g	376	7g	1g	0g	3g
Cornmeal Porridge (condensed milk & sugar)	21g	134	5g	4g	2g	0g
Cornmeal Porridge (with water)	11g	55	1g	1g	0g	0g
Crunchy Clusters	73g	378	9g	4g	2g	8g
Frosted Flakes	87g	350	5g	1g	0g	2g
Fruit & Fibre	70g	348	8g	6g	3g	9g
Granola	63g	448	10g	17g	3g	6g
Grapenuts	81g	365	11g	2g	0g	12g
Honey Nut Flakes	87g	384	5g	4g	1g	4g
Honey Puffed Wheat	87g	355	5g	1g	0g	3g
Instant Oats (uncooked)	65g	352	11g	7g	1g	9g
Malted Wheats	76g	339	9g	2g	0g	9g
Muesli	73g	366	9g	6g	1g	9g
Muesli (no added sugar)	71g	357	10g	6g	1g	9g
Multigrain Hoops	81g	368	8g	4g	1g	6g
Oat Biscuit	69g	358	12g	2g	1g	10g
Oat Flakes	60g	374	11g	8g	2g	9g
Porridge (with semi-skimmed milk)	12g	84	5g	2g	1g	1g
Porridge (with water)	9g	47	1g	1g	0g	1g
Porridge Oats (uncooked)	71g	381	11g	8g	1g	8g
Raisin Bites	75g	337	9g	2g	0g	11g
Rice Snaps	91g	374	6g	1g	0g	1g
Special Flakes with Berries	77g	380	13g	2g	1g	3g
Spelt Muesli	62g	380	9g	9g	1g	7g
Wheat Biscuit	73g	332	11g	2g	0g	10g
Wheat Pillow	71g	333	11g	3g	0g	12g

20cm Side Plate

Toast with Choc Spread
& Butter

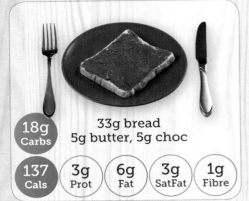

18g Carbs

33g bread
5g butter, 5g choc

137 Cals | **3g** Prot | **6g** Fat | **3g** SatFat | **1g** Fibre

Toast with Honey
& Butter

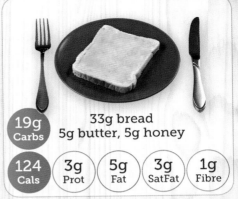

19g Carbs

33g bread
5g butter, 5g honey

124 Cals | **3g** Prot | **5g** Fat | **3g** SatFat | **1g** Fibre

Toast with Jam
& Butter

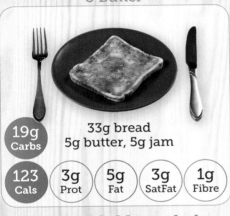

19g Carbs

33g bread
5g butter, 5g jam

123 Cals | **3g** Prot | **5g** Fat | **3g** SatFat | **1g** Fibre

Toast with Lemon Curd
& Butter

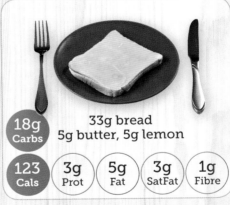

18g Carbs

33g bread
5g butter, 5g lemon

123 Cals | **3g** Prot | **5g** Fat | **3g** SatFat | **1g** Fibre

Toast with Marmalade
& Butter

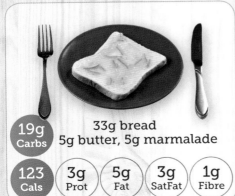

19g Carbs

33g bread
5g butter, 5g marmalade

123 Cals | **3g** Prot | **5g** Fat | **3g** SatFat | **1g** Fibre

Toast with Peanut Butter
& Butter

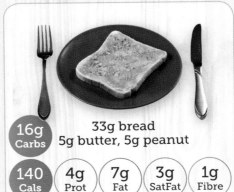

16g Carbs

33g bread
5g butter, 5g peanut

140 Cals | **4g** Prot | **7g** Fat | **3g** SatFat | **1g** Fibre

26cm Dinner Plate

Low-carb Cooked Breakfast

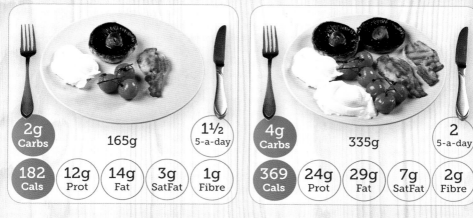

2g Carbs | 165g | **1½** 5-a-day
182 Cals | **12g** Prot | **14g** Fat | **3g** SatFat | **1g** Fibre

4g Carbs | 335g | **2** 5-a-day
369 Cals | **24g** Prot | **29g** Fat | **7g** SatFat | **2g** Fibre

Kippers, Spinach & Peppers

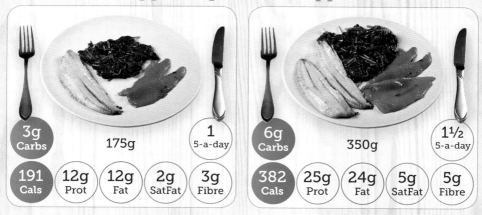

3g Carbs | 175g | **1** 5-a-day
191 Cals | **12g** Prot | **12g** Fat | **2g** SatFat | **3g** Fibre

6g Carbs | 350g | **1½** 5-a-day
382 Cals | **25g** Prot | **24g** Fat | **5g** SatFat | **5g** Fibre

Scrambled Eggs, Tomatoes & Halloumi

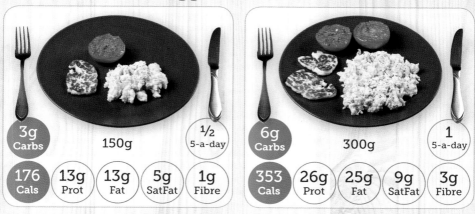

3g Carbs | 150g | **½** 5-a-day
176 Cals | **13g** Prot | **13g** Fat | **5g** SatFat | **1g** Fibre

6g Carbs | 300g | **1** 5-a-day
353 Cals | **26g** Prot | **25g** Fat | **9g** SatFat | **3g** Fibre

26cm Dinner Plate

Pancake (plain)

Pancake with Choc Spread

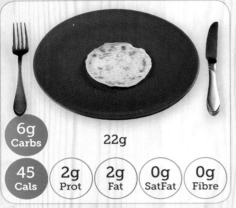

6g Carbs

22g

45 Cals | **2g** Prot | **2g** Fat | **0g** SatFat | **0g** Fibre

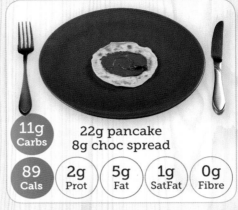

11g Carbs

22g pancake
8g choc spread

89 Cals | **2g** Prot | **5g** Fat | **1g** SatFat | **0g** Fibre

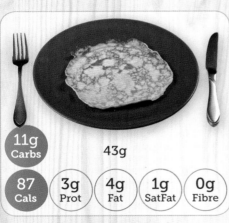

11g Carbs

43g

87 Cals | **3g** Prot | **4g** Fat | **1g** SatFat | **0g** Fibre

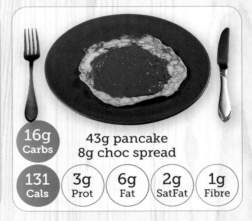

16g Carbs

43g pancake
8g choc spread

131 Cals | **3g** Prot | **6g** Fat | **2g** SatFat | **1g** Fibre

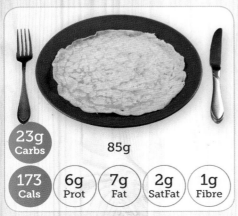

23g Carbs

85g

173 Cals | **6g** Prot | **7g** Fat | **2g** SatFat | **1g** Fibre

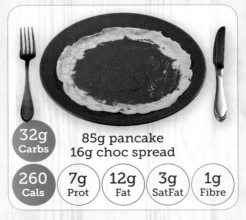

32g Carbs

85g pancake
16g choc spread

260 Cals | **7g** Prot | **12g** Fat | **3g** SatFat | **1g** Fibre

Pancake with Maple Syrup

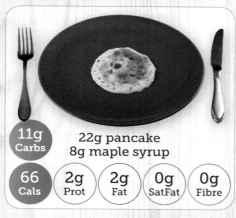

11g Carbs

22g pancake
8g maple syrup

66 Cals | **2g** Prot | **2g** Fat | **0g** SatFat | **0g** Fibre

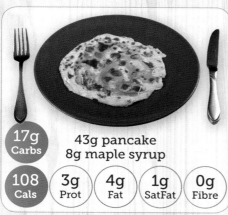

17g Carbs

43g pancake
8g maple syrup

108 Cals | **3g** Prot | **4g** Fat | **1g** SatFat | **0g** Fibre

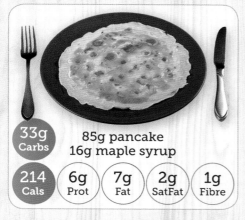

33g Carbs

85g pancake
16g maple syrup

214 Cals | **6g** Prot | **7g** Fat | **2g** SatFat | **1g** Fibre

Pancake with Sugar & Lemon

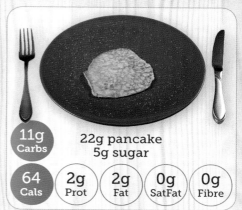

11g Carbs

22g pancake
5g sugar

64 Cals | **2g** Prot | **2g** Fat | **0g** SatFat | **0g** Fibre

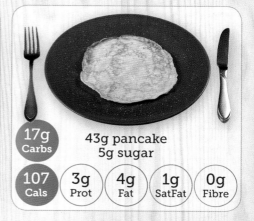

17g Carbs

43g pancake
5g sugar

107 Cals | **3g** Prot | **4g** Fat | **1g** SatFat | **0g** Fibre

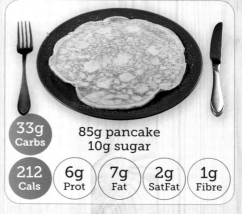

33g Carbs

85g pancake
10g sugar

212 Cals | **6g** Prot | **7g** Fat | **2g** SatFat | **1g** Fibre

20cm Side Plate / 26cm Dinner Plate

Breakfast Tart

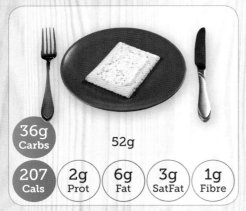

36g Carbs

52g

207 Cals | **2g** Prot | **6g** Fat | **3g** SatFat | **1g** Fibre

Scotch Pancake

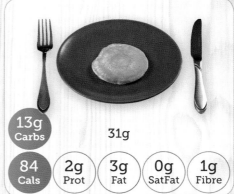

13g Carbs

31g

84 Cals | **2g** Prot | **3g** Fat | **0g** SatFat | **1g** Fibre

Eggy Bread

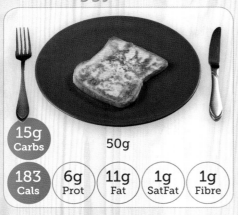

15g Carbs

50g

183 Cals | **6g** Prot | **11g** Fat | **1g** SatFat | **1g** Fibre

Fried Bread (in oil)

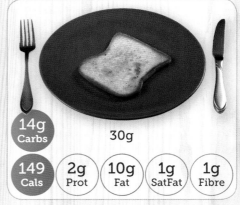

14g Carbs

30g

149 Cals | **2g** Prot | **10g** Fat | **1g** SatFat | **1g** Fibre

Waffle (sweet)

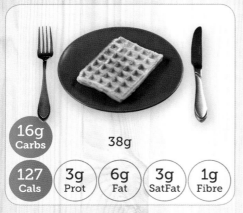

16g Carbs

38g

127 Cals | **3g** Prot | **6g** Fat | **3g** SatFat | **1g** Fibre

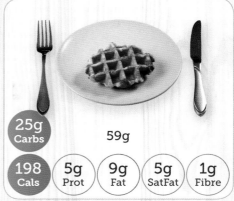

25g Carbs

59g

198 Cals | **5g** Prot | **9g** Fat | **5g** SatFat | **1g** Fibre

Bakewell Tart

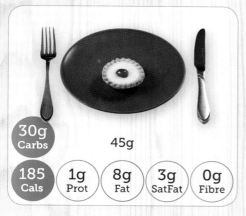

30g Carbs

45g

185 Cals | 1g Prot | 8g Fat | 3g SatFat | 0g Fibre

Baklava

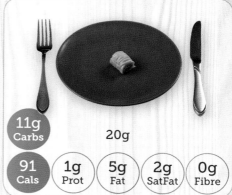

11g Carbs

20g

91 Cals | 1g Prot | 5g Fat | 2g SatFat | 0g Fibre

Carrot Cake

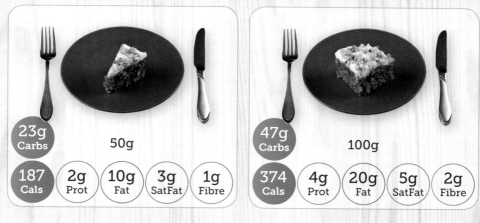

23g Carbs

50g

187 Cals | 2g Prot | 10g Fat | 3g SatFat | 1g Fibre

47g Carbs

100g

374 Cals | 4g Prot | 20g Fat | 5g SatFat | 2g Fibre

Chocolate Cake

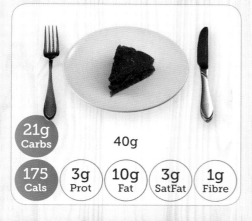

21g Carbs

40g

175 Cals | 3g Prot | 10g Fat | 3g SatFat | 1g Fibre

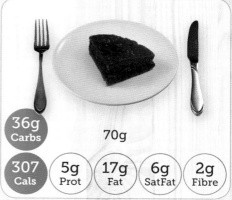

36g Carbs

70g

307 Cals | 5g Prot | 17g Fat | 6g SatFat | 2g Fibre

20cm Side Plate

Coffee & Walnut Cake

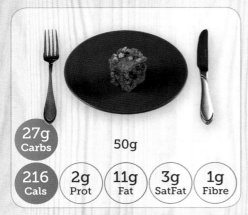

27g Carbs

50g

216 Cals | **2g** Prot | **11g** Fat | **3g** SatFat | **1g** Fibre

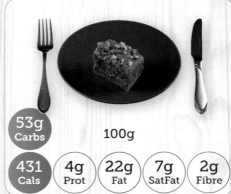

53g Carbs

100g

431 Cals | **4g** Prot | **22g** Fat | **7g** SatFat | **2g** Fibre

Fruit Cake

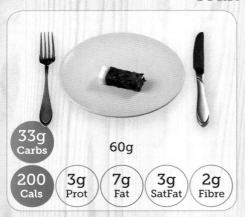

33g Carbs

60g

200 Cals | **3g** Prot | **7g** Fat | **3g** SatFat | **2g** Fibre

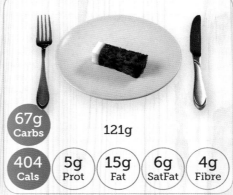

67g Carbs

121g

404 Cals | **5g** Prot | **15g** Fat | **6g** SatFat | **4g** Fibre

Ginger Cake

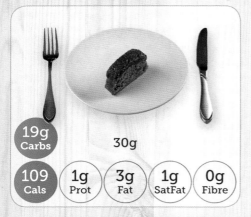

19g Carbs

30g

109 Cals | **1g** Prot | **3g** Fat | **1g** SatFat | **0g** Fibre

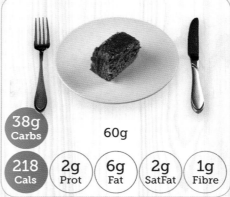

38g Carbs

60g

218 Cals | **2g** Prot | **6g** Fat | **2g** SatFat | **1g** Fibre

Malt Loaf

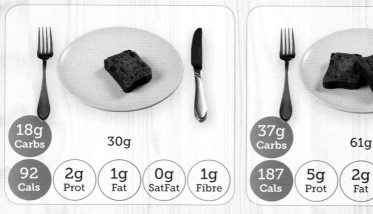

18g Carbs		30g		
92 Cals	2g Prot	1g Fat	0g SatFat	1g Fibre

37g Carbs		61g		
187 Cals	5g Prot	2g Fat	0g SatFat	3g Fibre

Swiss Roll

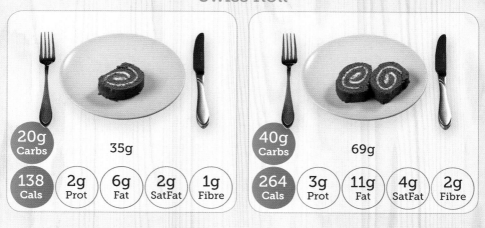

20g Carbs		35g		
138 Cals	2g Prot	6g Fat	2g SatFat	1g Fibre

40g Carbs		69g		
264 Cals	3g Prot	11g Fat	4g SatFat	2g Fibre

Victoria Sponge

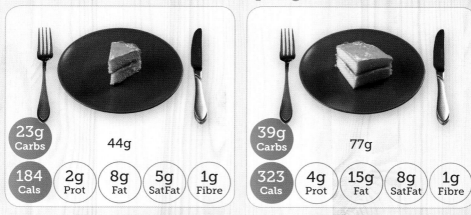

23g Carbs		44g		
184 Cals	2g Prot	8g Fat	5g SatFat	1g Fibre

39g Carbs		77g		
323 Cals	4g Prot	15g Fat	8g SatFat	1g Fibre

Apple Danish

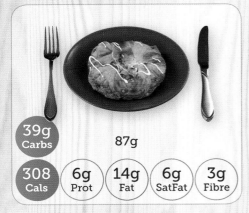

39g Carbs   87g

308 Cals | **6g** Prot | **14g** Fat | **6g** SatFat | **3g** Fibre

Chocolate Chip Twist

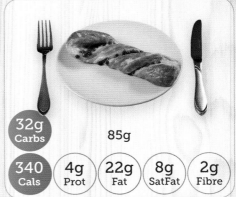

32g Carbs   85g

340 Cals | **4g** Prot | **22g** Fat | **8g** SatFat | **2g** Fibre

Cinnamon Swirl

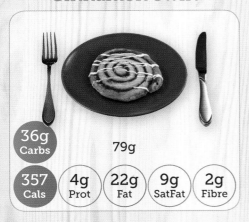

36g Carbs   79g

357 Cals | **4g** Prot | **22g** Fat | **9g** SatFat | **2g** Fibre

Fruit Trellis

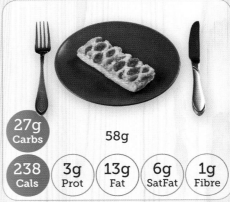

27g Carbs   58g

238 Cals | **3g** Prot | **13g** Fat | **6g** SatFat | **1g** Fibre

Pain aux Raisins

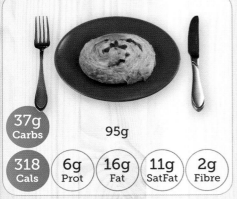

37g Carbs   95g

318 Cals | **6g** Prot | **16g** Fat | **11g** SatFat | **2g** Fibre

Pecan Plait

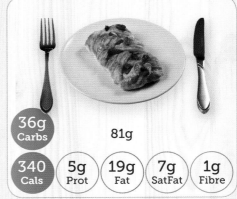

36g Carbs   81g

340 Cals | **5g** Prot | **19g** Fat | **7g** SatFat | **1g** Fibre

Chocolate Éclair

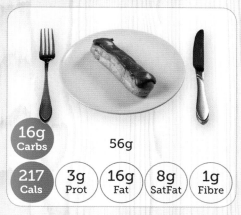

16g Carbs

56g

217 Cals | **3g** Prot | **16g** Fat | **8g** SatFat | **1g** Fibre

Corn Flake Cake

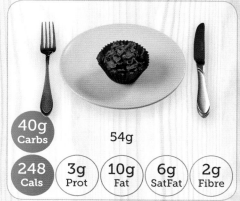

40g Carbs

54g

248 Cals | **3g** Prot | **10g** Fat | **6g** SatFat | **2g** Fibre

Cup Cake

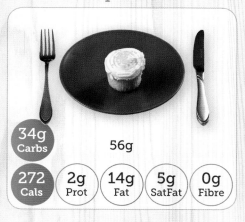

34g Carbs

56g

272 Cals | **2g** Prot | **14g** Fat | **5g** SatFat | **0g** Fibre

Custard Slice

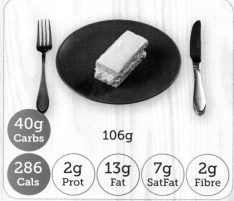

40g Carbs

106g

286 Cals | **2g** Prot | **13g** Fat | **7g** SatFat | **2g** Fibre

Custard Tart

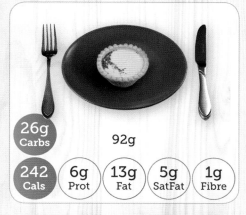

26g Carbs

92g

242 Cals | **6g** Prot | **13g** Fat | **5g** SatFat | **1g** Fibre

Mini Battenburg

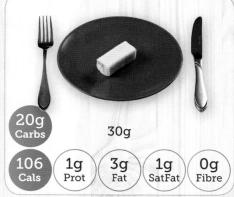

20g Carbs

30g

106 Cals | **1g** Prot | **3g** Fat | **1g** SatFat | **0g** Fibre

20cm Side Plate

Choc Ring Doughnut

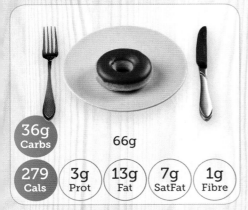

36g Carbs

66g

279 Cals | **3g** Prot | **13g** Fat | **7g** SatFat | **1g** Fibre

Glazed Ring Doughnut

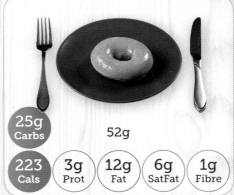

25g Carbs

52g

223 Cals | **3g** Prot | **12g** Fat | **6g** SatFat | **1g** Fibre

Jam Doughnut

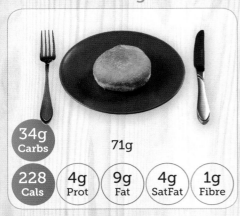

34g Carbs

71g

228 Cals | **4g** Prot | **9g** Fat | **4g** SatFat | **1g** Fibre

Mini Doughnut

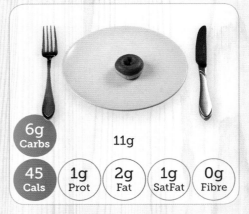

6g Carbs

11g

45 Cals | **1g** Prot | **2g** Fat | **1g** SatFat | **0g** Fibre

Sprinkle Ring Doughnut

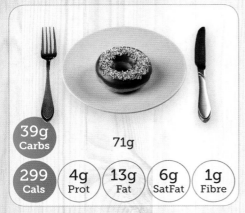

39g Carbs

71g

299 Cals | **4g** Prot | **13g** Fat | **6g** SatFat | **1g** Fibre

Sugar Ring Doughnut

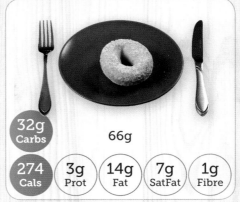

32g Carbs

66g

274 Cals | **3g** Prot | **14g** Fat | **7g** SatFat | **1g** Fibre

Fresh Cream Doughnut

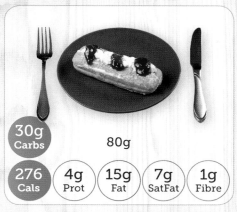

30g Carbs

80g

276 Cals | **4g** Prot | **15g** Fat | **7g** SatFat | **1g** Fibre

Yum Yum

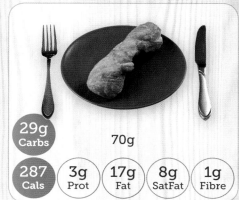

29g Carbs

70g

287 Cals | **3g** Prot | **17g** Fat | **8g** SatFat | **1g** Fibre

Blueberry Muffin

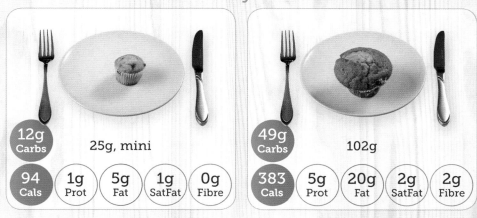

12g Carbs

25g, mini

94 Cals | **1g** Prot | **5g** Fat | **1g** SatFat | **0g** Fibre

49g Carbs

102g

383 Cals | **5g** Prot | **20g** Fat | **2g** SatFat | **2g** Fibre

Chocolate Muffin

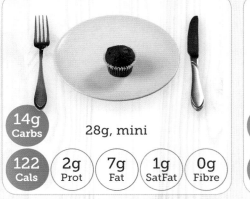

14g Carbs

28g, mini

122 Cals | **2g** Prot | **7g** Fat | **1g** SatFat | **0g** Fibre

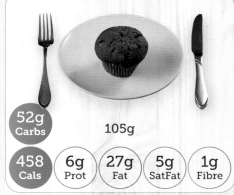

52g Carbs

105g

458 Cals | **6g** Prot | **27g** Fat | **5g** SatFat | **1g** Fibre

Flapjack

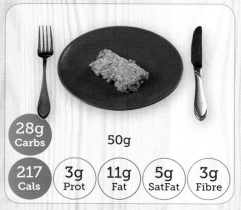

28g Carbs

50g

217 Cals | **3g** Prot | **11g** Fat | **5g** SatFat | **3g** Fibre

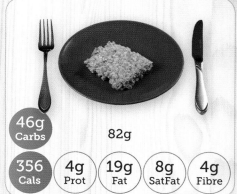

46g Carbs

82g

356 Cals | **4g** Prot | **19g** Fat | **8g** SatFat | **4g** Fibre

Meringue Nest

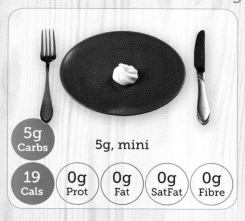

5g Carbs

5g, mini

19 Cals | **0g** Prot | **0g** Fat | **0g** SatFat | **0g** Fibre

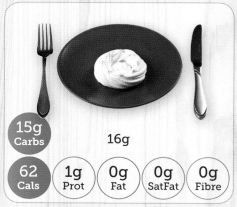

15g Carbs

16g

62 Cals | **1g** Prot | **0g** Fat | **0g** SatFat | **0g** Fibre

Mince Pie

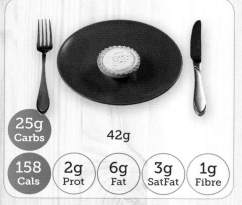

25g Carbs

42g

158 Cals | **2g** Prot | **6g** Fat | **3g** SatFat | **1g** Fibre

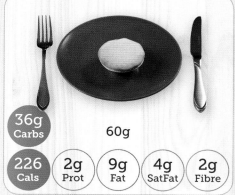

36g Carbs

60g

226 Cals | **2g** Prot | **9g** Fat | **4g** SatFat | **2g** Fibre

Belgian Bun

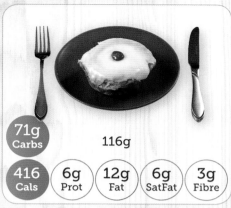

71g Carbs

116g

416 Cals | **6g** Prot | **12g** Fat | **6g** SatFat | **3g** Fibre

Iced Bun

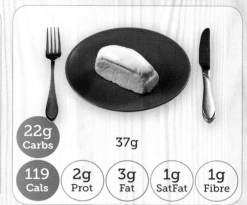

22g Carbs

37g

119 Cals | **2g** Prot | **3g** Fat | **1g** SatFat | **1g** Fibre

Hot Cross Bun

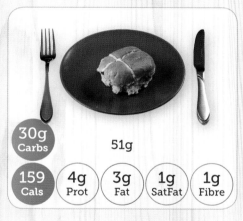

30g Carbs

51g

159 Cals | **4g** Prot | **3g** Fat | **1g** SatFat | **1g** Fibre

Cheese Scone

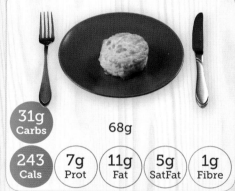

31g Carbs

68g

243 Cals | **7g** Prot | **11g** Fat | **5g** SatFat | **1g** Fibre

Fruit Scone

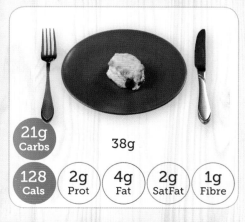

21g Carbs

38g

128 Cals | **2g** Prot | **4g** Fat | **2g** SatFat | **1g** Fibre

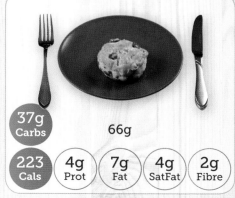

37g Carbs

66g

223 Cals | **4g** Prot | **7g** Fat | **4g** SatFat | **2g** Fibre

	Carbs	Cals	Prot	Fat	SatFat	Fibre
Flour (per 100g weight)						
Chickpea	57g	353	23g	5g	1g	10g
Cornflour	92g	354	1g	1g	0g	0g
Fufu	81g	350	5g	0g	0g	1g
Gari	95g	361	1g	0g	0g	5g
Granary	69g	334	10g	1g	0g	3g
Plain White	81g	352	9g	1g	0g	4g
Rye	74g	319	7g	2g	0g	14g
Self-Raising	80g	348	9g	2g	0g	4g
Wholemeal	70g	327	12g	2g	0g	10g
Baking (per 100g weight)						
Choux Pastry (raw)	20g	203	6g	12g	4g	1g
Cocoa Powder	12g	312	19g	22g	13g	16g
Custard Powder	92g	354	1g	1g	0g	0g
Desiccated Coconut	6g	604	6g	62g	53g	18g
Egg	0g	131	13g	9g	3g	0g
Egg White	0g	43	11g	0g	0g	0g
Egg Yolk	0g	347	16g	31g	9g	0g
Filo Pastry (raw)	59g	278	8g	3g	0g	3g
Marzipan	68g	389	5g	13g	1g	2g
Oatmeal	71g	381	11g	8g	1g	8g
Puff Pastry (raw)	34g	384	5g	26g	13g	3g
Shortcrust Pastry (raw)	39g	453	6g	31g	12g	3g
Stem Ginger	71g	292	1g	1g	0g	2g
Sugar (per 100g weight)						
Caster	100g	400	0g	0g	0g	0g
Dark Muscovado	95g	384	0g	0g	0g	1g
Demerara	100g	394	1g	0g	0g	0g
Granulated	100g	400	0g	0g	0g	0g
Icing	100g	393	0g	0g	0g	0g

26cm Dinner Plate

Brie

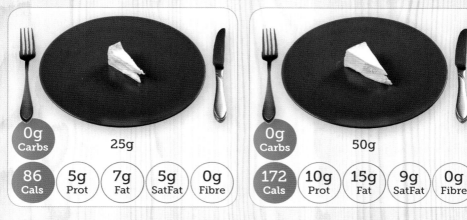

0g Carbs		25g			
86 Cals	5g Prot	7g Fat	5g SatFat	0g Fibre	

0g Carbs		50g			
172 Cals	10g Prot	15g Fat	9g SatFat	0g Fibre	

Camembert

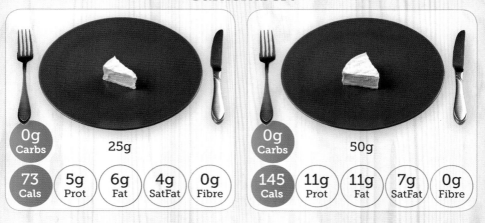

0g Carbs		25g			
73 Cals	5g Prot	6g Fat	4g SatFat	0g Fibre	

0g Carbs		50g			
145 Cals	11g Prot	11g Fat	7g SatFat	0g Fibre	

Cheddar (reduced fat)

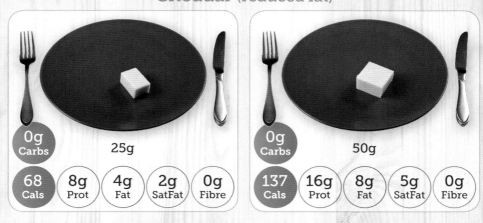

0g Carbs		25g			
68 Cals	8g Prot	4g Fat	2g SatFat	0g Fibre	

0g Carbs		50g			
137 Cals	16g Prot	8g Fat	5g SatFat	0g Fibre	

26cm Dinner Plate

Cheddar

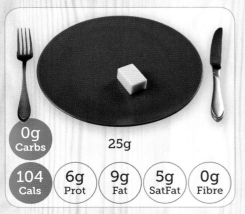

0g Carbs

25g

104 Cals | **6g** Prot | **9g** Fat | **5g** SatFat | **0g** Fibre

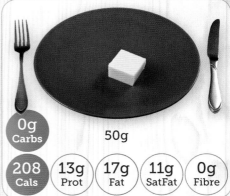

0g Carbs

50g

208 Cals | **13g** Prot | **17g** Fat | **11g** SatFat | **0g** Fibre

Cheddar (grated)

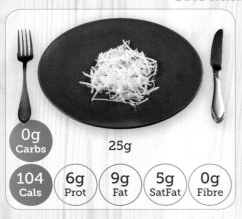

0g Carbs

25g

104 Cals | **6g** Prot | **9g** Fat | **5g** SatFat | **0g** Fibre

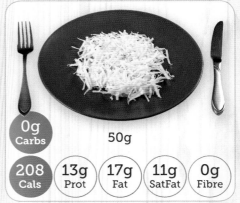

0g Carbs

50g

208 Cals | **13g** Prot | **17g** Fat | **11g** SatFat | **0g** Fibre

Cheddar (sliced)

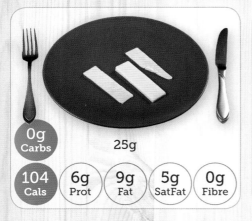

0g Carbs

25g

104 Cals | **6g** Prot | **9g** Fat | **5g** SatFat | **0g** Fibre

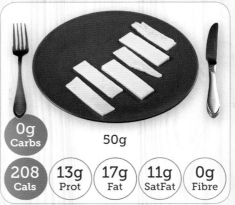

0g Carbs

50g

208 Cals | **13g** Prot | **17g** Fat | **11g** SatFat | **0g** Fibre

Cottage Cheese

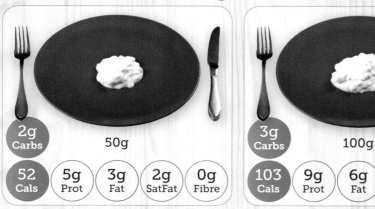

2g Carbs	50g			
52 Cals	5g Prot	3g Fat	2g SatFat	0g Fibre

3g Carbs	100g			
103 Cals	9g Prot	6g Fat	3g SatFat	0g Fibre

Cream Cheese

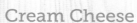
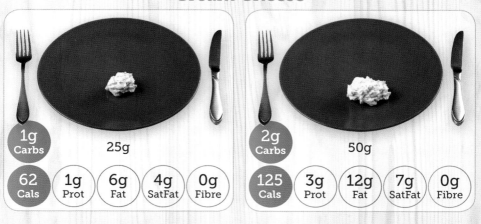

1g Carbs	25g			
62 Cals	1g Prot	6g Fat	4g SatFat	0g Fibre

2g Carbs	50g			
125 Cals	3g Prot	12g Fat	7g SatFat	0g Fibre

Edam

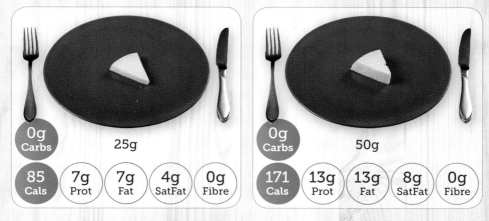

0g Carbs	25g			
85 Cals	7g Prot	7g Fat	4g SatFat	0g Fibre

0g Carbs	50g			
171 Cals	13g Prot	13g Fat	8g SatFat	0g Fibre

26cm Dinner Plate

Feta

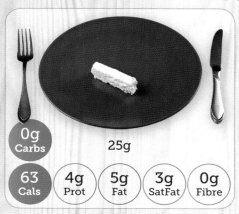

0g Carbs

25g

63 Cals | **4g** Prot | **5g** Fat | **3g** SatFat | **0g** Fibre

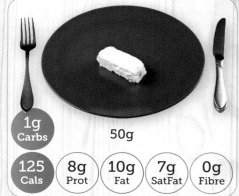

1g Carbs

50g

125 Cals | **8g** Prot | **10g** Fat | **7g** SatFat | **0g** Fibre

Goat's Cheese

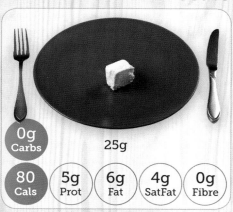

0g Carbs

25g

80 Cals | **5g** Prot | **6g** Fat | **4g** SatFat | **0g** Fibre

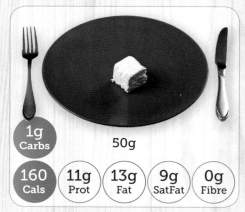

1g Carbs

50g

160 Cals | **11g** Prot | **13g** Fat | **9g** SatFat | **0g** Fibre

Halloumi

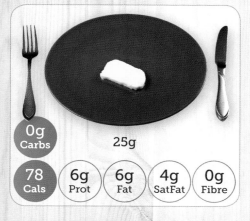

0g Carbs

25g

78 Cals | **6g** Prot | **6g** Fat | **4g** SatFat | **0g** Fibre

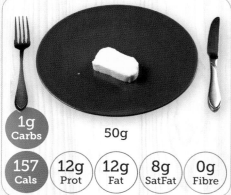

1g Carbs

50g

157 Cals | **12g** Prot | **12g** Fat | **8g** SatFat | **0g** Fibre

Mozzarella

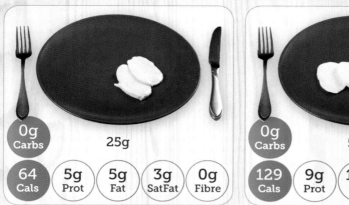

0g
Carbs

25g

64
Cals

5g
Prot

5g
Fat

3g
SatFat

0g
Fibre

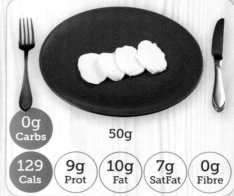

0g
Carbs

50g

129
Cals

9g
Prot

10g
Fat

7g
SatFat

0g
Fibre

Parmesan

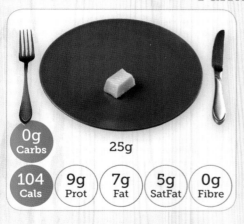

0g
Carbs

25g

104
Cals

9g
Prot

7g
Fat

5g
SatFat

0g
Fibre

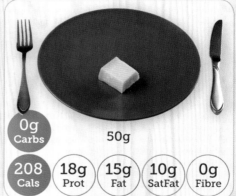

0g
Carbs

50g

208
Cals

18g
Prot

15g
Fat

10g
SatFat

0g
Fibre

Parmesan (grated)

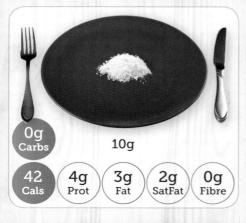

0g
Carbs

10g

42
Cals

4g
Prot

3g
Fat

2g
SatFat

0g
Fibre

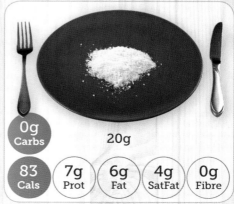

0g
Carbs

20g

83
Cals

7g
Prot

6g
Fat

4g
SatFat

0g
Fibre

Ricotta

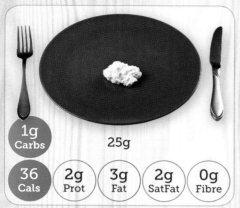

1g Carbs — 25g
36 Cals | 2g Prot | 3g Fat | 2g SatFat | 0g Fibre

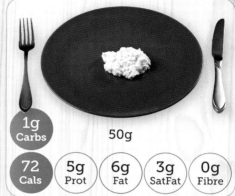

1g Carbs — 50g
72 Cals | 5g Prot | 6g Fat | 3g SatFat | 0g Fibre

Squirty Cheese

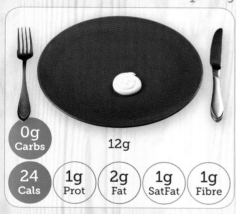

0g Carbs — 12g
24 Cals | 1g Prot | 2g Fat | 1g SatFat | 1g Fibre

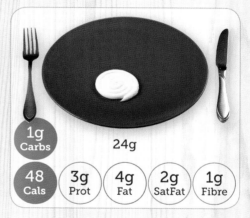

1g Carbs — 24g
48 Cals | 3g Prot | 4g Fat | 2g SatFat | 1g Fibre

Spreadable Cheese

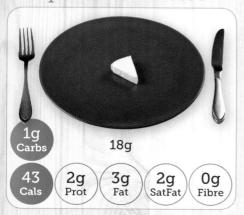

1g Carbs — 18g
43 Cals | 2g Prot | 3g Fat | 2g SatFat | 0g Fibre

Processed Cheese Slice

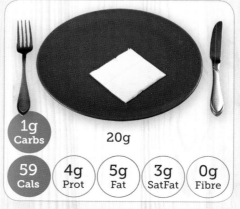

1g Carbs — 20g
59 Cals | 4g Prot | 5g Fat | 3g SatFat | 0g Fibre

Stilton

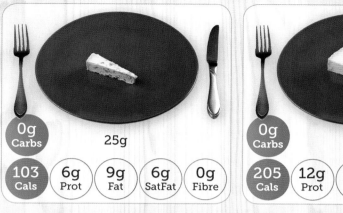

0g
Carbs

25g

103
Cals

6g
Prot

9g
Fat

6g
SatFat

0g
Fibre

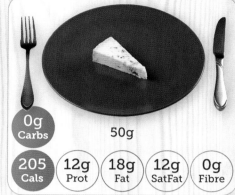

0g
Carbs

50g

205
Cals

12g
Prot

18g
Fat

12g
SatFat

0g
Fibre

Red Leicester

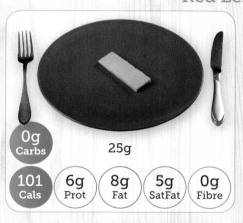

0g
Carbs

25g

101
Cals

6g
Prot

8g
Fat

5g
SatFat

0g
Fibre

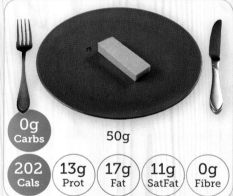

0g
Carbs

50g

202
Cals

13g
Prot

17g
Fat

11g
SatFat

0g
Fibre

Wensleydale with Cranberries

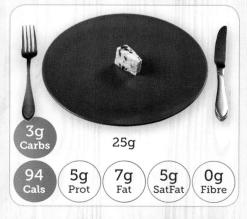

3g
Carbs

25g

94
Cals

5g
Prot

7g
Fat

5g
SatFat

0g
Fibre

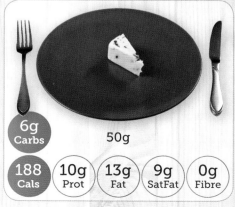

6g
Carbs

50g

188
Cals

10g
Prot

13g
Fat

9g
SatFat

0g
Fibre

22cm Large Bowl

Apple Pie

Apple & Rhubarb Crumble

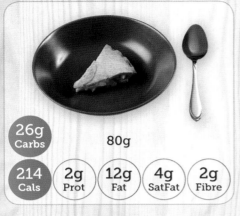

26g Carbs 80g

214 Cals | **2g Prot** | **12g Fat** | **4g SatFat** | **2g Fibre**

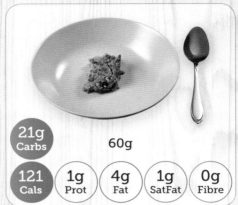

21g Carbs 60g

121 Cals | **1g Prot** | **4g Fat** | **1g SatFat** | **0g Fibre**

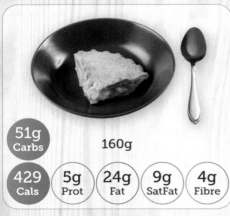

51g Carbs 160g

429 Cals | **5g Prot** | **24g Fat** | **9g SatFat** | **4g Fibre**

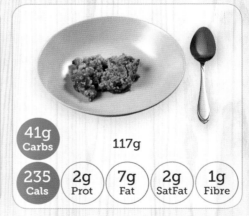

41g Carbs 117g

235 Cals | **2g Prot** | **7g Fat** | **2g SatFat** | **1g Fibre**

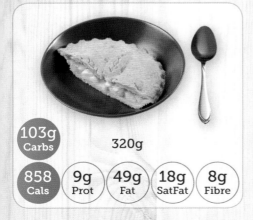

103g Carbs 320g

858 Cals | **9g Prot** | **49g Fat** | **18g SatFat** | **8g Fibre**

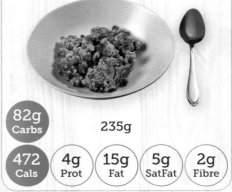

82g Carbs 235g

472 Cals | **4g Prot** | **15g Fat** | **5g SatFat** | **2g Fibre**

Apple Strudel

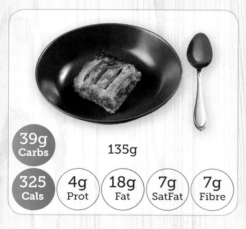

13g Carbs

45g

108 Cals | **1g** Prot | **6g** Fat | **2g** SatFat | **2g** Fibre

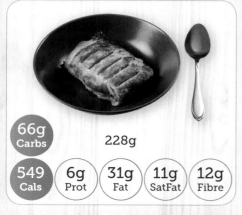

39g Carbs

135g

325 Cals | **4g** Prot | **18g** Fat | **7g** SatFat | **7g** Fibre

66g Carbs

228g

549 Cals | **6g** Prot | **31g** Fat | **11g** SatFat | **12g** Fibre

Banoffee Pie

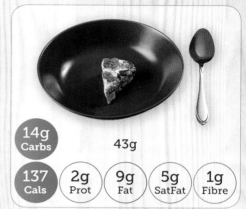

14g Carbs

43g

137 Cals | **2g** Prot | **9g** Fat | **5g** SatFat | **1g** Fibre

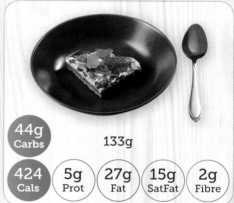

44g Carbs

133g

424 Cals | **5g** Prot | **27g** Fat | **15g** SatFat | **2g** Fibre

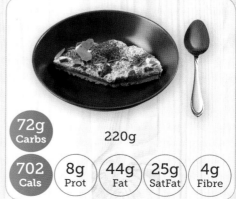

72g Carbs

220g

702 Cals | **8g** Prot | **44g** Fat | **25g** SatFat | **4g** Fibre

Black Forest Gateau

Bread & Butter Pudding

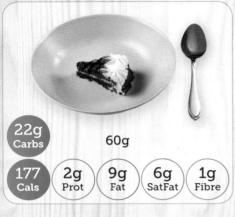

22g Carbs — 60g

177 Cals | **2g** Prot | **9g** Fat | **6g** SatFat | **1g** Fibre

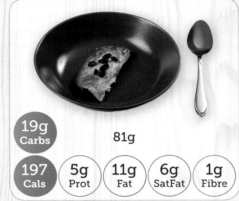

19g Carbs — 81g

197 Cals | **5g** Prot | **11g** Fat | **6g** SatFat | **1g** Fibre

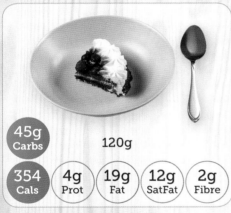

45g Carbs — 120g

354 Cals | **4g** Prot | **19g** Fat | **12g** SatFat | **2g** Fibre

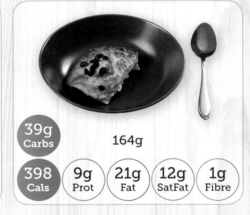

39g Carbs — 164g

398 Cals | **9g** Prot | **21g** Fat | **12g** SatFat | **1g** Fibre

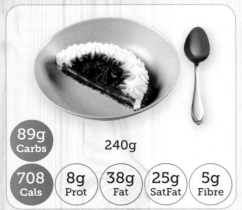

89g Carbs — 240g

708 Cals | **8g** Prot | **38g** Fat | **25g** SatFat | **5g** Fibre

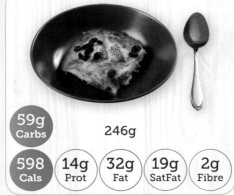

59g Carbs — 246g

598 Cals | **14g** Prot | **32g** Fat | **19g** SatFat | **2g** Fibre

Brownie

Cheesecake

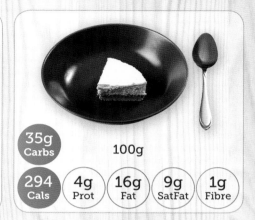

Brownie

24g Carbs — 45g
228 Cals | 3g Prot | 14g Fat | 7g SatFat | 1g Fibre

Cheesecake

35g Carbs — 100g
294 Cals | 4g Prot | 16g Fat | 9g SatFat | 1g Fibre

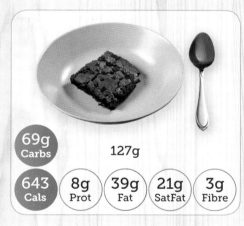

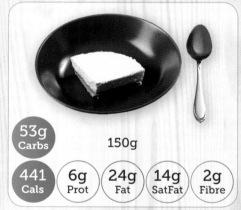

Brownie

69g Carbs — 127g
643 Cals | 8g Prot | 39g Fat | 21g SatFat | 3g Fibre

Cheesecake

53g Carbs — 150g
441 Cals | 6g Prot | 24g Fat | 14g SatFat | 2g Fibre

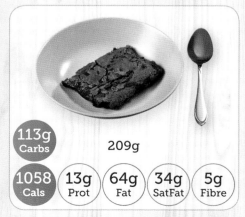

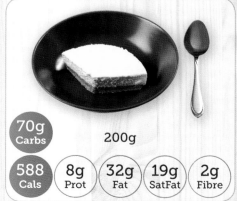

Brownie

113g Carbs — 209g
1058 Cals | 13g Prot | 64g Fat | 34g SatFat | 5g Fibre

Cheesecake

70g Carbs — 200g
588 Cals | 8g Prot | 32g Fat | 19g SatFat | 2g Fibre

22cm Large Bowl

Chocolate Mousse

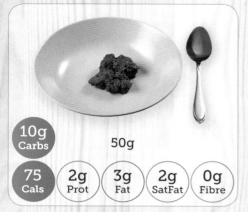

10g **Carbs**

50g

75 **Cals**

2g Prot

3g Fat

2g SatFat

0g Fibre

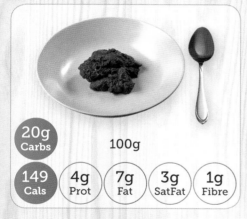

20g **Carbs**

100g

149 **Cals**

4g Prot

7g Fat

3g SatFat

1g Fibre

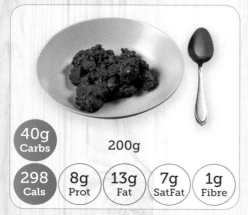

40g **Carbs**

200g

298 **Cals**

8g Prot

13g Fat

7g SatFat

1g Fibre

Chocolate Torte

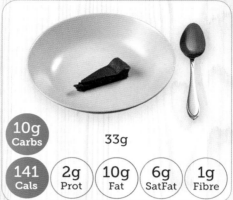

10g **Carbs**

33g

141 **Cals**

2g Prot

10g Fat

6g SatFat

1g Fibre

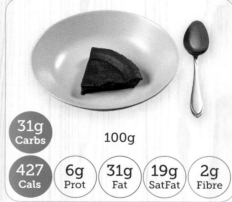

31g **Carbs**

100g

427 **Cals**

6g Prot

31g Fat

19g SatFat

2g Fibre

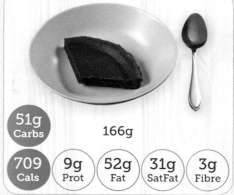

51g **Carbs**

166g

709 **Cals**

9g Prot

52g Fat

31g SatFat

3g Fibre

Christmas Pudding

Custard
(with semi-skimmed milk)

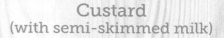

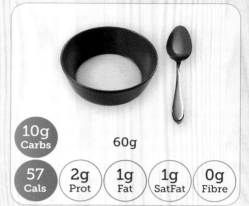

20g Carbs — 35g

100 Cals	1g Prot	2g Fat	1g SatFat	1g Fibre

10g Carbs — 60g

57 Cals	2g Prot	1g Fat	1g SatFat	0g Fibre

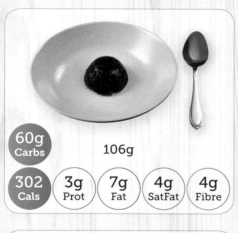

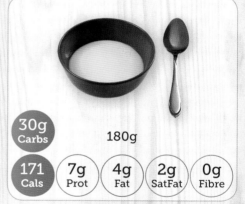

60g Carbs — 106g

302 Cals	3g Prot	7g Fat	4g SatFat	4g Fibre

30g Carbs — 180g

171 Cals	7g Prot	4g Fat	2g SatFat	0g Fibre

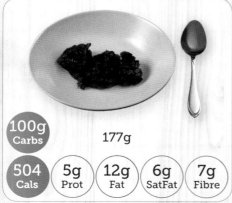

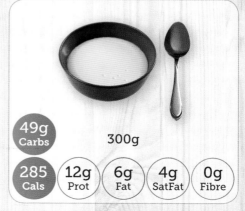

100g Carbs — 177g

504 Cals	5g Prot	12g Fat	6g SatFat	7g Fibre

49g Carbs — 300g

285 Cals	12g Prot	6g Fat	4g SatFat	0g Fibre

Ice Cream (chocolate)   Ice Cream (vanilla)

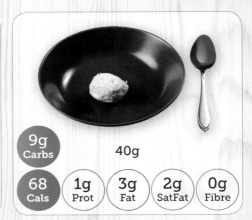

10g Carbs — 40g — **9g** Carbs — 40g

| **83** Cals | **2g** Prot | **4g** Fat | **3g** SatFat | **0g** Fibre | **68** Cals | **1g** Prot | **3g** Fat | **2g** SatFat | **0g** Fibre |

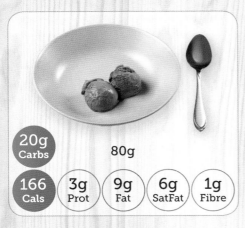
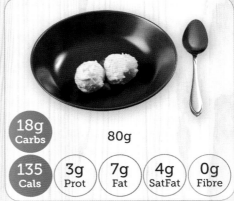

20g Carbs — 80g — **18g** Carbs — 80g

| **166** Cals | **3g** Prot | **9g** Fat | **6g** SatFat | **1g** Fibre | **135** Cals | **3g** Prot | **7g** Fat | **4g** SatFat | **0g** Fibre |

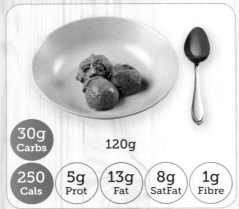
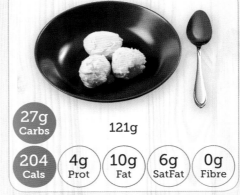

30g Carbs — 120g — **27g** Carbs — 121g

| **250** Cals | **5g** Prot | **13g** Fat | **8g** SatFat | **1g** Fibre | **204** Cals | **4g** Prot | **10g** Fat | **6g** SatFat | **0g** Fibre |

Sorbet (lemon)

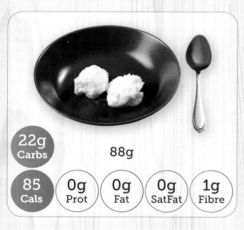

11g Carbs
45g

44 Cals | **0g Prot** | **0g Fat** | **0g SatFat** | **0g Fibre**

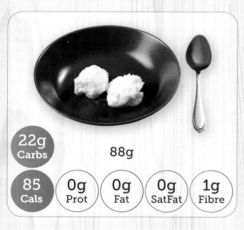

22g Carbs
88g

85 Cals | **0g Prot** | **0g Fat** | **0g SatFat** | **1g Fibre**

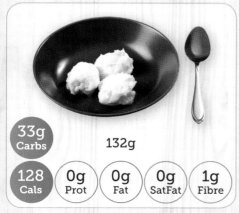

33g Carbs
132g

128 Cals | **0g Prot** | **0g Fat** | **0g SatFat** | **1g Fibre**

Sorbet (raspberry)

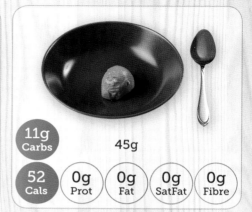

11g Carbs
45g

52 Cals | **0g Prot** | **0g Fat** | **0g SatFat** | **0g Fibre**

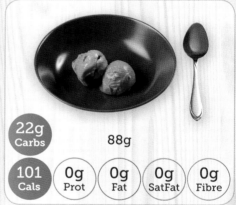

22g Carbs
88g

101 Cals | **0g Prot** | **0g Fat** | **0g SatFat** | **0g Fibre**

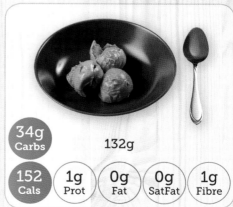

34g Carbs
132g

152 Cals | **1g Prot** | **0g Fat** | **0g SatFat** | **1g Fibre**

22cm Large Bowl

Choc Ice

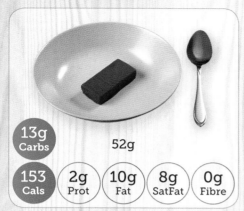

13g Carbs

52g

153 Cals | **2g** Prot | **10g** Fat | **8g** SatFat | **0g** Fibre

Crème Brûlée

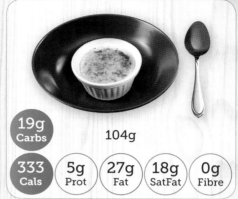

19g Carbs

104g

333 Cals | **5g** Prot | **27g** Fat | **18g** SatFat | **0g** Fibre

Chocolate & Nut Cone

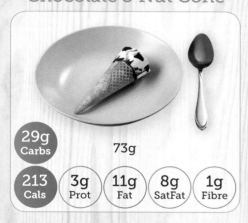

29g Carbs

73g

213 Cals | **3g** Prot | **11g** Fat | **8g** SatFat | **1g** Fibre

Panna Cotta

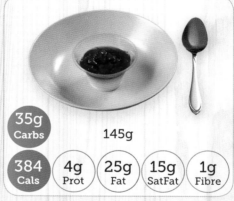

35g Carbs

145g

384 Cals | **4g** Prot | **25g** Fat | **15g** SatFat | **1g** Fibre

Ice Cream Lolly

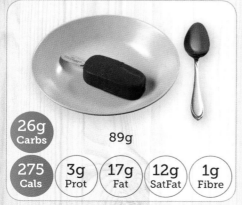

26g Carbs

89g

275 Cals | **3g** Prot | **17g** Fat | **12g** SatFat | **1g** Fibre

Strawberry Tartlet

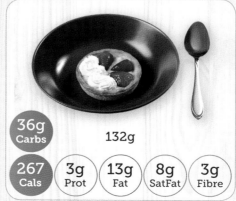

36g Carbs

132g

267 Cals | **3g** Prot | **13g** Fat | **8g** SatFat | **3g** Fibre

Jelly

Jelly (sugar free)

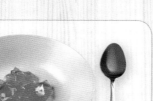

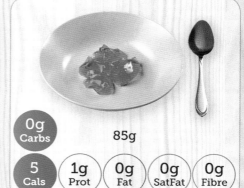

13g Carbs — 85g

52 Cals | **1g** Prot | **0g** Fat | **0g** SatFat | **0g** Fibre

0g Carbs — 85g

5 Cals | **1g** Prot | **0g** Fat | **0g** SatFat | **0g** Fibre

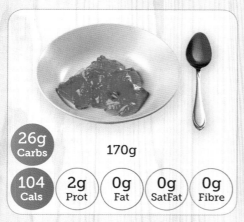

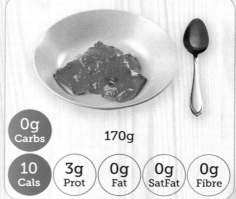

26g Carbs — 170g

104 Cals | **2g** Prot | **0g** Fat | **0g** SatFat | **0g** Fibre

0g Carbs — 170g

10 Cals | **3g** Prot | **0g** Fat | **0g** SatFat | **0g** Fibre

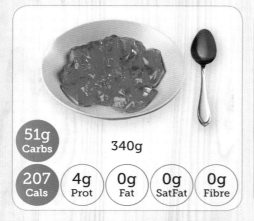

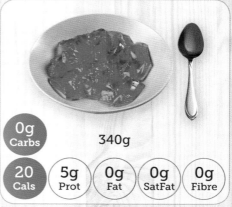

51g Carbs — 340g

207 Cals | **4g** Prot | **0g** Fat | **0g** SatFat | **0g** Fibre

0g Carbs — 340g

20 Cals | **5g** Prot | **0g** Fat | **0g** SatFat | **0g** Fibre

Lemon Meringue Pie

Profiteroles

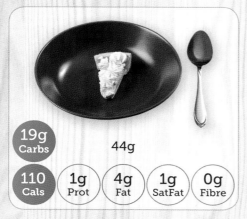

19g Carbs   44g

110 Cals   **1g** Prot   **4g** Fat   **1g** SatFat   **0g** Fibre

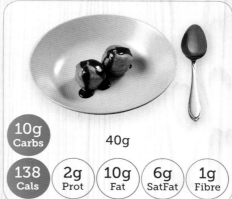

10g Carbs   40g

138 Cals   **2g** Prot   **10g** Fat   **6g** SatFat   **1g** Fibre

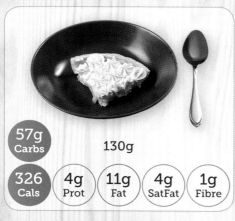

57g Carbs   130g

326 Cals   **4g** Prot   **11g** Fat   **4g** SatFat   **1g** Fibre

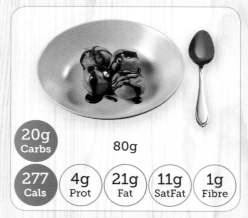

20g Carbs   80g

277 Cals   **4g** Prot   **21g** Fat   **11g** SatFat   **1g** Fibre

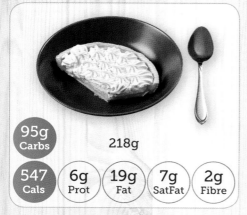

95g Carbs   218g

547 Cals   **6g** Prot   **19g** Fat   **7g** SatFat   **2g** Fibre

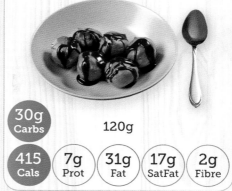

30g Carbs   120g

415 Cals   **7g** Prot   **31g** Fat   **17g** SatFat   **2g** Fibre

Rice Pudding

Roulade

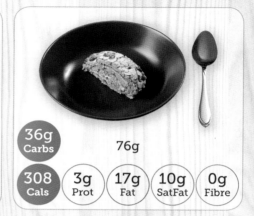

23g Carbs
140g

119 Cals | **5g** Prot | **2g** Fat | **1g** SatFat | **0g** Fibre

36g Carbs
76g

308 Cals | **3g** Prot | **17g** Fat | **10g** SatFat | **0g** Fibre

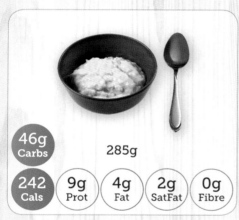
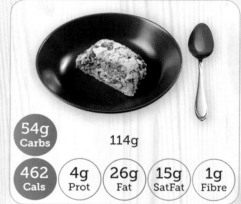

46g Carbs
285g

242 Cals | **9g** Prot | **4g** Fat | **2g** SatFat | **0g** Fibre

54g Carbs
114g

462 Cals | **4g** Prot | **26g** Fat | **15g** SatFat | **1g** Fibre

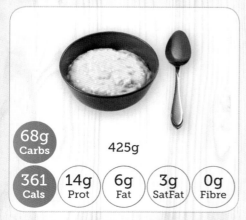
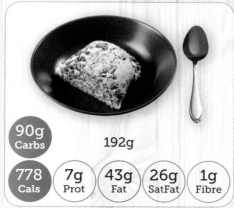

68g Carbs
425g

361 Cals | **14g** Prot | **6g** Fat | **3g** SatFat | **0g** Fibre

90g Carbs
192g

778 Cals | **7g** Prot | **43g** Fat | **26g** SatFat | **1g** Fibre

22cm Large Bowl

Spotted Dick

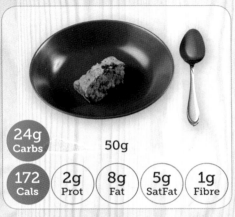

24g Carbs

50g

172 Cals · **2g** Prot · **8g** Fat · **5g** SatFat · **1g** Fibre

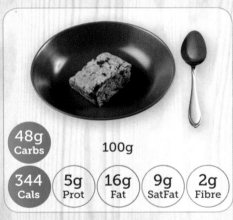

48g Carbs

100g

344 Cals · **5g** Prot · **16g** Fat · **9g** SatFat · **2g** Fibre

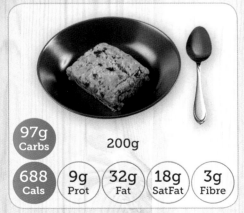

97g Carbs

200g

688 Cals · **9g** Prot · **32g** Fat · **18g** SatFat · **3g** Fibre

Sticky Toffee Pudding

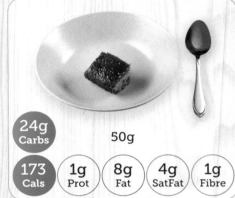

24g Carbs

50g

173 Cals · **1g** Prot · **8g** Fat · **4g** SatFat · **1g** Fibre

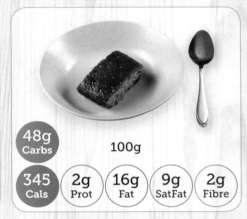

48g Carbs

100g

345 Cals · **2g** Prot · **16g** Fat · **9g** SatFat · **2g** Fibre

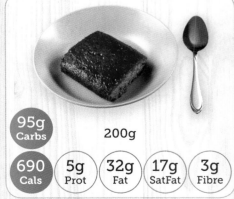

95g Carbs

200g

690 Cals · **5g** Prot · **32g** Fat · **17g** SatFat · **3g** Fibre

Strawberry Delight

Summer Pudding

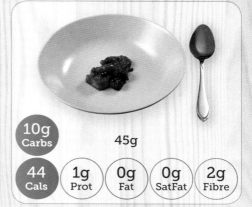

8g Carbs   50g

58 Cals	2g Prot	2g Fat	2g SatFat	0g Fibre

10g Carbs   45g

44 Cals	1g Prot	0g Fat	0g SatFat	2g Fibre

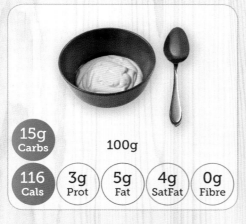

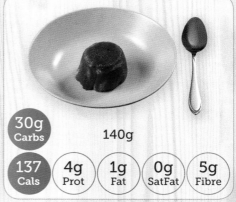

15g Carbs   100g

116 Cals	3g Prot	5g Fat	4g SatFat	0g Fibre

30g Carbs   140g

137 Cals	4g Prot	1g Fat	0g SatFat	5g Fibre

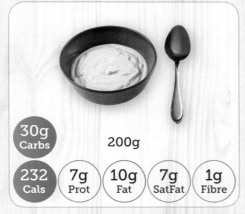

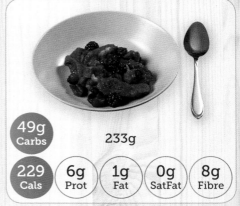

30g Carbs   200g

232 Cals	7g Prot	10g Fat	7g SatFat	1g Fibre

49g Carbs   233g

229 Cals	6g Prot	1g Fat	0g SatFat	8g Fibre

Tiramisu

Trifle

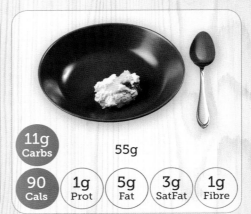

Tiramisu

12g Carbs — 45g
110 Cals | 2g Prot | 6g Fat | 4g SatFat | 0g Fibre

Trifle

11g Carbs — 55g
90 Cals | 1g Prot | 5g Fat | 3g SatFat | 1g Fibre

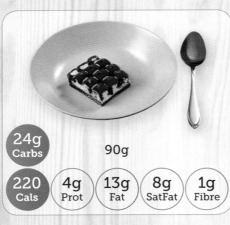

24g Carbs — 90g
220 Cals | 4g Prot | 13g Fat | 8g SatFat | 1g Fibre

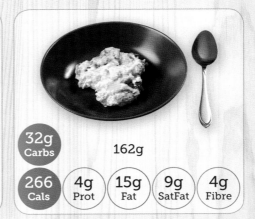

32g Carbs — 162g
266 Cals | 4g Prot | 15g Fat | 9g SatFat | 4g Fibre

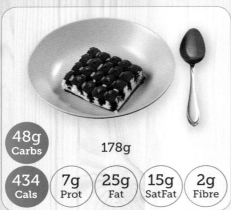

48g Carbs — 178g
434 Cals | 7g Prot | 25g Fat | 15g SatFat | 2g Fibre

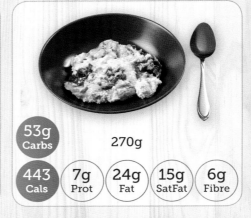

53g Carbs — 270g
443 Cals | 7g Prot | 24g Fat | 15g SatFat | 6g Fibre

Apple Juice

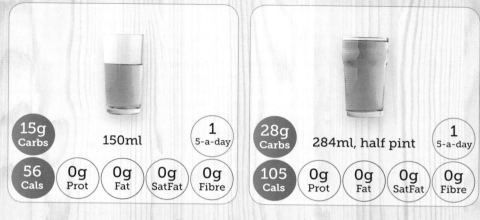

15g Carbs · 150ml · **1** 5-a-day
56 Cals · **0g** Prot · **0g** Fat · **0g** SatFat · **0g** Fibre

28g Carbs · 284ml, half pint · **1** 5-a-day
105 Cals · **0g** Prot · **0g** Fat · **0g** SatFat · **0g** Fibre

Cranberry Juice

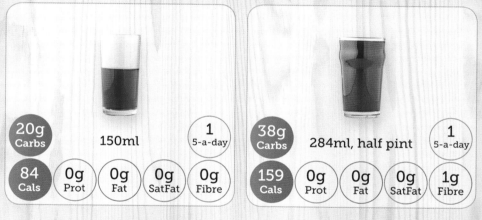

20g Carbs · 150ml · **1** 5-a-day
84 Cals · **0g** Prot · **0g** Fat · **0g** SatFat · **0g** Fibre

38g Carbs · 284ml, half pint · **1** 5-a-day
159 Cals · **0g** Prot · **0g** Fat · **0g** SatFat · **1g** Fibre

Grapefruit Juice

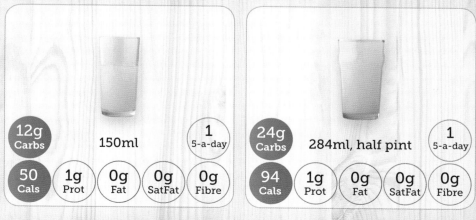

12g Carbs · 150ml · **1** 5-a-day
50 Cals · **1g** Prot · **0g** Fat · **0g** SatFat · **0g** Fibre

24g Carbs · 284ml, half pint · **1** 5-a-day
94 Cals · **1g** Prot · **0g** Fat · **0g** SatFat · **0g** Fibre

Orange Juice

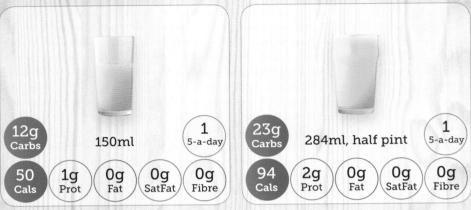

12g Carbs — 150ml — **1** 5-a-day
50 Cals — **1g** Prot — **0g** Fat — **0g** SatFat — **0g** Fibre

23g Carbs — 284ml, half pint — **1** 5-a-day
94 Cals — **2g** Prot — **0g** Fat — **0g** SatFat — **0g** Fibre

Pineapple Juice

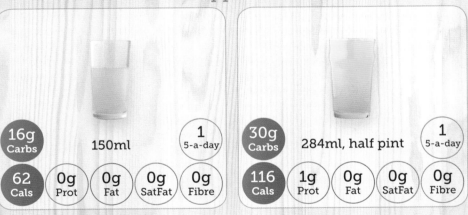

16g Carbs — 150ml — **1** 5-a-day
62 Cals — **0g** Prot — **0g** Fat — **0g** SatFat — **0g** Fibre

30g Carbs — 284ml, half pint — **1** 5-a-day
116 Cals — **1g** Prot — **0g** Fat — **0g** SatFat — **0g** Fibre

Tomato Juice

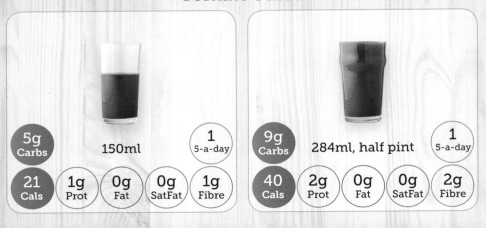

5g Carbs — 150ml — **1** 5-a-day
21 Cals — **1g** Prot — **0g** Fat — **0g** SatFat — **1g** Fibre

9g Carbs — 284ml, half pint — **1** 5-a-day
40 Cals — **2g** Prot — **0g** Fat — **0g** SatFat — **2g** Fibre

Smoothie (strawberry & banana)

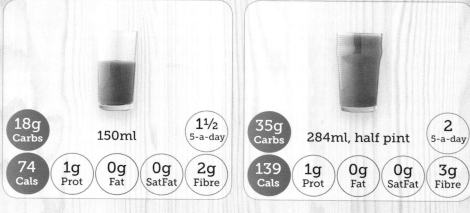

18g Carbs — 150ml — **1½** 5-a-day
74 Cals | **1g** Prot | **0g** Fat | **0g** SatFat | **2g** Fibre

35g Carbs — 284ml, half pint — **2** 5-a-day
139 Cals | **1g** Prot | **0g** Fat | **0g** SatFat | **3g** Fibre

Squash

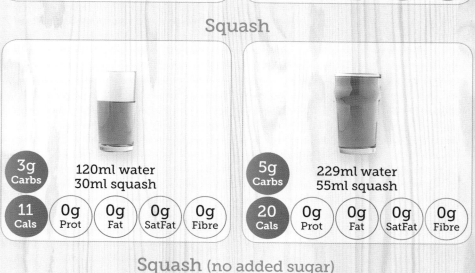

3g Carbs — 120ml water / 30ml squash
11 Cals | **0g** Prot | **0g** Fat | **0g** SatFat | **0g** Fibre

5g Carbs — 229ml water / 55ml squash
20 Cals | **0g** Prot | **0g** Fat | **0g** SatFat | **0g** Fibre

Squash (no added sugar)

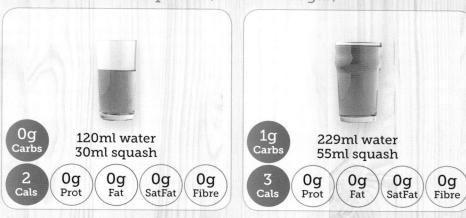

0g Carbs — 120ml water / 30ml squash
2 Cals | **0g** Prot | **0g** Fat | **0g** SatFat | **0g** Fibre

1g Carbs — 229ml water / 55ml squash
3 Cals | **0g** Prot | **0g** Fat | **0g** SatFat | **0g** Fibre

Cola

Diet Cola

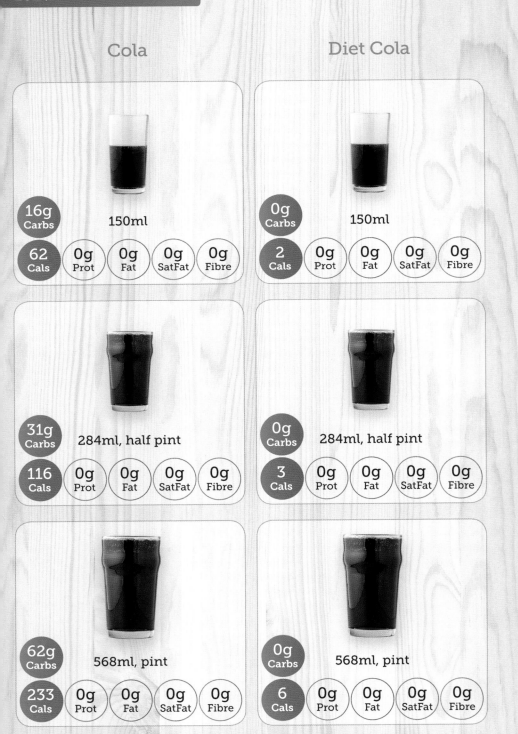

Cola

16g Carbs — 150ml
62 Cals | 0g Prot | 0g Fat | 0g SatFat | 0g Fibre

31g Carbs — 284ml, half pint
116 Cals | 0g Prot | 0g Fat | 0g SatFat | 0g Fibre

62g Carbs — 568ml, pint
233 Cals | 0g Prot | 0g Fat | 0g SatFat | 0g Fibre

Diet Cola

0g Carbs — 150ml
2 Cals | 0g Prot | 0g Fat | 0g SatFat | 0g Fibre

0g Carbs — 284ml, half pint
3 Cals | 0g Prot | 0g Fat | 0g SatFat | 0g Fibre

0g Carbs — 568ml, pint
6 Cals | 0g Prot | 0g Fat | 0g SatFat | 0g Fibre

Lemonade (sparkling)

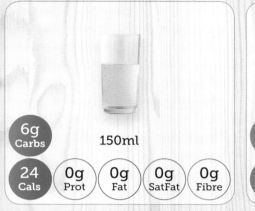

6g Carbs
150ml

24 Cals | **0g** Prot | **0g** Fat | **0g** SatFat | **0g** Fibre

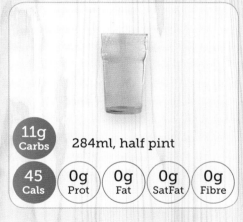

11g Carbs
284ml, half pint

45 Cals | **0g** Prot | **0g** Fat | **0g** SatFat | **0g** Fibre

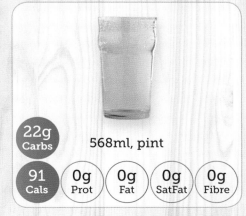

22g Carbs
568ml, pint

91 Cals | **0g** Prot | **0g** Fat | **0g** SatFat | **0g** Fibre

Lucozade Energy

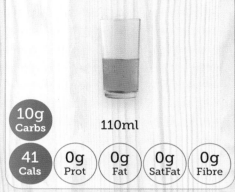

10g Carbs
110ml

41 Cals | **0g** Prot | **0g** Fat | **0g** SatFat | **0g** Fibre

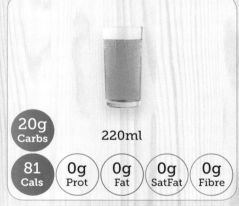

20g Carbs
220ml

81 Cals | **0g** Prot | **0g** Fat | **0g** SatFat | **0g** Fibre

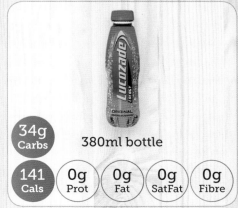

34g Carbs
380ml bottle

141 Cals | **0g** Prot | **0g** Fat | **0g** SatFat | **0g** Fibre

Iced Tea

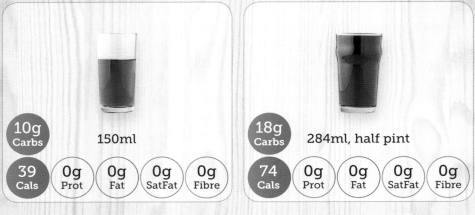

10g Carbs — 150ml

39 Cals | **0g** Prot | **0g** Fat | **0g** SatFat | **0g** Fibre

18g Carbs — 284ml, half pint

74 Cals | **0g** Prot | **0g** Fat | **0g** SatFat | **0g** Fibre

Lemonade (fresh)

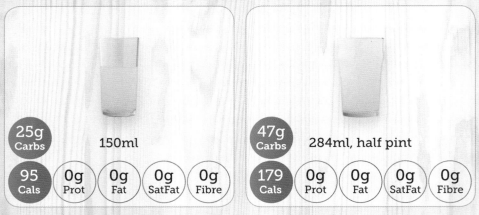

25g Carbs — 150ml

95 Cals | **0g** Prot | **0g** Fat | **0g** SatFat | **0g** Fibre

47g Carbs — 284ml, half pint

179 Cals | **0g** Prot | **0g** Fat | **0g** SatFat | **0g** Fibre

Malt Drink

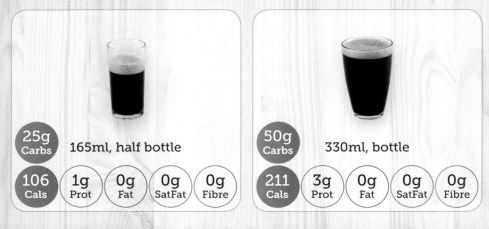

25g Carbs — 165ml, half bottle

106 Cals | **1g** Prot | **0g** Fat | **0g** SatFat | **0g** Fibre

50g Carbs — 330ml, bottle

211 Cals | **3g** Prot | **0g** Fat | **0g** SatFat | **0g** Fibre

Cappuccino
(whole milk)

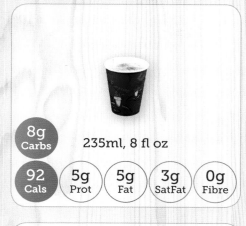

8g Carbs

235ml, 8 fl oz

92 Cals | **5g** Prot | **5g** Fat | **3g** SatFat | **0g** Fibre

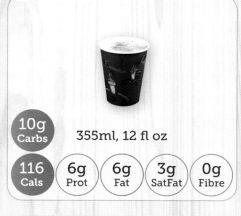

10g Carbs

355ml, 12 fl oz

116 Cals | **6g** Prot | **6g** Fat | **3g** SatFat | **0g** Fibre

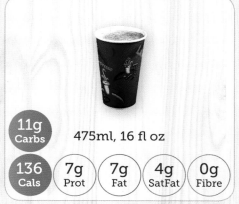

11g Carbs

475ml, 16 fl oz

136 Cals | **7g** Prot | **7g** Fat | **4g** SatFat | **0g** Fibre

Cappuccino
(skimmed milk)

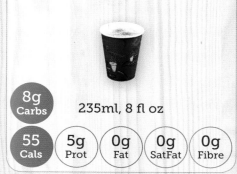

8g Carbs

235ml, 8 fl oz

55 Cals | **5g** Prot | **0g** Fat | **0g** SatFat | **0g** Fibre

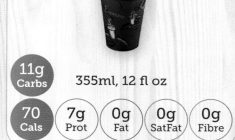

11g Carbs

355ml, 12 fl oz

70 Cals | **7g** Prot | **0g** Fat | **0g** SatFat | **0g** Fibre

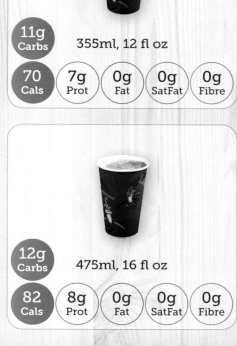

12g Carbs

475ml, 16 fl oz

82 Cals | **8g** Prot | **0g** Fat | **0g** SatFat | **0g** Fibre

Hot Chocolate
(whole milk)

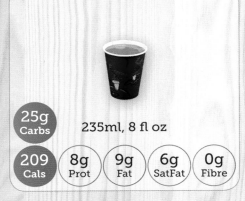

25g Carbs

235ml, 8 fl oz

209 Cals | **8g** Prot | **9g** Fat | **6g** SatFat | **0g** Fibre

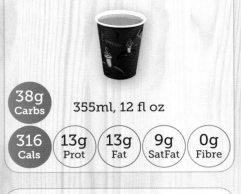

38g Carbs

355ml, 12 fl oz

316 Cals | **13g** Prot | **13g** Fat | **9g** SatFat | **0g** Fibre

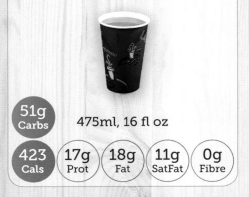

51g Carbs

475ml, 16 fl oz

423 Cals | **17g** Prot | **18g** Fat | **11g** SatFat | **0g** Fibre

Hot Chocolate
(skimmed milk)

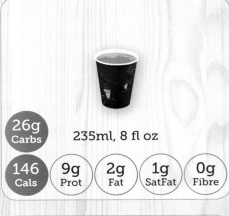

26g Carbs

235ml, 8 fl oz

146 Cals | **9g** Prot | **2g** Fat | **1g** SatFat | **0g** Fibre

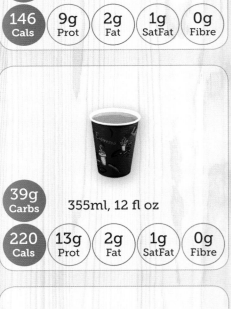

39g Carbs

355ml, 12 fl oz

220 Cals | **13g** Prot | **2g** Fat | **1g** SatFat | **0g** Fibre

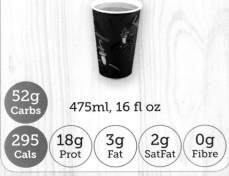

52g Carbs

475ml, 16 fl oz

295 Cals | **18g** Prot | **3g** Fat | **2g** SatFat | **0g** Fibre

Latte
(whole milk)

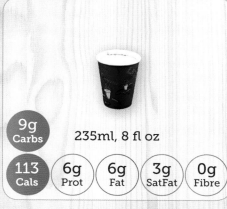

9g Carbs   235ml, 8 fl oz

113 Cals | **6g** Prot | **6g** Fat | **3g** SatFat | **0g** Fibre

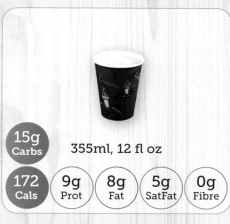

15g Carbs   355ml, 12 fl oz

172 Cals | **9g** Prot | **8g** Fat | **5g** SatFat | **0g** Fibre

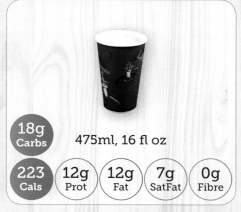

18g Carbs   475ml, 16 fl oz

223 Cals | **12g** Prot | **12g** Fat | **7g** SatFat | **0g** Fibre

Latte
(skimmed milk)

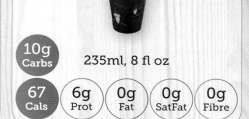

10g Carbs   235ml, 8 fl oz

67 Cals | **6g** Prot | **0g** Fat | **0g** SatFat | **0g** Fibre

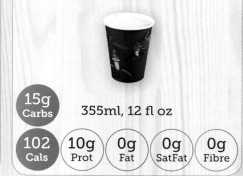

15g Carbs   355ml, 12 fl oz

102 Cals | **10g** Prot | **0g** Fat | **0g** SatFat | **0g** Fibre

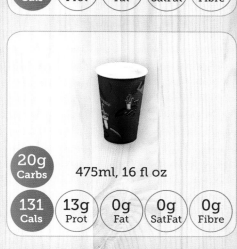

20g Carbs   475ml, 16 fl oz

131 Cals | **13g** Prot | **0g** Fat | **0g** SatFat | **0g** Fibre

Cup of Coffee (black)

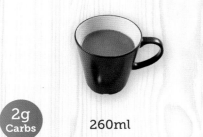

1g Carbs
260ml

5 Cals | **1g** Prot | **0g** Fat | **0g** SatFat | **0g** Fibre

Cup of Coffee (with milk)

2g Carbs
260ml

18 Cals | **2g** Prot | **1g** Fat | **0g** SatFat | **0g** Fibre

Cup of Tea (with milk)

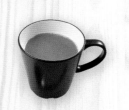

2g Carbs
260ml

18 Cals | **1g** Prot | **1g** Fat | **0g** SatFat | **0g** Fibre

Espresso

0g Carbs
60ml

1 Cals | **0g** Prot | **0g** Fat | **0g** SatFat | **0g** Fibre

Hot Malt Drink

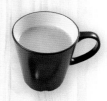

32g Carbs
260ml

218 Cals | **11g** Prot | **5g** Fat | **3g** SatFat | **1g** Fibre

Teaspoon of Sugar

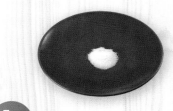

5g Carbs
5g, 1 tsp

20 Cals | **0g** Prot | **0g** Fat | **0g** SatFat | **0g** Fibre

Ale (4% ABV)

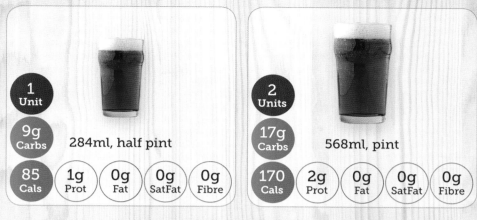

1 Unit
9g Carbs
85 Cals | **1g** Prot | **0g** Fat | **0g** SatFat | **0g** Fibre

284ml, half pint

2 Units
17g Carbs
170 Cals | **2g** Prot | **0g** Fat | **0g** SatFat | **0g** Fibre

568ml, pint

Lager (4% ABV)

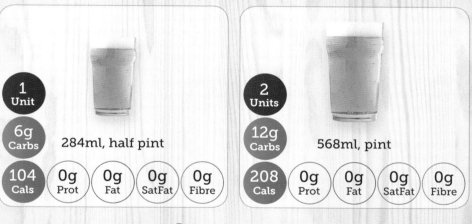

1 Unit
6g Carbs
104 Cals | **0g** Prot | **0g** Fat | **0g** SatFat | **0g** Fibre

284ml, half pint

2 Units
12g Carbs
208 Cals | **0g** Prot | **0g** Fat | **0g** SatFat | **0g** Fibre

568ml, pint

Stout (4% ABV)

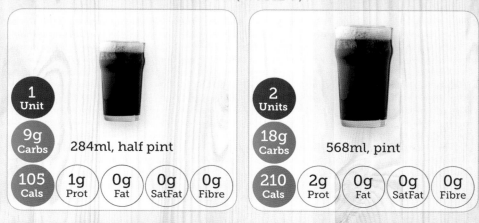

1 Unit
9g Carbs
105 Cals | **1g** Prot | **0g** Fat | **0g** SatFat | **0g** Fibre

284ml, half pint

2 Units
18g Carbs
210 Cals | **2g** Prot | **0g** Fat | **0g** SatFat | **0g** Fibre

568ml, pint

Cider (dry, 5% ABV)

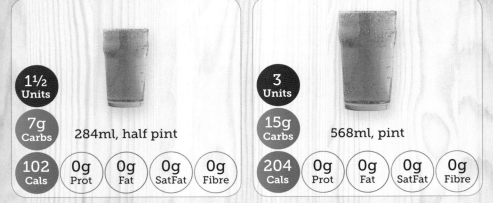

1½ Units
7g Carbs
102 Cals · 0g Prot · 0g Fat · 0g SatFat · 0g Fibre

284ml, half pint

3 Units
15g Carbs
204 Cals · 0g Prot · 0g Fat · 0g SatFat · 0g Fibre

568ml, pint

Cider (sweet, 5% ABV)

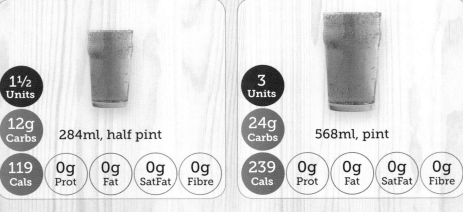

1½ Units
12g Carbs
119 Cals · 0g Prot · 0g Fat · 0g SatFat · 0g Fibre

284ml, half pint

3 Units
24g Carbs
239 Cals · 0g Prot · 0g Fat · 0g SatFat · 0g Fibre

568ml, pint

WKD Vodka Blue   WKD Iron Brew

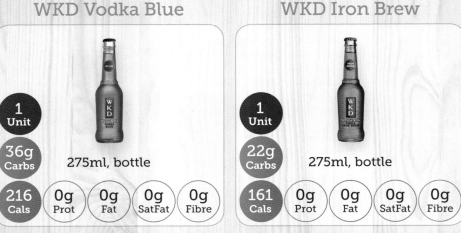

1 Unit
36g Carbs
216 Cals · 0g Prot · 0g Fat · 0g SatFat · 0g Fibre

275ml, bottle

1 Unit
22g Carbs
161 Cals · 0g Prot · 0g Fat · 0g SatFat · 0g Fibre

275ml, bottle

Red Wine

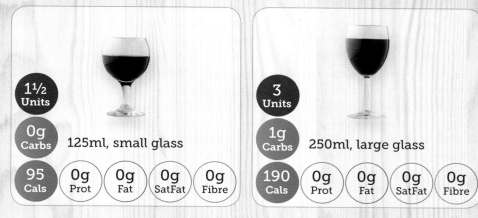

1½ Units — **0g Carbs** — **95 Cals** — 0g Prot — 0g Fat — 0g SatFat — 0g Fibre
125ml, small glass

3 Units — **1g Carbs** — **190 Cals** — 0g Prot — 0g Fat — 0g SatFat — 0g Fibre
250ml, large glass

White Wine (dry)

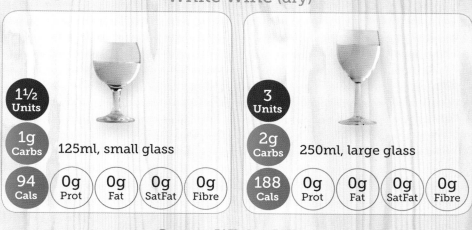

1½ Units — **1g Carbs** — **94 Cals** — 0g Prot — 0g Fat — 0g SatFat — 0g Fibre
125ml, small glass

3 Units — **2g Carbs** — **188 Cals** — 0g Prot — 0g Fat — 0g SatFat — 0g Fibre
250ml, large glass

Sweet White Wine

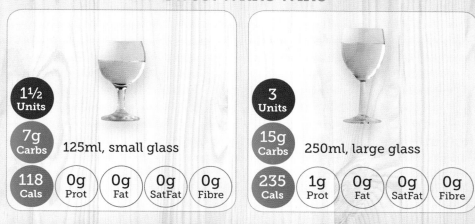

1½ Units — **7g Carbs** — **118 Cals** — 0g Prot — 0g Fat — 0g SatFat — 0g Fibre
125ml, small glass

3 Units — **15g Carbs** — **235 Cals** — 1g Prot — 0g Fat — 0g SatFat — 0g Fibre
250ml, large glass

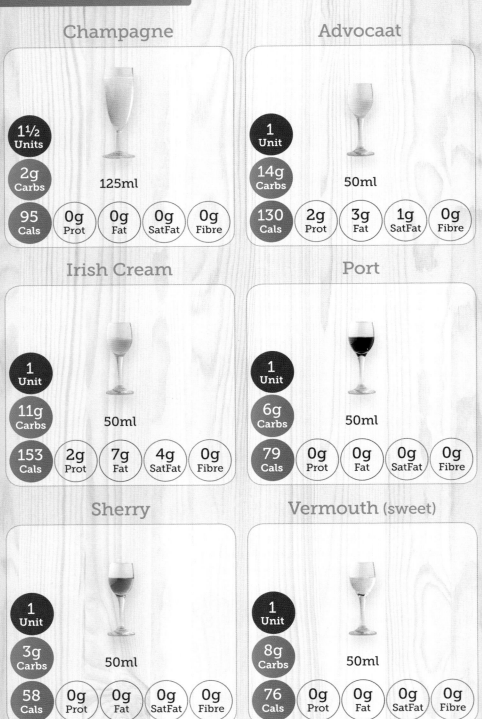

Champagne

1½ Units
2g Carbs
95 Cals
0g Prot
0g Fat
0g SatFat
0g Fibre

125ml

Advocaat

1 Unit
14g Carbs
130 Cals
2g Prot
3g Fat
1g SatFat
0g Fibre

50ml

Irish Cream

1 Unit
11g Carbs
153 Cals
2g Prot
7g Fat
4g SatFat
0g Fibre

50ml

Port

1 Unit
6g Carbs
79 Cals
0g Prot
0g Fat
0g SatFat
0g Fibre

50ml

Sherry

1 Unit
3g Carbs
58 Cals
0g Prot
0g Fat
0g SatFat
0g Fibre

50ml

Vermouth (sweet)

1 Unit
8g Carbs
76 Cals
0g Prot
0g Fat
0g SatFat
0g Fibre

50ml

Brandy

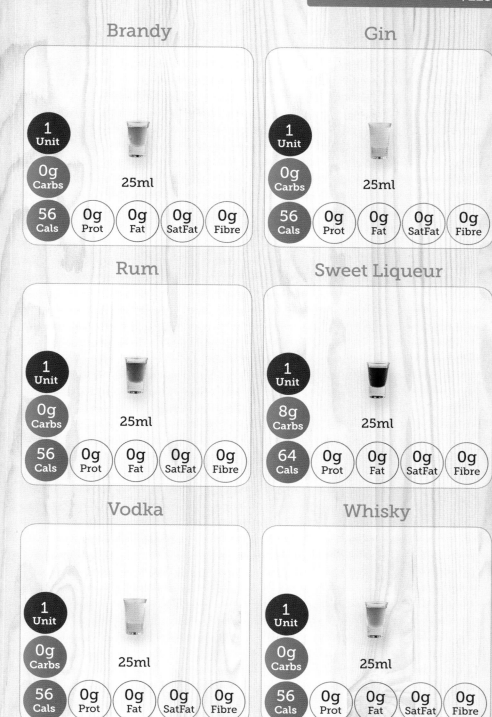

1 Unit
0g Carbs
25ml
56 Cals | 0g Prot | 0g Fat | 0g SatFat | 0g Fibre

Gin

1 Unit
0g Carbs
25ml
56 Cals | 0g Prot | 0g Fat | 0g SatFat | 0g Fibre

Rum

1 Unit
0g Carbs
25ml
56 Cals | 0g Prot | 0g Fat | 0g SatFat | 0g Fibre

Sweet Liqueur

1 Unit
8g Carbs
25ml
64 Cals | 0g Prot | 0g Fat | 0g SatFat | 0g Fibre

Vodka

1 Unit
0g Carbs
25ml
56 Cals | 0g Prot | 0g Fat | 0g SatFat | 0g Fibre

Whisky

1 Unit
0g Carbs
25ml
56 Cals | 0g Prot | 0g Fat | 0g SatFat | 0g Fibre

26cm Dinner Plate

Boiled Egg

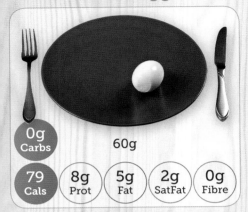

0g Carbs

60g

79 Cals | **8g** Prot | **5g** Fat | **2g** SatFat | **0g** Fibre

Scrambled Egg
(with milk)

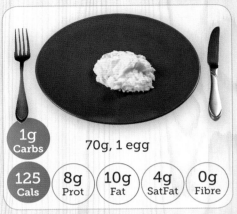

1g Carbs

70g, 1 egg

125 Cals | **8g** Prot | **10g** Fat | **4g** SatFat | **0g** Fibre

Fried Egg

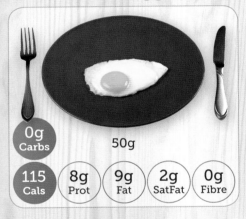

0g Carbs

50g

115 Cals | **8g** Prot | **9g** Fat | **2g** SatFat | **0g** Fibre

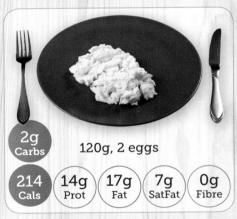

2g Carbs

120g, 2 eggs

214 Cals | **14g** Prot | **17g** Fat | **7g** SatFat | **0g** Fibre

Poached Egg

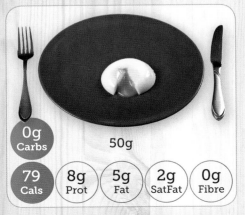

0g Carbs

50g

79 Cals | **8g** Prot | **5g** Fat | **2g** SatFat | **0g** Fibre

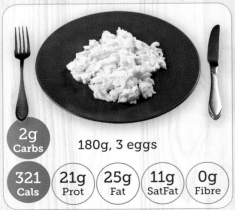

2g Carbs

180g, 3 eggs

321 Cals | **21g** Prot | **25g** Fat | **11g** SatFat | **0g** Fibre

Omelette (plain)

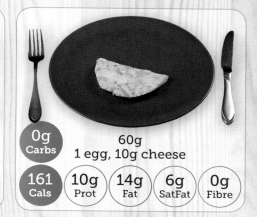

0g Carbs

50g, 1 egg

| **96** Cals | 5g Prot | 8g Fat | 2g SatFat | 0g Fibre |

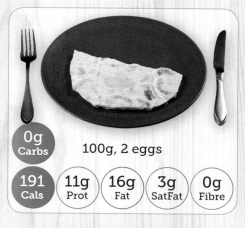

0g Carbs

100g, 2 eggs

| **191** Cals | 11g Prot | 16g Fat | 3g SatFat | 0g Fibre |

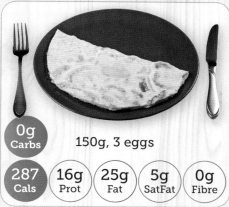

0g Carbs

150g, 3 eggs

| **287** Cals | 16g Prot | 25g Fat | 5g SatFat | 0g Fibre |

Omelette (cheese)

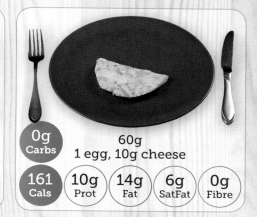

0g Carbs

60g
1 egg, 10g cheese

| **161** Cals | 10g Prot | 14g Fat | 6g SatFat | 0g Fibre |

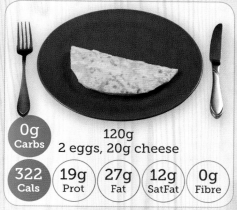

0g Carbs

120g
2 eggs, 20g cheese

| **322** Cals | 19g Prot | 27g Fat | 12g SatFat | 0g Fibre |

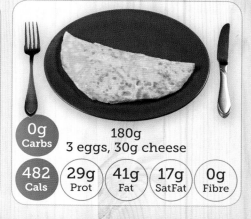

0g Carbs

180g
3 eggs, 30g cheese

| **482** Cals | 29g Prot | 41g Fat | 17g SatFat | 0g Fibre |

26cm Dinner Plate / 20cm Side Plate

Eggs Benedict

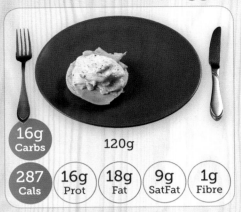

16g Carbs
120g
287 Cals | **16g** Prot | **18g** Fat | **9g** SatFat | **1g** Fibre

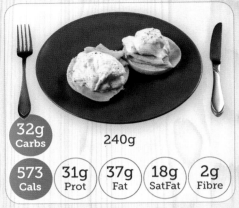

32g Carbs
240g
573 Cals | **31g** Prot | **37g** Fat | **18g** SatFat | **2g** Fibre

Eggs Florentine

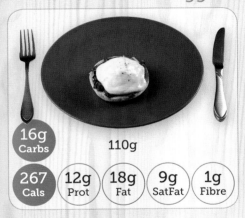

16g Carbs
110g
267 Cals | **12g** Prot | **18g** Fat | **9g** SatFat | **1g** Fibre

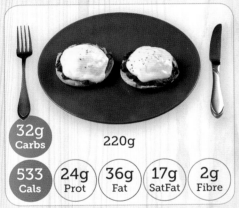

32g Carbs
220g
533 Cals | **24g** Prot | **36g** Fat | **17g** SatFat | **2g** Fibre

Scotch Egg

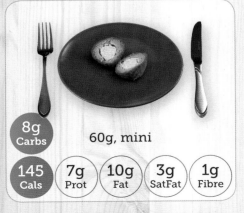

8g Carbs
60g, mini
145 Cals | **7g** Prot | **10g** Fat | **3g** SatFat | **1g** Fibre

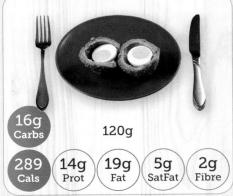

16g Carbs
120g
289 Cals | **14g** Prot | **19g** Fat | **5g** SatFat | **2g** Fibre

Apricots

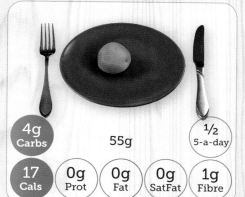

4g Carbs

55g

½ 5-a-day

17 Cals | 0g Prot | 0g Fat | 0g SatFat | 1g Fibre

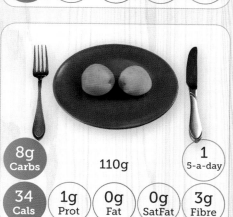

8g Carbs

110g

1 5-a-day

34 Cals | 1g Prot | 0g Fat | 0g SatFat | 3g Fibre

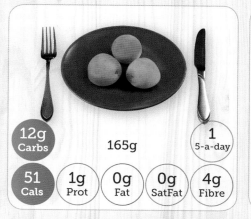

12g Carbs

165g

1 5-a-day

51 Cals | 1g Prot | 0g Fat | 0g SatFat | 4g Fibre

Apricots (tinned in juice)

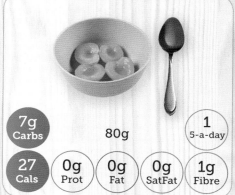

7g Carbs

80g

1 5-a-day

27 Cals | 0g Prot | 0g Fat | 0g SatFat | 1g Fibre

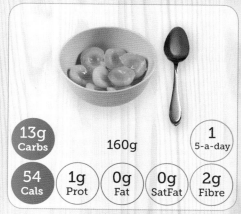

13g Carbs

160g

1 5-a-day

54 Cals | 1g Prot | 0g Fat | 0g SatFat | 2g Fibre

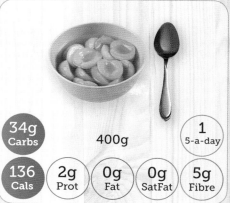

34g Carbs

400g

1 5-a-day

136 Cals | 2g Prot | 0g Fat | 0g SatFat | 5g Fibre

20cm Side Plate / 14cm Cereal Bowl

Apple

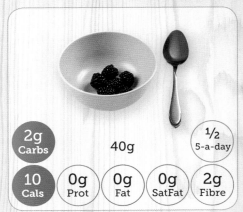

9g Carbs · 85g · ½ 5-a-day

37 Cals · 0g Prot · 0g Fat · 0g SatFat · 1g Fibre

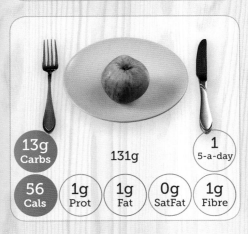

13g Carbs · 131g · 1 5-a-day

56 Cals · 1g Prot · 1g Fat · 0g SatFat · 1g Fibre

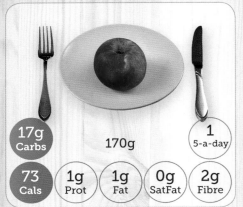

17g Carbs · 170g · 1 5-a-day

73 Cals · 1g Prot · 1g Fat · 0g SatFat · 2g Fibre

Blackberries

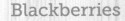

2g Carbs · 40g · ½ 5-a-day

10 Cals · 0g Prot · 0g Fat · 0g SatFat · 2g Fibre

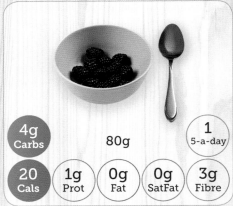

4g Carbs · 80g · 1 5-a-day

20 Cals · 1g Prot · 0g Fat · 0g SatFat · 3g Fibre

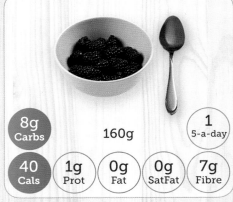

8g Carbs · 160g · 1 5-a-day

40 Cals · 1g Prot · 0g Fat · 0g SatFat · 7g Fibre

Banana (with skin)

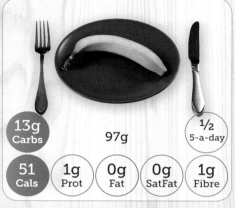

13g Carbs — 97g — ½ 5-a-day

51 Cals | 1g Prot | 0g Fat | 0g SatFat | 1g Fibre

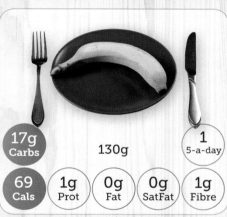

17g Carbs — 130g — 1 5-a-day

69 Cals | 1g Prot | 0g Fat | 0g SatFat | 1g Fibre

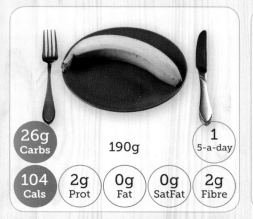

26g Carbs — 190g — 1 5-a-day

104 Cals | 2g Prot | 0g Fat | 0g SatFat | 2g Fibre

Banana (without skin)

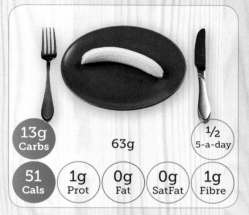

13g Carbs — 63g — ½ 5-a-day

51 Cals | 1g Prot | 0g Fat | 0g SatFat | 1g Fibre

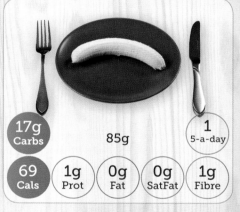

17g Carbs — 85g — 1 5-a-day

69 Cals | 1g Prot | 0g Fat | 0g SatFat | 1g Fibre

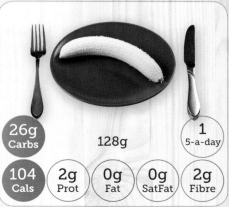

26g Carbs — 128g — 1 5-a-day

104 Cals | 2g Prot | 0g Fat | 0g SatFat | 2g Fibre

Blueberries

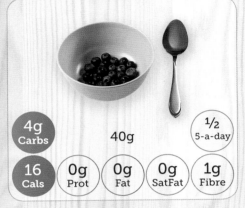

4g Carbs — 40g — ½ 5-a-day

16 Cals | 0g Prot | 0g Fat | 0g SatFat | 1g Fibre

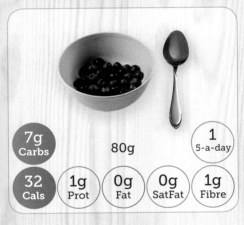

7g Carbs — 80g — 1 5-a-day

32 Cals | 1g Prot | 0g Fat | 0g SatFat | 1g Fibre

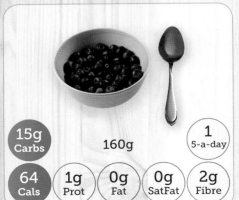

15g Carbs — 160g — 1 5-a-day

64 Cals | 1g Prot | 0g Fat | 0g SatFat | 2g Fibre

Cherries

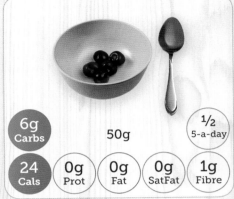

6g Carbs — 50g — ½ 5-a-day

24 Cals | 0g Prot | 0g Fat | 0g SatFat | 1g Fibre

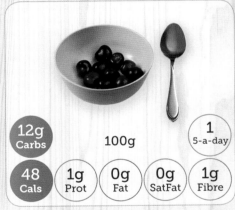

12g Carbs — 100g — 1 5-a-day

48 Cals | 1g Prot | 0g Fat | 0g SatFat | 1g Fibre

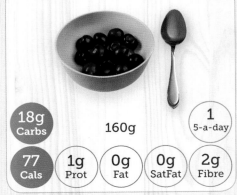

18g Carbs — 160g — 1 5-a-day

77 Cals | 1g Prot | 0g Fat | 0g SatFat | 2g Fibre

Clementine

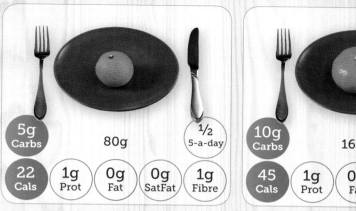

5g Carbs | 80g | ½ 5-a-day

22 Cals | 1g Prot | 0g Fat | 0g SatFat | 1g Fibre

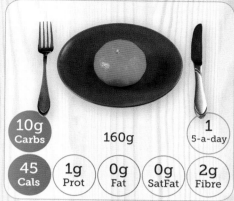

10g Carbs | 160g | 1 5-a-day

45 Cals | 1g Prot | 0g Fat | 0g SatFat | 2g Fibre

Cranberries

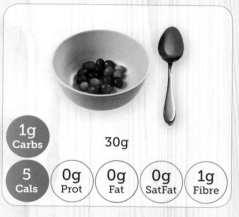

1g Carbs | 30g

5 Cals | 0g Prot | 0g Fat | 0g SatFat | 1g Fibre

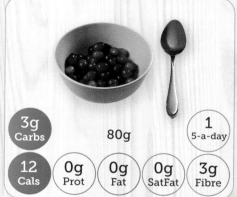

3g Carbs | 80g | 1 5-a-day

12 Cals | 0g Prot | 0g Fat | 0g SatFat | 3g Fibre

Figs

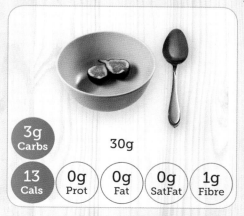

3g Carbs | 30g

13 Cals | 0g Prot | 0g Fat | 0g SatFat | 1g Fibre

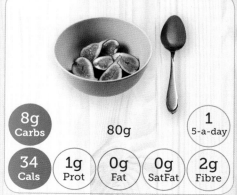

8g Carbs | 80g | 1 5-a-day

34 Cals | 1g Prot | 0g Fat | 0g SatFat | 2g Fibre

14cm Cereal Bowl / 20cm Side Plate

Fruit Cocktail (tinned in juice)

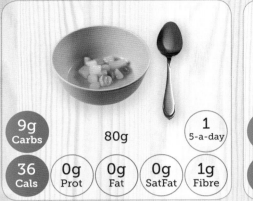

9g Carbs — 80g — **1** 5-a-day

36 Cals — **0g** Prot — **0g** Fat — **0g** SatFat — **1g** Fibre

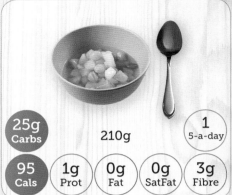

25g Carbs — 210g — **1** 5-a-day

95 Cals — **1g** Prot — **0g** Fat — **0g** SatFat — **3g** Fibre

Grapefruit

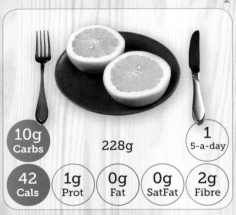

10g Carbs — 228g — **1** 5-a-day

42 Cals — **1g** Prot — **0g** Fat — **0g** SatFat — **2g** Fibre

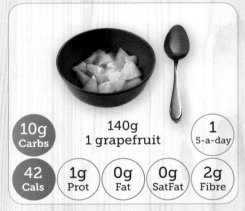

10g Carbs — 140g 1 grapefruit — **1** 5-a-day

42 Cals — **1g** Prot — **0g** Fat — **0g** SatFat — **2g** Fibre

Grapes (seedless)

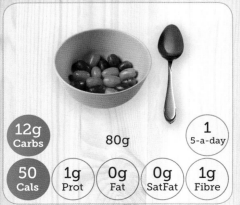

12g Carbs — 80g — **1** 5-a-day

50 Cals — **1g** Prot — **0g** Fat — **0g** SatFat — **1g** Fibre

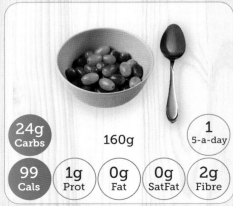

24g Carbs — 160g — **1** 5-a-day

99 Cals — **1g** Prot — **0g** Fat — **0g** SatFat — **2g** Fibre

Kiwi

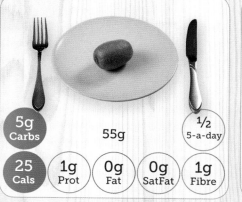

5g Carbs   55g   **½** 5-a-day

25 Cals   1g Prot   0g Fat   0g SatFat   1g Fibre

Mango

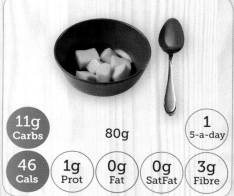

11g Carbs   80g   **1** 5-a-day

46 Cals   1g Prot   0g Fat   0g SatFat   3g Fibre

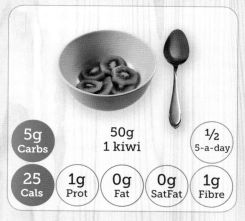

5g Carbs   50g 1 kiwi   **½** 5-a-day

25 Cals   1g Prot   0g Fat   0g SatFat   1g Fibre

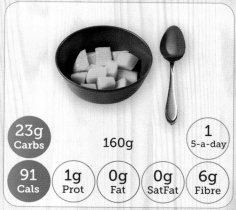

23g Carbs   160g   **1** 5-a-day

91 Cals   1g Prot   0g Fat   0g SatFat   6g Fibre

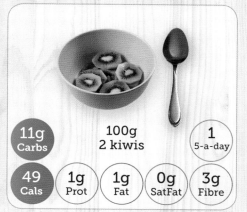

11g Carbs   100g 2 kiwis   **1** 5-a-day

49 Cals   1g Prot   1g Fat   0g SatFat   3g Fibre

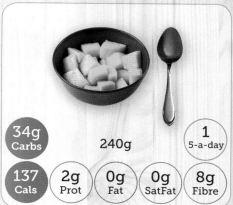

34g Carbs   240g   **1** 5-a-day

137 Cals   2g Prot   0g Fat   0g SatFat   8g Fibre

Melon (honeydew)　　　　Orange

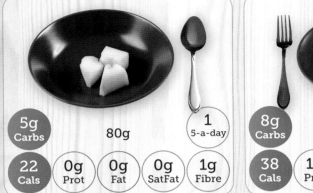

5g Carbs	80g	1 5-a-day

22 Cals	0g Prot	0g Fat	0g SatFat	1g Fibre

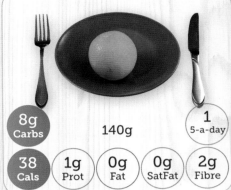

8g Carbs	140g	1 5-a-day

38 Cals	1g Prot	0g Fat	0g SatFat	2g Fibre

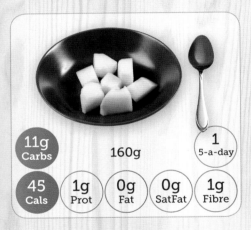

11g Carbs	160g	1 5-a-day

45 Cals	1g Prot	0g Fat	0g SatFat	1g Fibre

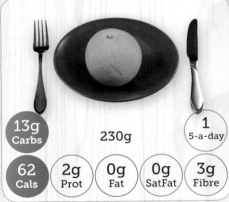

13g Carbs	230g	1 5-a-day

62 Cals	2g Prot	0g Fat	0g SatFat	3g Fibre

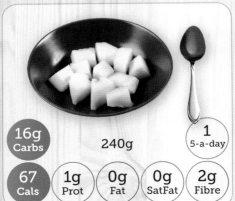

16g Carbs	240g	1 5-a-day

67 Cals	1g Prot	0g Fat	0g SatFat	2g Fibre

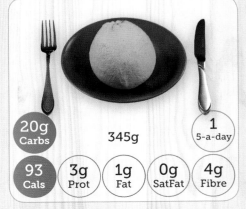

20g Carbs	345g	1 5-a-day

93 Cals	3g Prot	1g Fat	0g SatFat	4g Fibre

Papaya

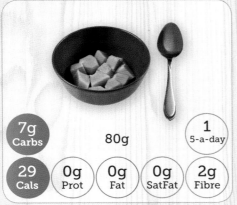

7g Carbs   80g   **1** 5-a-day

29 Cals   **0g** Prot   **0g** Fat   **0g** SatFat   **2g** Fibre

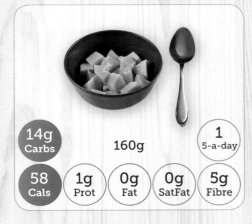

14g Carbs   160g   **1** 5-a-day

58 Cals   **1g** Prot   **0g** Fat   **0g** SatFat   **5g** Fibre

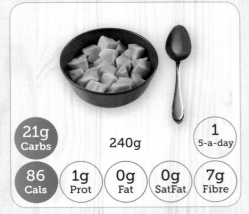

21g Carbs   240g   **1** 5-a-day

86 Cals   **1g** Prot   **0g** Fat   **0g** SatFat   **7g** Fibre

Pomegranate

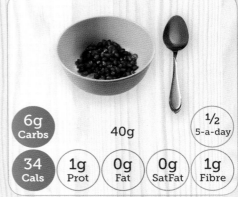

6g Carbs   40g   **½** 5-a-day

34 Cals   **1g** Prot   **0g** Fat   **0g** SatFat   **1g** Fibre

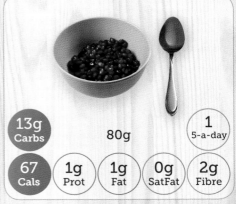

13g Carbs   80g   **1** 5-a-day

67 Cals   **1g** Prot   **1g** Fat   **0g** SatFat   **2g** Fibre

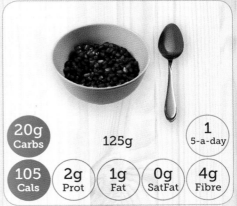

20g Carbs   125g   **1** 5-a-day

105 Cals   **2g** Prot   **1g** Fat   **0g** SatFat   **4g** Fibre

Peach

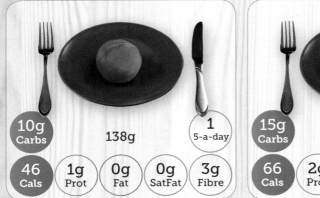

10g Carbs
138g
1 5-a-day
46 Cals
1g Prot
0g Fat
0g SatFat
3g Fibre

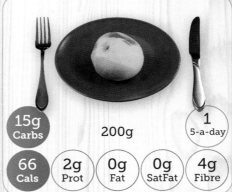

15g Carbs
200g
1 5-a-day
66 Cals
2g Prot
0g Fat
0g SatFat
4g Fibre

Peaches (tinned in juice)

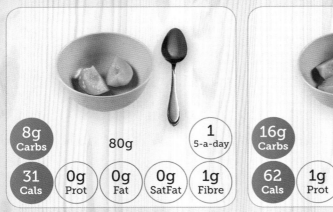

8g Carbs
80g
1 5-a-day
31 Cals
0g Prot
0g Fat
0g SatFat
1g Fibre

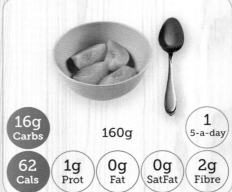

16g Carbs
160g
1 5-a-day
62 Cals
1g Prot
0g Fat
0g SatFat
2g Fibre

Nectarine

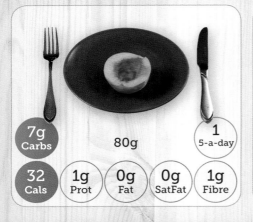

7g Carbs
80g
1 5-a-day
32 Cals
1g Prot
0g Fat
0g SatFat
1g Fibre

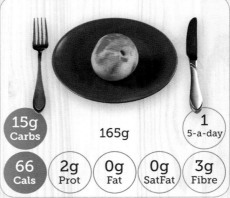

15g Carbs
165g
1 5-a-day
66 Cals
2g Prot
0g Fat
0g SatFat
3g Fibre

Pear

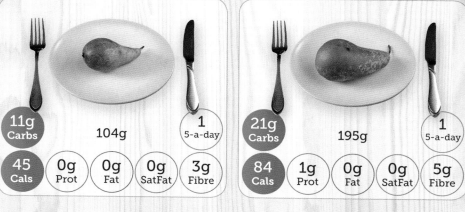

11g Carbs	104g	1 5-a-day

45 Cals	0g Prot	0g Fat	0g SatFat	3g Fibre

21g Carbs	195g	1 5-a-day

84 Cals	1g Prot	0g Fat	0g SatFat	5g Fibre

Pears (tinned in juice)

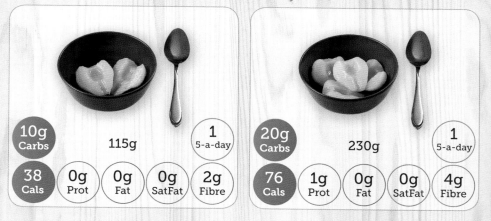

10g Carbs	115g	1 5-a-day

38 Cals	0g Prot	0g Fat	0g SatFat	2g Fibre

20g Carbs	230g	1 5-a-day

76 Cals	1g Prot	0g Fat	0g SatFat	4g Fibre

Persimmon

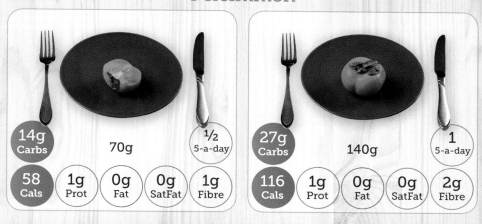

14g Carbs	70g	½ 5-a-day

58 Cals	1g Prot	0g Fat	0g SatFat	1g Fibre

27g Carbs	140g	1 5-a-day

116 Cals	1g Prot	0g Fat	0g SatFat	2g Fibre

20cm Side Plate / 14cm Cereal Bowl

Pineapple

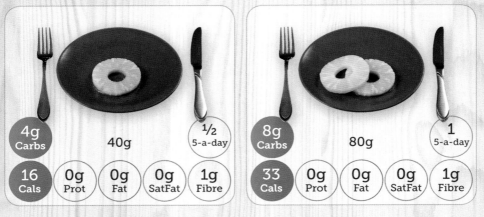

4g Carbs | 40g | **½** 5-a-day
16 Cals | **0g** Prot | **0g** Fat | **0g** SatFat | **1g** Fibre

8g Carbs | 80g | **1** 5-a-day
33 Cals | **0g** Prot | **0g** Fat | **0g** SatFat | **1g** Fibre

Pineapple (tinned in juice)

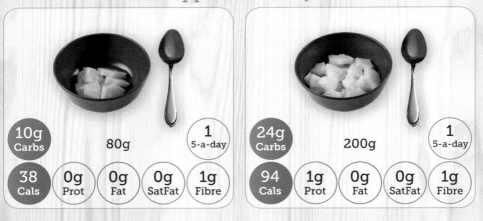

10g Carbs | 80g | **1** 5-a-day
38 Cals | **0g** Prot | **0g** Fat | **0g** SatFat | **1g** Fibre

24g Carbs | 200g | **1** 5-a-day
94 Cals | **1g** Prot | **0g** Fat | **0g** SatFat | **1g** Fibre

Plum

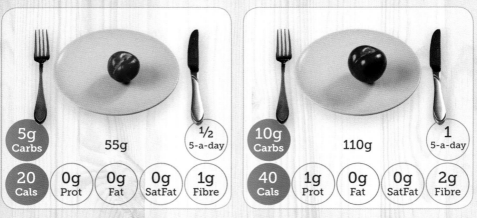

5g Carbs | 55g | **½** 5-a-day
20 Cals | **0g** Prot | **0g** Fat | **0g** SatFat | **1g** Fibre

10g Carbs | 110g | **1** 5-a-day
40 Cals | **1g** Prot | **0g** Fat | **0g** SatFat | **2g** Fibre

Raspberries

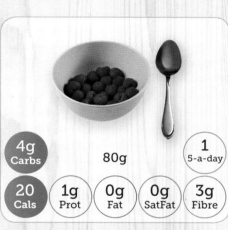

2g Carbs

40g

½ 5-a-day

10 Cals | 1g Prot | 0g Fat | 0g SatFat | 1g Fibre

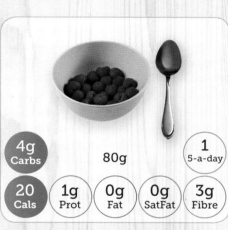

4g Carbs

80g

1 5-a-day

20 Cals | 1g Prot | 0g Fat | 0g SatFat | 3g Fibre

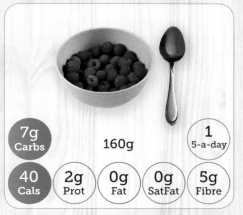

7g Carbs

160g

1 5-a-day

40 Cals | 2g Prot | 0g Fat | 0g SatFat | 5g Fibre

Rhubarb
(stewed with sugar)

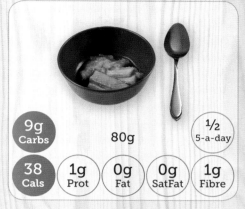

9g Carbs

80g

½ 5-a-day

38 Cals | 1g Prot | 0g Fat | 0g SatFat | 1g Fibre

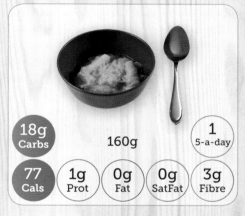

18g Carbs

160g

1 5-a-day

77 Cals | 1g Prot | 0g Fat | 0g SatFat | 3g Fibre

Satsuma

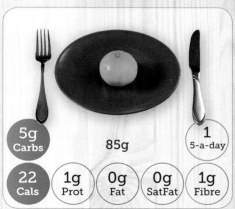

5g Carbs

85g

1 5-a-day

22 Cals | 1g Prot | 0g Fat | 0g SatFat | 1g Fibre

Strawberries

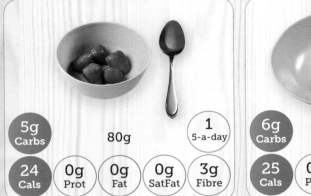

5g Carbs 80g **1** 5-a-day

24 Cals 0g Prot 0g Fat 0g SatFat 3g Fibre

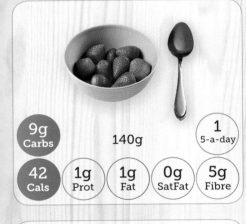

9g Carbs 140g **1** 5-a-day

42 Cals 1g Prot 1g Fat 0g SatFat 5g Fibre

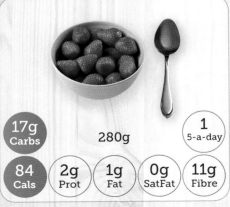

17g Carbs 280g **1** 5-a-day

84 Cals 2g Prot 1g Fat 0g SatFat 11g Fibre

Watermelon

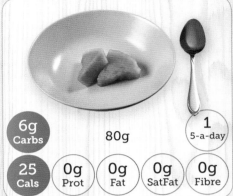

6g Carbs 80g **1** 5-a-day

25 Cals 0g Prot 0g Fat 0g SatFat 0g Fibre

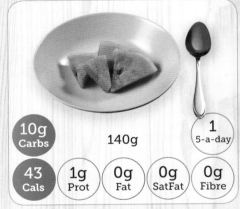

10g Carbs 140g **1** 5-a-day

43 Cals 1g Prot 0g Fat 0g SatFat 0g Fibre

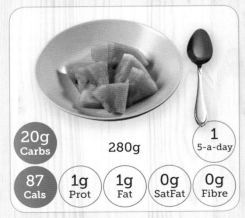

20g Carbs 280g **1** 5-a-day

87 Cals 1g Prot 1g Fat 0g SatFat 0g Fibre

Fruit (per 100g weight)

	Carbs	Cals	Prot	Fat	SatFat	Fibre
Apple (weighed whole)	10g	43	1g	0g	0g	1g
Apricot	7g	31	1g	0g	0g	2g
Banana (weighed with skin)	13g	51	1g	0g	0g	1g
Blackberries	5g	25	1g	0g	0g	4g
Blueberries	9g	40	1g	0g	0g	2g
Cherries	12g	48	1g	0g	0g	1g
Clementine (weighed with skin)	7g	28	1g	0g	0g	1g
Cranberries	3g	15	0g	0g	0g	4g
Figs	10g	43	1g	0g	0g	2g
Fruit Cocktail (tinned in juice)	12g	45	0g	0g	0g	1g
Gooseberries	9g	40	1g	0g	0g	3g
Grapefruit (flesh only)	7g	30	1g	0g	0g	2g
Grapes	15g	62	1g	0g	0g	1g
Kiwi (weighed with skin)	9g	42	1g	0g	0g	2g
Mango (flesh only)	14g	57	1g	0g	0g	4g
Melon, Honeydew (flesh only)	7g	28	1g	0g	0g	1g
Nectarine (weighed with skin)	9g	40	1g	0g	0g	2g
Orange (weighed with skin)	6g	27	1g	0g	0g	1g
Papaya (flesh only)	9g	36	1g	0g	0g	3g
Peach	8g	33	1g	0g	0g	2g
Peaches (tinned in juice)	10g	39	1g	0g	0g	1g
Pear	11g	43	0g	0g	0g	3g
Persimmon	20g	83	1g	0g	0g	2g
Pineapple (flesh only)	10g	41	0g	0g	0g	2g
Plum	9g	36	1g	0g	0g	2g
Pomegranate Seeds	16g	84	2g	1g	0g	3g
Raspberries	5g	25	1g	0g	0g	3g
Rhubarb (raw)	1g	7	1g	0g	0g	2g
Strawberries	6g	30	1g	1g	0g	4g
Watermelon (flesh only)	7g	31	1g	0g	0g	0g

14cm Cereal Bowl

Apple Rings

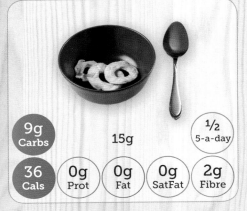

9g Carbs   15g   ½ 5-a-day

36 Cals   0g Prot   0g Fat   0g SatFat   2g Fibre

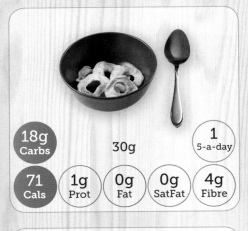

18g Carbs   30g   1 5-a-day

71 Cals   1g Prot   0g Fat   0g SatFat   4g Fibre

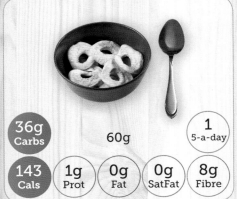

36g Carbs   60g   1 5-a-day

143 Cals   1g Prot   0g Fat   0g SatFat   8g Fibre

Apricots

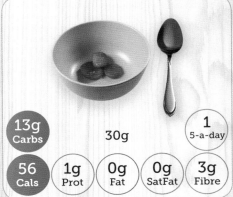

13g Carbs   30g   1 5-a-day

56 Cals   1g Prot   0g Fat   0g SatFat   3g Fibre

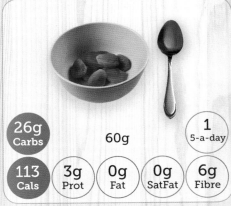

26g Carbs   60g   1 5-a-day

113 Cals   3g Prot   0g Fat   0g SatFat   6g Fibre

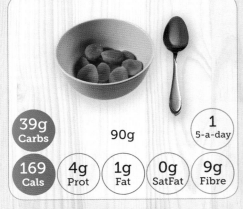

39g Carbs   90g   1 5-a-day

169 Cals   4g Prot   1g Fat   0g SatFat   9g Fibre

Banana Chips

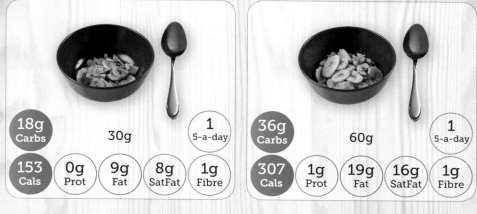

18g Carbs	30g			**1** 5-a-day
153 Cals	**0g** Prot	**9g** Fat	**8g** SatFat	**1g** Fibre

36g Carbs	60g			**1** 5-a-day
307 Cals	**1g** Prot	**19g** Fat	**16g** SatFat	**1g** Fibre

Cranberries

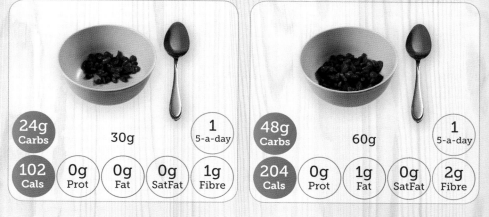

24g Carbs	30g			**1** 5-a-day
102 Cals	**0g** Prot	**0g** Fat	**0g** SatFat	**1g** Fibre

48g Carbs	60g			**1** 5-a-day
204 Cals	**0g** Prot	**1g** Fat	**0g** SatFat	**2g** Fibre

Dates

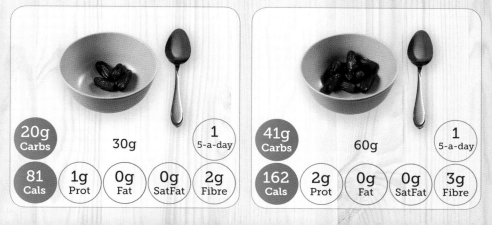

20g Carbs	30g			**1** 5-a-day
81 Cals	**1g** Prot	**0g** Fat	**0g** SatFat	**2g** Fibre

41g Carbs	60g			**1** 5-a-day
162 Cals	**2g** Prot	**0g** Fat	**0g** SatFat	**3g** Fibre

Figs

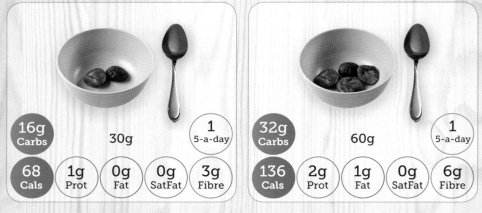

16g Carbs | 30g | **1** 5-a-day

68 Cals | **1g** Prot | **0g** Fat | **0g** SatFat | **3g** Fibre

32g Carbs | 60g | **1** 5-a-day

136 Cals | **2g** Prot | **1g** Fat | **0g** SatFat | **6g** Fibre

Pineapple

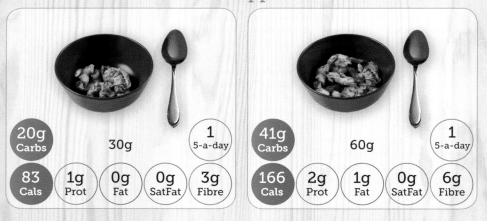

20g Carbs | 30g | **1** 5-a-day

83 Cals | **1g** Prot | **0g** Fat | **0g** SatFat | **3g** Fibre

41g Carbs | 60g | **1** 5-a-day

166 Cals | **2g** Prot | **1g** Fat | **0g** SatFat | **6g** Fibre

Prunes

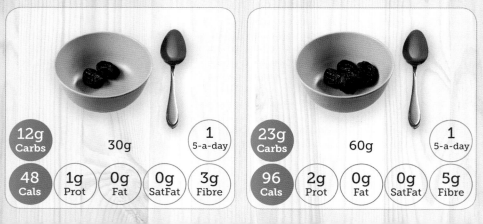

12g Carbs | 30g | **1** 5-a-day

48 Cals | **1g** Prot | **0g** Fat | **0g** SatFat | **3g** Fibre

23g Carbs | 60g | **1** 5-a-day

96 Cals | **2g** Prot | **0g** Fat | **0g** SatFat | **5g** Fibre

Raisins

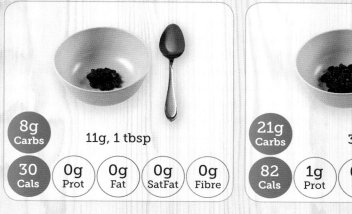

8g Carbs	11g, 1 tbsp	

30 Cals	0g Prot	0g Fat	0g SatFat	0g Fibre

21g Carbs	30g	1 5-a-day

82 Cals	1g Prot	0g Fat	0g SatFat	1g Fibre

Sultanas

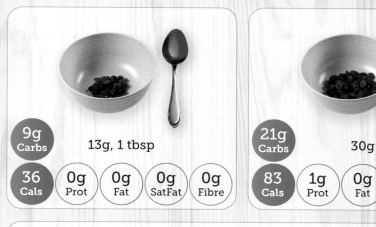

9g Carbs	13g, 1 tbsp	

36 Cals	0g Prot	0g Fat	0g SatFat	0g Fibre

21g Carbs	30g	1 5-a-day

83 Cals	1g Prot	0g Fat	0g SatFat	1g Fibre

Dried Fruit (per 100g weight)

	Carbs	Cals	Prot	Fat	SatFat	Fibre
Apple	60g	238	2g	1g	0g	13g
Apricots	43g	188	5g	1g	0g	10g
Cranberries	80g	340	0g	1g	0g	4g
Dates	68g	270	3g	0g	0g	5g
Figs	53g	227	4g	2g	0g	10g
Prunes	38g	160	3g	1g	0g	9g
Raisins	69g	272	2g	0g	0g	3g
Sultanas	69g	275	3g	0g	0g	3g

14cm Cereal Bowl

Fibre Flakes GF

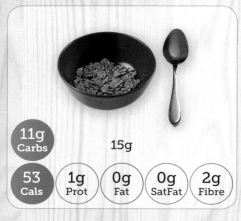

11g Carbs

15g

53 Cals | **1g** Prot | **0g** Fat | **0g** SatFat | **2g** Fibre

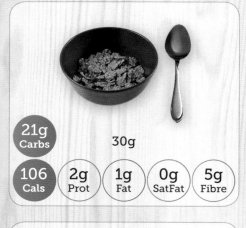

21g Carbs

30g

106 Cals | **2g** Prot | **1g** Fat | **0g** SatFat | **5g** Fibre

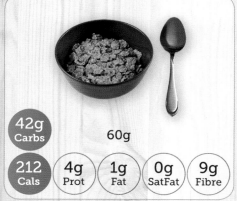

42g Carbs

60g

212 Cals | **4g** Prot | **1g** Fat | **0g** SatFat | **9g** Fibre

Special Flakes GF

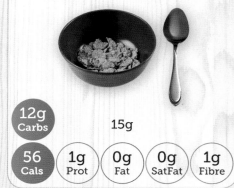

12g Carbs

15g

56 Cals | **1g** Prot | **0g** Fat | **0g** SatFat | **1g** Fibre

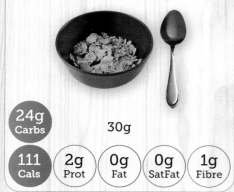

24g Carbs

30g

111 Cals | **2g** Prot | **0g** Fat | **0g** SatFat | **1g** Fibre

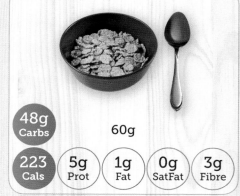

48g Carbs

60g

223 Cals | **5g** Prot | **1g** Fat | **0g** SatFat | **3g** Fibre

Muesli 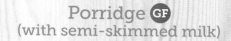 GF

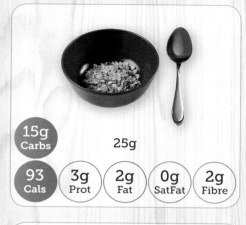

15g Carbs

25g

93 Cals | **3g** Prot | **2g** Fat | **0g** SatFat | **2g** Fibre

Porridge GF
(with semi-skimmed milk)

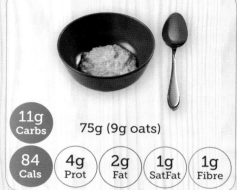

11g Carbs

75g (9g oats)

84 Cals | **4g** Prot | **2g** Fat | **1g** SatFat | **1g** Fibre

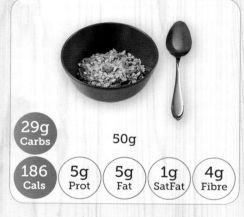

29g Carbs

50g

186 Cals | **5g** Prot | **5g** Fat | **1g** SatFat | **4g** Fibre

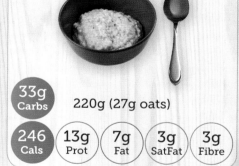

33g Carbs

220g (27g oats)

246 Cals | **13g** Prot | **7g** Fat | **3g** SatFat | **3g** Fibre

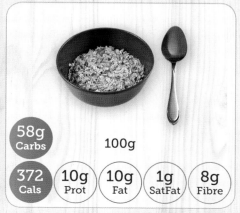

58g Carbs

100g

372 Cals | **10g** Prot | **10g** Fat | **1g** SatFat | **8g** Fibre

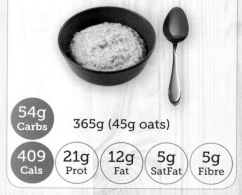

54g Carbs

365g (45g oats)

409 Cals | **21g** Prot | **12g** Fat | **5g** SatFat | **5g** Fibre

Brown Bread 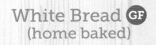 GF
(home baked)

White Bread GF
(home baked)

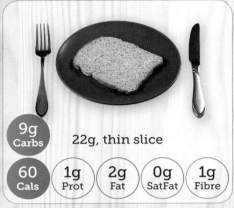

9g Carbs

22g, thin slice

60 Cals | **1g** Prot | **2g** Fat | **0g** SatFat | **1g** Fibre

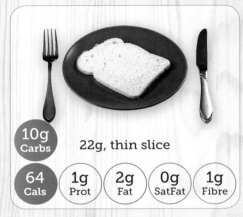

10g Carbs

22g, thin slice

64 Cals | **1g** Prot | **2g** Fat | **0g** SatFat | **1g** Fibre

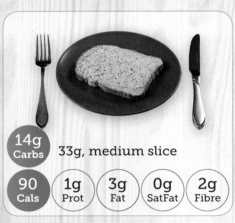

14g Carbs

33g, medium slice

90 Cals | **1g** Prot | **3g** Fat | **0g** SatFat | **2g** Fibre

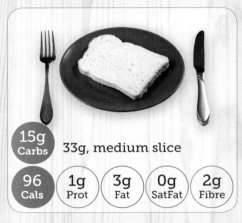

15g Carbs

33g, medium slice

96 Cals | **1g** Prot | **3g** Fat | **0g** SatFat | **2g** Fibre

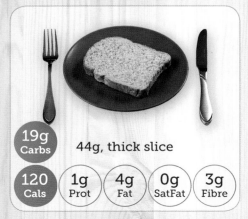

19g Carbs

44g, thick slice

120 Cals | **1g** Prot | **4g** Fat | **0g** SatFat | **3g** Fibre

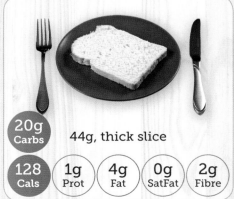

20g Carbs

44g, thick slice

128 Cals | **1g** Prot | **4g** Fat | **0g** SatFat | **2g** Fibre

Brown Bread (sliced) GF

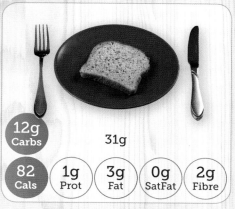

12g Carbs

31g

82 Cals | 1g Prot | 3g Fat | 0g SatFat | 2g Fibre

White Bread (sliced) GF

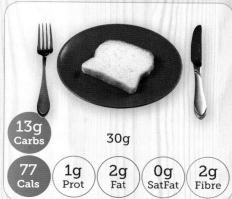

13g Carbs

30g

77 Cals | 1g Prot | 2g Fat | 0g SatFat | 2g Fibre

Fibre Roll GF

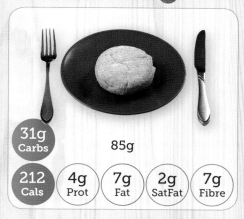

31g Carbs

85g

212 Cals | 4g Prot | 7g Fat | 2g SatFat | 7g Fibre

White Roll GF

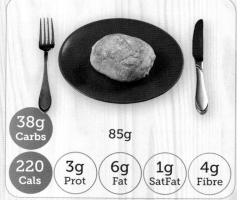

38g Carbs

85g

220 Cals | 3g Prot | 6g Fat | 1g SatFat | 4g Fibre

Brown Roll (part baked) GF

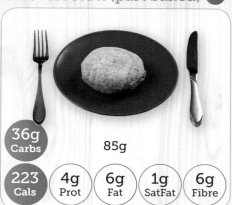

36g Carbs

85g

223 Cals | 4g Prot | 6g Fat | 1g SatFat | 6g Fibre

White Roll (part baked) GF

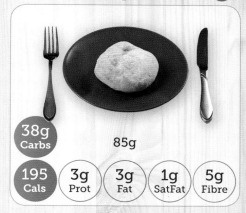

38g Carbs

85g

195 Cals | 3g Prot | 3g Fat | 1g SatFat | 5g Fibre

20cm Side Plate / 26cm Dinner Plate

Breadstick GF

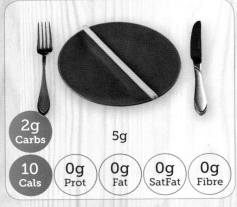

2g Carbs   5g

10 Cals | **0g** Prot | **0g** Fat | **0g** SatFat | **0g** Fibre

Crispbread GF

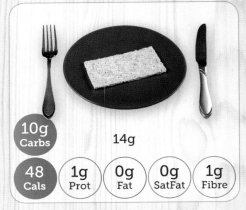

10g Carbs   14g

48 Cals | **1g** Prot | **0g** Fat | **0g** SatFat | **1g** Fibre

Naan Bread GF

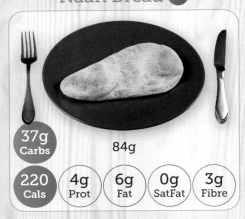

37g Carbs   84g

220 Cals | **4g** Prot | **6g** Fat | **0g** SatFat | **3g** Fibre

Pitta Bread GF

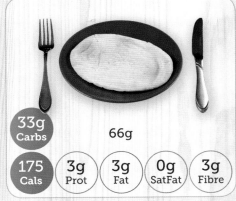

33g Carbs   66g

175 Cals | **3g** Prot | **3g** Fat | **0g** SatFat | **3g** Fibre

Pizza Base GF

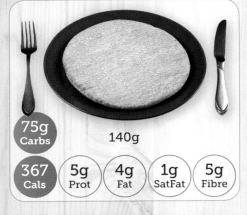

75g Carbs   140g

367 Cals | **5g** Prot | **4g** Fat | **1g** SatFat | **5g** Fibre

Rice Cake GF

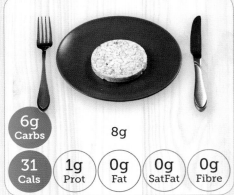

6g Carbs   8g

31 Cals | **1g** Prot | **0g** Fat | **0g** SatFat | **0g** Fibre

Chocolate Chip Cookie GF

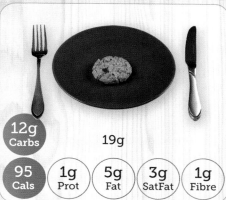

12g Carbs 19g

95 Cals | 1g Prot | 5g Fat | 3g SatFat | 1g Fibre

Chocolate Digestive GF

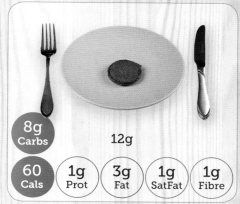

8g Carbs 12g

60 Cals | 1g Prot | 3g Fat | 1g SatFat | 1g Fibre

Digestive GF

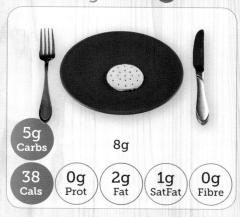

5g Carbs 8g

38 Cals | 0g Prot | 2g Fat | 1g SatFat | 0g Fibre

Savoury Biscuit GF

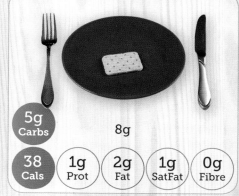

5g Carbs 8g

38 Cals | 1g Prot | 2g Fat | 1g SatFat | 0g Fibre

Sweet Biscuit GF

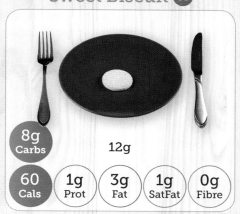

8g Carbs 12g

60 Cals | 1g Prot | 3g Fat | 1g SatFat | 0g Fibre

Tea Biscuit GF

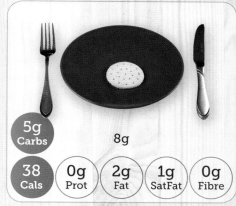

5g Carbs 8g

38 Cals | 0g Prot | 2g Fat | 1g SatFat | 0g Fibre

26cm Dinner Plate

Pasta Twists GF

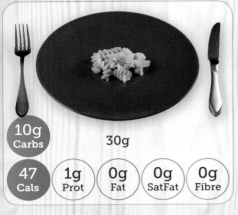

10g Carbs   30g

47 Cals	1g Prot	0g Fat	0g SatFat	0g Fibre

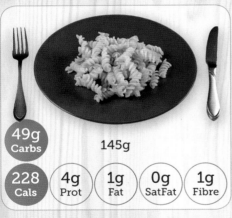

49g Carbs   145g

228 Cals	4g Prot	1g Fat	0g SatFat	1g Fibre

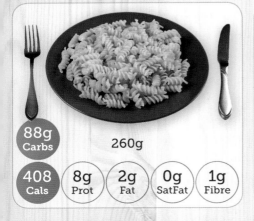

88g Carbs   260g

408 Cals	8g Prot	2g Fat	0g SatFat	1g Fibre

Penne (fibre) GF

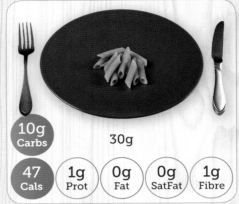

10g Carbs   30g

47 Cals	1g Prot	0g Fat	0g SatFat	1g Fibre

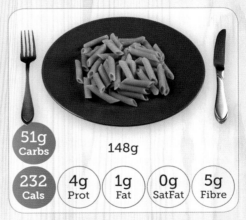

51g Carbs   148g

232 Cals	4g Prot	1g Fat	0g SatFat	5g Fibre

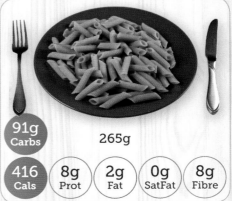

91g Carbs   265g

416 Cals	8g Prot	2g Fat	0g SatFat	8g Fibre

Spaghetti GF

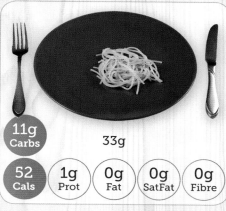

11g Carbs — 33g

52 Cals | **1g** Prot | **0g** Fat | **0g** SatFat | **0g** Fibre

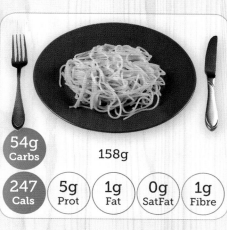

54g Carbs — 158g

247 Cals | **5g** Prot | **1g** Fat | **0g** SatFat | **1g** Fibre

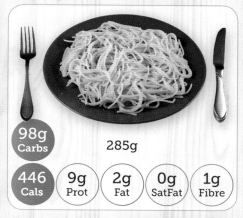

98g Carbs — 285g

446 Cals | **9g** Prot | **2g** Fat | **0g** SatFat | **1g** Fibre

Tagliatelle GF

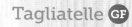

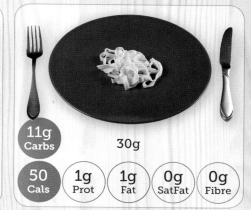

11g Carbs — 30g

50 Cals | **1g** Prot | **1g** Fat | **0g** SatFat | **0g** Fibre

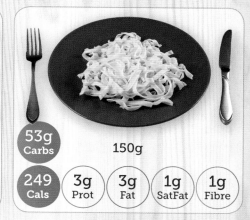

53g Carbs — 150g

249 Cals | **3g** Prot | **3g** Fat | **1g** SatFat | **1g** Fibre

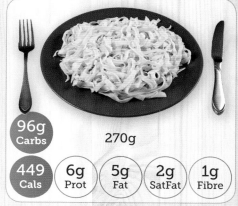

96g Carbs — 270g

449 Cals | **6g** Prot | **5g** Fat | **2g** SatFat | **1g** Fibre

Beans on Toast (with butter)

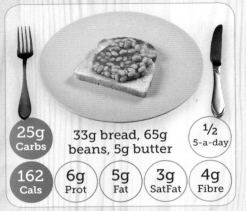

25g Carbs — 33g bread, 65g beans, 5g butter — **½** 5-a-day

162 Cals — **6g** Prot — **5g** Fat — **3g** SatFat — **4g** Fibre

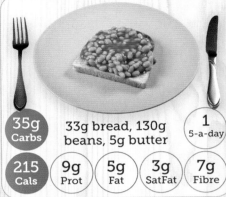

35g Carbs — 33g bread, 130g beans, 5g butter — **1** 5-a-day

215 Cals — **9g** Prot — **5g** Fat — **3g** SatFat — **7g** Fibre

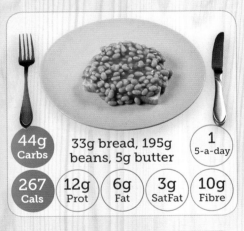

44g Carbs — 33g bread, 195g beans, 5g butter — **1** 5-a-day

267 Cals — **12g** Prot — **6g** Fat — **3g** SatFat — **10g** Fibre

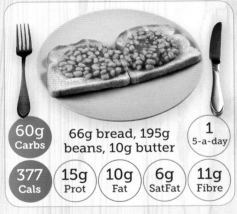

60g Carbs — 66g bread, 195g beans, 10g butter — **1** 5-a-day

377 Cals — **15g** Prot — **10g** Fat — **6g** SatFat — **11g** Fibre

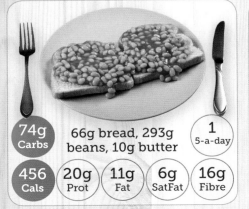

74g Carbs — 66g bread, 293g beans, 10g butter — **1** 5-a-day

456 Cals — **20g** Prot — **11g** Fat — **6g** SatFat — **16g** Fibre

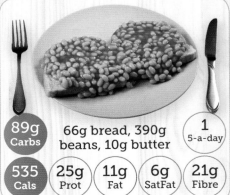

89g Carbs — 66g bread, 390g beans, 10g butter — **1** 5-a-day

535 Cals — **25g** Prot — **11g** Fat — **6g** SatFat — **21g** Fibre

Chicken Goujons, Potato Smiles & Peas

Fish Fingers, Chips & Baked Beans

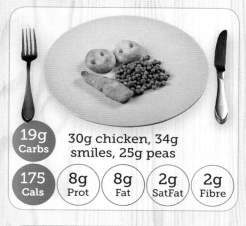

19g Carbs — 30g chicken, 34g smiles, 25g peas

175 Cals — **8g** Prot — **8g** Fat — **2g** SatFat — **2g** Fibre

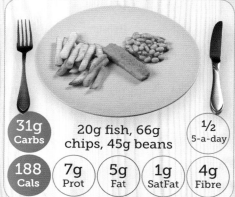

31g Carbs — 20g fish, 66g chips, 45g beans — **½** 5-a-day

188 Cals — **7g** Prot — **5g** Fat — **1g** SatFat — **4g** Fibre

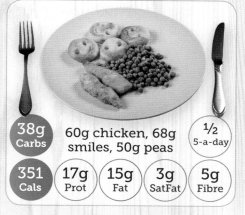

38g Carbs — 60g chicken, 68g smiles, 50g peas — **½** 5-a-day

351 Cals — **17g** Prot — **15g** Fat — **3g** SatFat — **5g** Fibre

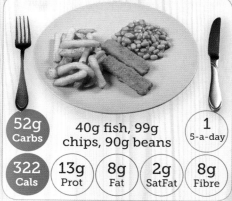

52g Carbs — 40g fish, 99g chips, 90g beans — **1** 5-a-day

322 Cals — **13g** Prot — **8g** Fat — **2g** SatFat — **8g** Fibre

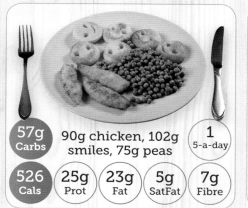

57g Carbs — 90g chicken, 102g smiles, 75g peas — **1** 5-a-day

526 Cals — **25g** Prot — **23g** Fat — **5g** SatFat — **7g** Fibre

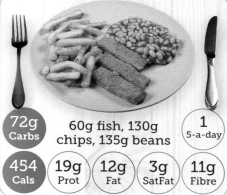

72g Carbs — 60g fish, 130g chips, 135g beans — **1** 5-a-day

454 Cals — **19g** Prot — **12g** Fat — **3g** SatFat — **11g** Fibre

Beef Stew & Dumplings

Corned Beef Hash

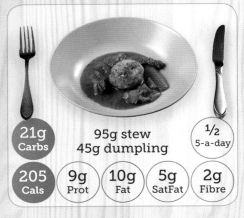

21g Carbs

95g stew
45g dumpling

½ 5-a-day

205 Cals | **9g** Prot | **10g** Fat | **5g** SatFat | **2g** Fibre

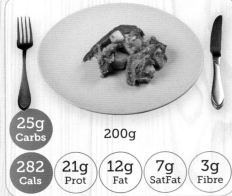

25g Carbs

200g

282 Cals | **21g** Prot | **12g** Fat | **7g** SatFat | **3g** Fibre

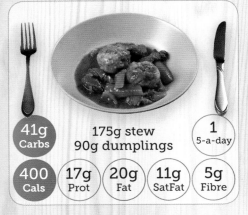

41g Carbs

175g stew
90g dumplings

1 5-a-day

400 Cals | **17g** Prot | **20g** Fat | **11g** SatFat | **5g** Fibre

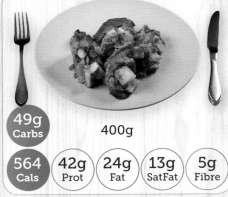

49g Carbs

400g

564 Cals | **42g** Prot | **24g** Fat | **13g** SatFat | **5g** Fibre

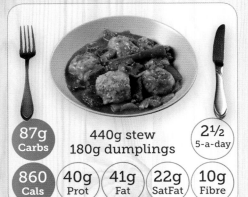

87g Carbs

440g stew
180g dumplings

2½ 5-a-day

860 Cals | **40g** Prot | **41g** Fat | **22g** SatFat | **10g** Fibre

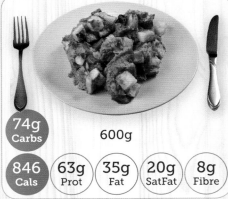

74g Carbs

600g

846 Cals | **63g** Prot | **35g** Fat | **20g** SatFat | **8g** Fibre

Chilli con Carne (with White Rice)

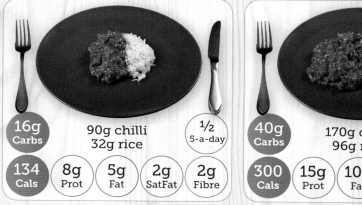

16g Carbs

90g chilli
32g rice

½ 5-a-day

134 Cals | **8g** Prot | **5g** Fat | **2g** SatFat | **2g** Fibre

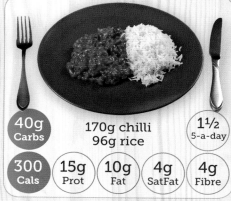

40g Carbs

170g chilli
96g rice

1½ 5-a-day

300 Cals | **15g** Prot | **10g** Fat | **4g** SatFat | **4g** Fibre

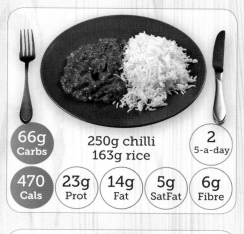

66g Carbs

250g chilli
163g rice

2 5-a-day

470 Cals | **23g** Prot | **14g** Fat | **5g** SatFat | **6g** Fibre

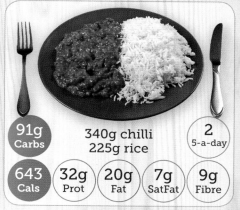

91g Carbs

340g chilli
225g rice

2 5-a-day

643 Cals | **32g** Prot | **20g** Fat | **7g** SatFat | **9g** Fibre

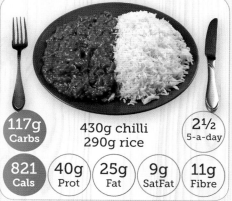

117g Carbs

430g chilli
290g rice

2½ 5-a-day

821 Cals | **40g** Prot | **25g** Fat | **9g** SatFat | **11g** Fibre

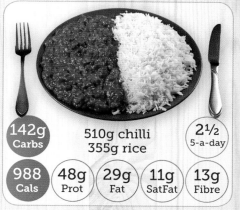

142g Carbs

510g chilli
355g rice

2½ 5-a-day

988 Cals | **48g** Prot | **29g** Fat | **11g** SatFat | **13g** Fibre

Curry, Chicken (with White Rice)

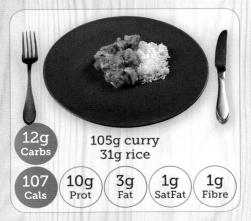

12g Carbs
105g curry
31g rice

107 Cals | **10g** Prot | **3g** Fat | **1g** SatFat | **1g** Fibre

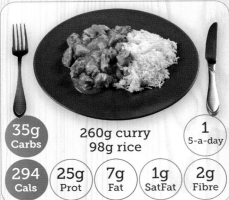

35g Carbs
260g curry
98g rice
1 5-a-day

294 Cals | **25g** Prot | **7g** Fat | **1g** SatFat | **2g** Fibre

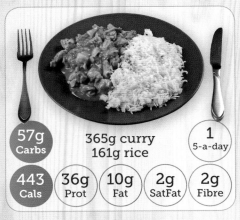

57g Carbs
365g curry
161g rice
1 5-a-day

443 Cals | **36g** Prot | **10g** Fat | **2g** SatFat | **2g** Fibre

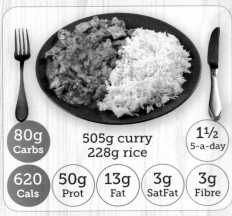

80g Carbs
505g curry
228g rice
1½ 5-a-day

620 Cals | **50g** Prot | **13g** Fat | **3g** SatFat | **3g** Fibre

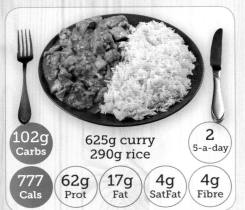

102g Carbs
625g curry
290g rice
2 5-a-day

777 Cals | **62g** Prot | **17g** Fat | **4g** SatFat | **4g** Fibre

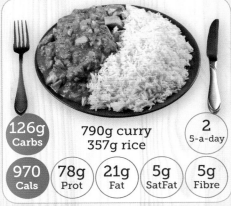

126g Carbs
790g curry
357g rice
2 5-a-day

970 Cals | **78g** Prot | **21g** Fat | **5g** SatFat | **5g** Fibre

Curry, Lentil (with Brown Rice)

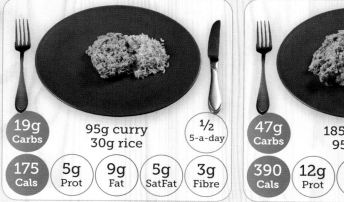

19g Carbs
95g curry
30g rice
½ 5-a-day
175 Cals
5g Prot
9g Fat
5g SatFat
3g Fibre

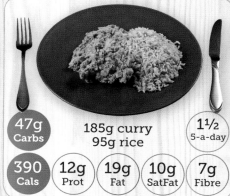

47g Carbs
185g curry
95g rice
1½ 5-a-day
390 Cals
12g Prot
19g Fat
10g SatFat
7g Fibre

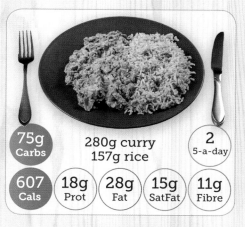

75g Carbs
280g curry
157g rice
2 5-a-day
607 Cals
18g Prot
28g Fat
15g SatFat
11g Fibre

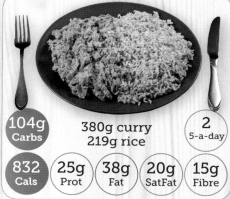

104g Carbs
380g curry
219g rice
2 5-a-day
832 Cals
25g Prot
38g Fat
20g SatFat
15g Fibre

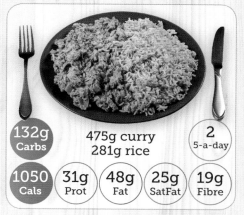

132g Carbs
475g curry
281g rice
2 5-a-day
1050 Cals
31g Prot
48g Fat
25g SatFat
19g Fibre

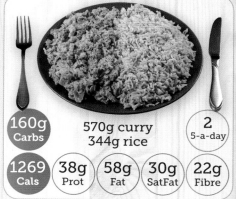

160g Carbs
570g curry
344g rice
2 5-a-day
1269 Cals
38g Prot
58g Fat
30g SatFat
22g Fibre

Curry, Vegetable & Potato (with White Rice)

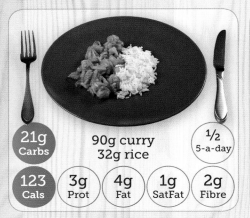

21g Carbs

90g curry
32g rice

½ 5-a-day

123 Cals | **3g** Prot | **4g** Fat | **1g** SatFat | **2g** Fibre

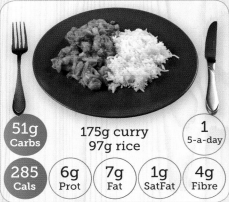

51g Carbs

175g curry
97g rice

1 5-a-day

285 Cals | **6g** Prot | **7g** Fat | **1g** SatFat | **4g** Fibre

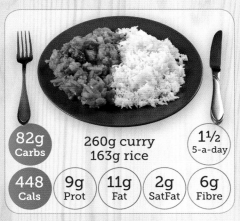

82g Carbs

260g curry
163g rice

1½ 5-a-day

448 Cals | **9g** Prot | **11g** Fat | **2g** SatFat | **6g** Fibre

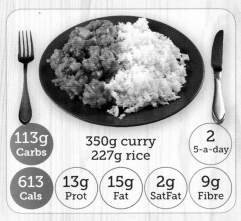

113g Carbs

350g curry
227g rice

2 5-a-day

613 Cals | **13g** Prot | **15g** Fat | **2g** SatFat | **9g** Fibre

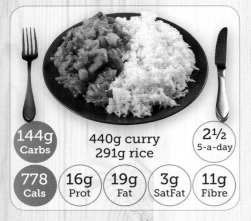

144g Carbs

440g curry
291g rice

2½ 5-a-day

778 Cals | **16g** Prot | **19g** Fat | **3g** SatFat | **11g** Fibre

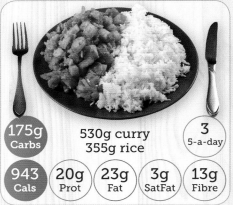

175g Carbs

530g curry
355g rice

3 5-a-day

943 Cals | **20g** Prot | **23g** Fat | **3g** SatFat | **13g** Fibre

Fish Pie

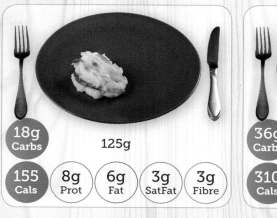

18g Carbs

125g

155 Cals | **8g** Prot | **6g** Fat | **3g** SatFat | **3g** Fibre

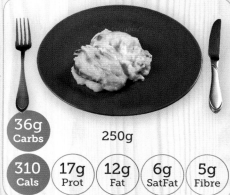

36g Carbs

250g

310 Cals | **17g** Prot | **12g** Fat | **6g** SatFat | **5g** Fibre

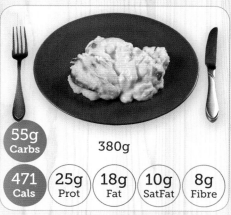

55g Carbs

380g

471 Cals | **25g** Prot | **18g** Fat | **10g** SatFat | **8g** Fibre

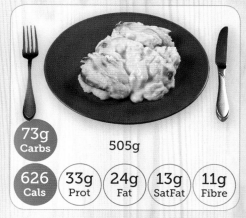

73g Carbs

505g

626 Cals | **33g** Prot | **24g** Fat | **13g** SatFat | **11g** Fibre

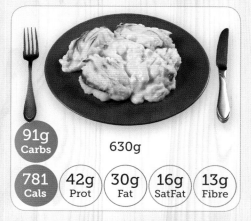

91g Carbs

630g

781 Cals | **42g** Prot | **30g** Fat | **16g** SatFat | **13g** Fibre

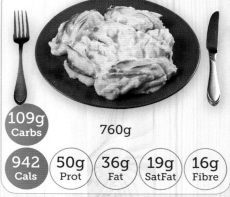

109g Carbs

760g

942 Cals | **50g** Prot | **36g** Fat | **19g** SatFat | **16g** Fibre

Fish Stew with Jollof Rice

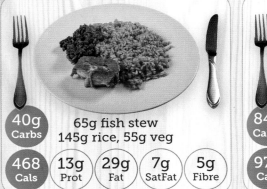

40g Carbs

65g fish stew
145g rice, 55g veg

468 Cals | **13g Prot** | **29g Fat** | **7g SatFat** | **5g Fibre**

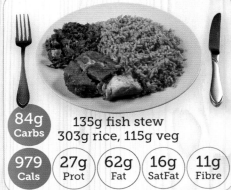

84g Carbs

135g fish stew
303g rice, 115g veg

979 Cals | **27g Prot** | **62g Fat** | **16g SatFat** | **11g Fibre**

Caribbean Dumplings

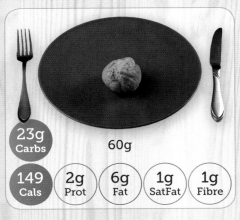

23g Carbs

60g

149 Cals | **2g Prot** | **6g Fat** | **1g SatFat** | **1g Fibre**

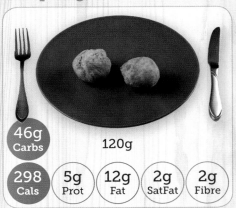

46g Carbs

120g

298 Cals | **5g Prot** | **12g Fat** | **2g SatFat** | **2g Fibre**

Jamaican Beef Patty

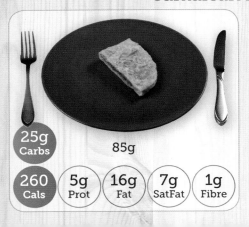

25g Carbs

85g

260 Cals | **5g Prot** | **16g Fat** | **7g SatFat** | **1g Fibre**

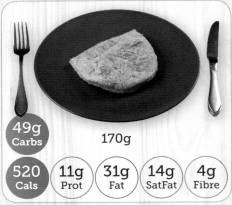

49g Carbs

170g

520 Cals | **11g Prot** | **31g Fat** | **14g SatFat** | **4g Fibre**

Goat & Potato Curry (with Rice & Peas)

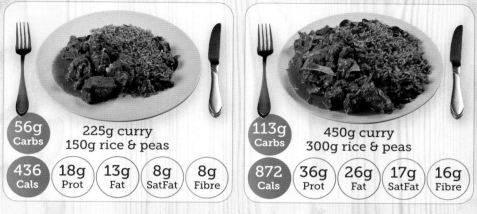

56g Carbs

225g curry
150g rice & peas

436 Cals | **18g** Prot | **13g** Fat | **8g** SatFat | **8g** Fibre

113g Carbs

450g curry
300g rice & peas

872 Cals | **36g** Prot | **26g** Fat | **17g** SatFat | **16g** Fibre

Jerk Chicken (with Rice & Peas)

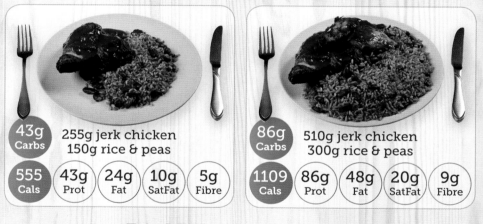

43g Carbs

255g jerk chicken
150g rice & peas

555 Cals | **43g** Prot | **24g** Fat | **10g** SatFat | **5g** Fibre

86g Carbs

510g jerk chicken
300g rice & peas

1109 Cals | **86g** Prot | **48g** Fat | **20g** SatFat | **9g** Fibre

Fried Fish (with Rice & Peas)

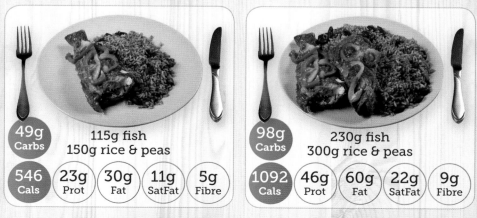

49g Carbs

115g fish
150g rice & peas

546 Cals | **23g** Prot | **30g** Fat | **11g** SatFat | **5g** Fibre

98g Carbs

230g fish
300g rice & peas

1092 Cals | **46g** Prot | **60g** Fat | **22g** SatFat | **9g** Fibre

Lasagne

Veggie Lasagne

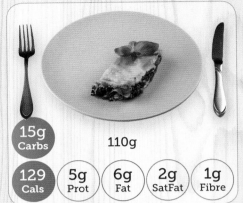

25g Carbs · 165g · ½ 5-a-day
297 Cals | 16g Prot | 16g Fat | 7g SatFat | 2g Fibre

15g Carbs · 110g
129 Cals | 5g Prot | 6g Fat | 2g SatFat | 1g Fibre

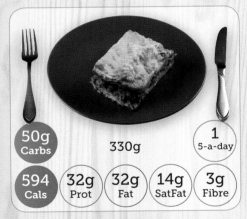
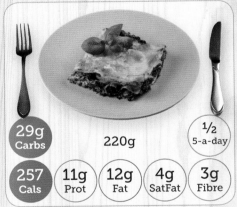

50g Carbs · 330g · 1 5-a-day
594 Cals | 32g Prot | 32g Fat | 14g SatFat | 3g Fibre

29g Carbs · 220g · ½ 5-a-day
257 Cals | 11g Prot | 12g Fat | 4g SatFat | 3g Fibre

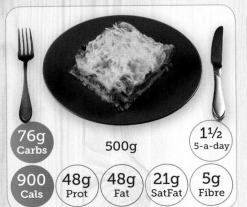
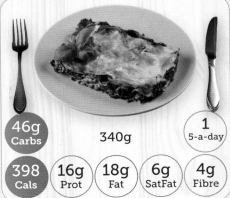

76g Carbs · 500g · 1½ 5-a-day
900 Cals | 48g Prot | 48g Fat | 21g SatFat | 5g Fibre

46g Carbs · 340g · 1 5-a-day
398 Cals | 16g Prot | 18g Fat | 6g SatFat | 4g Fibre

Mushroom Risotto

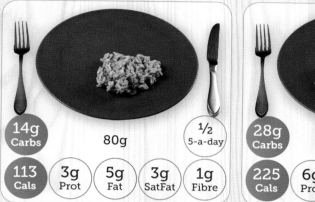

14g Carbs — 80g — ½ 5-a-day
113 Cals | 3g Prot | 5g Fat | 3g SatFat | 1g Fibre

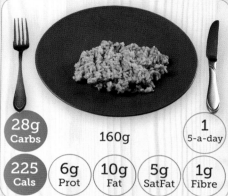

28g Carbs — 160g — 1 5-a-day
225 Cals | 6g Prot | 10g Fat | 5g SatFat | 1g Fibre

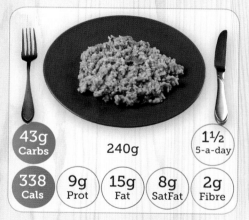

43g Carbs — 240g — 1½ 5-a-day
338 Cals | 9g Prot | 15g Fat | 8g SatFat | 2g Fibre

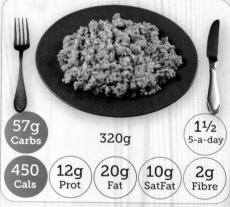

57g Carbs — 320g — 1½ 5-a-day
450 Cals | 12g Prot | 20g Fat | 10g SatFat | 2g Fibre

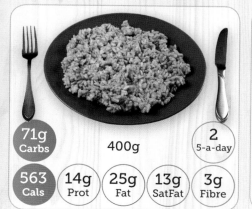

71g Carbs — 400g — 2 5-a-day
563 Cals | 14g Prot | 25g Fat | 13g SatFat | 3g Fibre

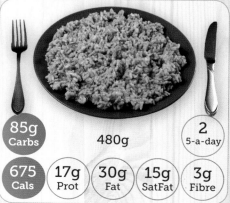

85g Carbs — 480g — 2 5-a-day
675 Cals | 17g Prot | 30g Fat | 15g SatFat | 3g Fibre

Macaroni Cheese

Penne Arrabbiata

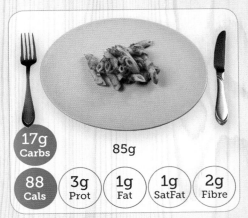

Macaroni Cheese
- 32g Carbs
- 163g
- 298 Cals
- 13g Prot
- 14g Fat
- 7g SatFat
- 2g Fibre

Penne Arrabbiata
- 17g Carbs
- 85g
- 88 Cals
- 3g Prot
- 1g Fat
- 1g SatFat
- 2g Fibre

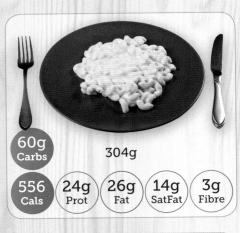
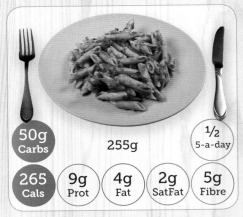

Macaroni Cheese
- 60g Carbs
- 304g
- 556 Cals
- 24g Prot
- 26g Fat
- 14g SatFat
- 3g Fibre

Penne Arrabbiata
- 50g Carbs
- 255g
- ½ 5-a-day
- 265 Cals
- 9g Prot
- 4g Fat
- 2g SatFat
- 5g Fibre

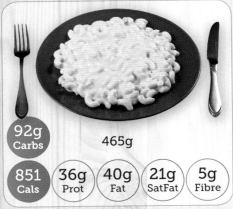
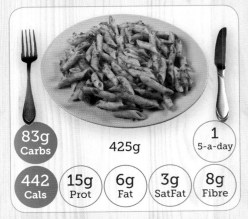

Macaroni Cheese
- 92g Carbs
- 465g
- 851 Cals
- 36g Prot
- 40g Fat
- 21g SatFat
- 5g Fibre

Penne Arrabbiata
- 83g Carbs
- 425g
- 1 5-a-day
- 442 Cals
- 15g Prot
- 6g Fat
- 3g SatFat
- 8g Fibre

Pasta Bake
(tuna, sweetcorn & cheese)

Pasta Meal (chicken,
broccoli & mascarpone)

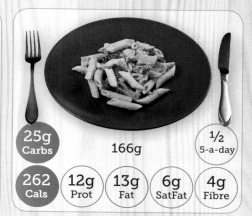

16g Carbs — 143g — **154** Cals — **11g** Prot — **5g** Fat — **3g** SatFat — **2g** Fibre

25g Carbs — 166g — **½** 5-a-day — **262** Cals — **12g** Prot — **13g** Fat — **6g** SatFat — **4g** Fibre

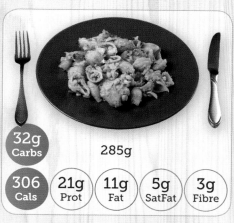
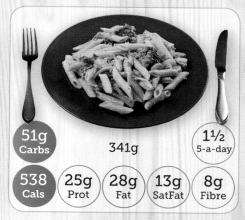

32g Carbs — 285g — **306** Cals — **21g** Prot — **11g** Fat — **5g** SatFat — **3g** Fibre

51g Carbs — 341g — **1½** 5-a-day — **538** Cals — **25g** Prot — **28g** Fat — **13g** SatFat — **8g** Fibre

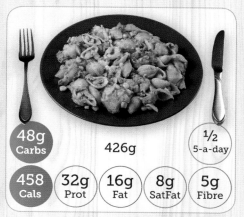
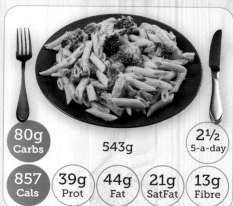

48g Carbs — 426g — **½** 5-a-day — **458** Cals — **32g** Prot — **16g** Fat — **8g** SatFat — **5g** Fibre

80g Carbs — 543g — **2½** 5-a-day — **857** Cals — **39g** Prot — **44g** Fat — **21g** SatFat — **13g** Fibre

26cm Dinner Plate

Chicken & Bacon Pie

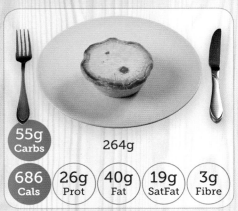

55g Carbs

264g

686 Cals | **26g** Prot | **40g** Fat | **19g** SatFat | **3g** Fibre

Steak Pie

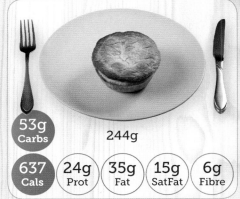

53g Carbs

244g

637 Cals | **24g** Prot | **35g** Fat | **15g** SatFat | **6g** Fibre

Steak & Potato Pie

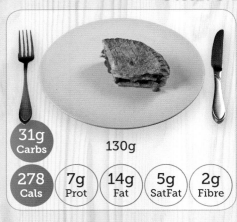

31g Carbs

130g

278 Cals | **7g** Prot | **14g** Fat | **5g** SatFat | **2g** Fibre

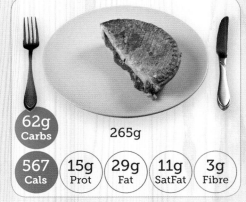

62g Carbs

265g

567 Cals | **15g** Prot | **29g** Fat | **11g** SatFat | **3g** Fibre

Steak & Kidney Pudding

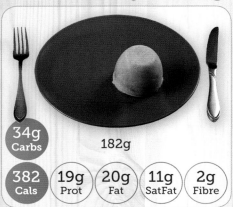

34g Carbs

182g

382 Cals | **19g** Prot | **20g** Fat | **11g** SatFat | **2g** Fibre

Top Crust Pie

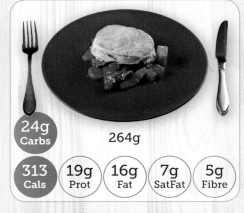

24g Carbs

264g

313 Cals | **19g** Prot | **16g** Fat | **7g** SatFat | **5g** Fibre

Pizza (chicken, deep pan, oven baked)

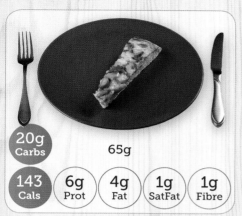

20g Carbs
65g
143 Cals | **6g** Prot | **4g** Fat | **1g** SatFat | **1g** Fibre

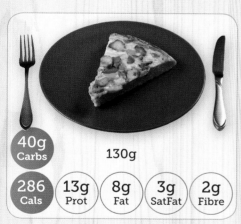

40g Carbs
130g
286 Cals | **13g** Prot | **8g** Fat | **3g** SatFat | **2g** Fibre

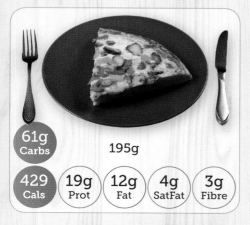

61g Carbs
195g
429 Cals | **19g** Prot | **12g** Fat | **4g** SatFat | **3g** Fibre

Pizza (pepperoni, thin crust, oven baked)

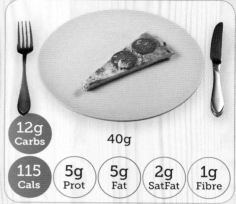

12g Carbs
40g
115 Cals | **5g** Prot | **5g** Fat | **2g** SatFat | **1g** Fibre

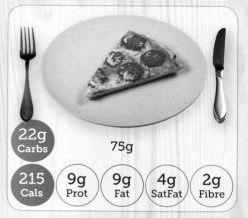

22g Carbs
75g
215 Cals | **9g** Prot | **9g** Fat | **4g** SatFat | **2g** Fibre

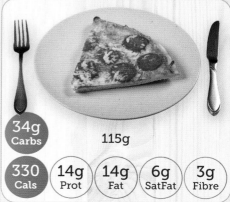

34g Carbs
115g
330 Cals | **14g** Prot | **14g** Fat | **6g** SatFat | **3g** Fibre

Quiche Lorraine

Salmon Frittata

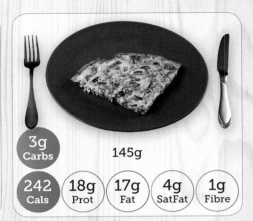

Quiche Lorraine

20g Carbs — 100g — 269 Cals — 9g Prot — 18g Fat — 8g SatFat — 1g Fibre

Salmon Frittata

3g Carbs — 145g — 242 Cals — 18g Prot — 17g Fat — 4g SatFat — 1g Fibre

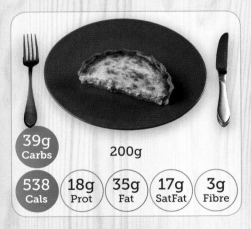

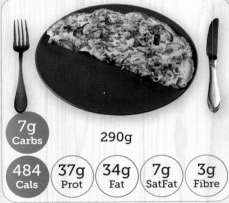

Quiche Lorraine

39g Carbs — 200g — 538 Cals — 18g Prot — 35g Fat — 17g SatFat — 3g Fibre

Salmon Frittata

7g Carbs — 290g — 484 Cals — 37g Prot — 34g Fat — 7g SatFat — 3g Fibre

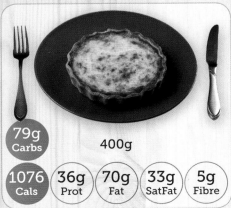

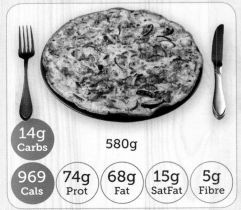

Quiche Lorraine

79g Carbs — 400g — 1076 Cals — 36g Prot — 70g Fat — 33g SatFat — 5g Fibre

Salmon Frittata

14g Carbs — 580g — 969 Cals — 74g Prot — 68g Fat — 15g SatFat — 5g Fibre

Chicken Caesar Salad

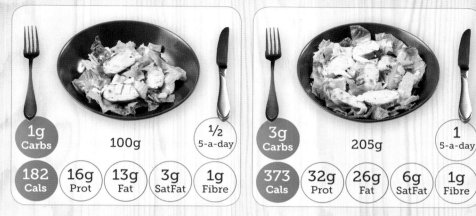

1g Carbs   100g   **½** 5-a-day

182 Cals | **16g** Prot | **13g** Fat | **3g** SatFat | **1g** Fibre

3g Carbs   205g   **1** 5-a-day

373 Cals | **32g** Prot | **26g** Fat | **6g** SatFat | **1g** Fibre

Greek Salad

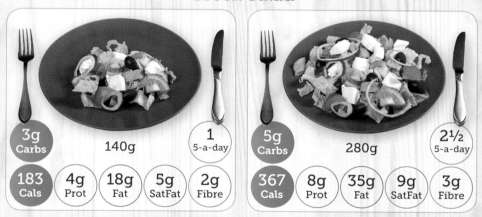

3g Carbs   140g   **1** 5-a-day

183 Cals | **4g** Prot | **18g** Fat | **5g** SatFat | **2g** Fibre

5g Carbs   280g   **2½** 5-a-day

367 Cals | **8g** Prot | **35g** Fat | **9g** SatFat | **3g** Fibre

Tuna Niçoise Salad

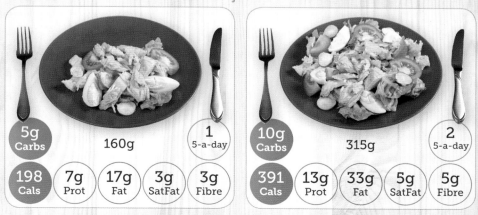

5g Carbs   160g   **1** 5-a-day

198 Cals | **7g** Prot | **17g** Fat | **3g** SatFat | **3g** Fibre

10g Carbs   315g   **2** 5-a-day

391 Cals | **13g** Prot | **33g** Fat | **5g** SatFat | **5g** Fibre

26cm Dinner Plate

Sausage & Mash (with butter)

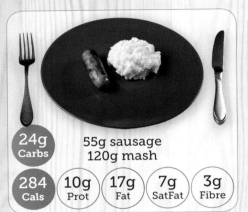

24g Carbs
284 Cals | **10g** Prot | **17g** Fat | **7g** SatFat | **3g** Fibre

55g sausage
120g mash

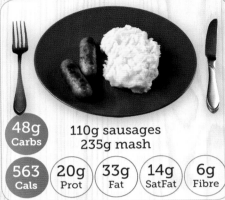

48g Carbs
563 Cals | **20g** Prot | **33g** Fat | **14g** SatFat | **6g** Fibre

110g sausages
235g mash

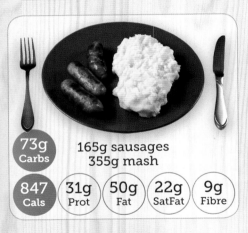

73g Carbs
847 Cals | **31g** Prot | **50g** Fat | **22g** SatFat | **9g** Fibre

165g sausages
355g mash

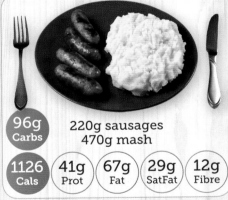

96g Carbs
1126 Cals | **41g** Prot | **67g** Fat | **29g** SatFat | **12g** Fibre

220g sausages
470g mash

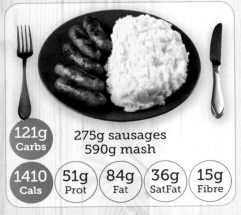

121g Carbs
1410 Cals | **51g** Prot | **84g** Fat | **36g** SatFat | **15g** Fibre

275g sausages
590g mash

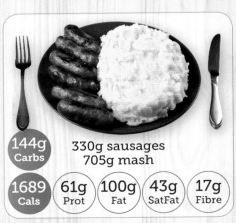

144g Carbs
1689 Cals | **61g** Prot | **100g** Fat | **43g** SatFat | **17g** Fibre

330g sausages
705g mash

Shepherd's Pie

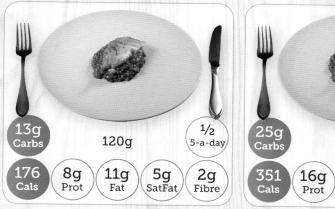

13g Carbs
120g
1/2 5-a-day
176 Cals | 8g Prot | 11g Fat | 5g SatFat | 2g Fibre

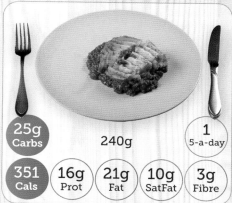

25g Carbs
240g
1 5-a-day
351 Cals | 16g Prot | 21g Fat | 10g SatFat | 3g Fibre

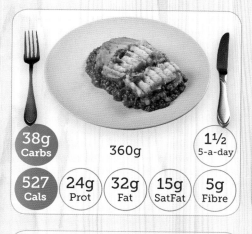

38g Carbs
360g
1 1/2 5-a-day
527 Cals | 24g Prot | 32g Fat | 15g SatFat | 5g Fibre

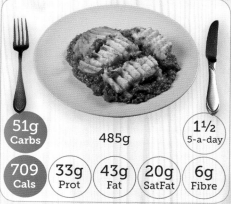

51g Carbs
485g
1 1/2 5-a-day
709 Cals | 33g Prot | 43g Fat | 20g SatFat | 6g Fibre

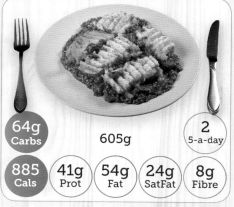

64g Carbs
605g
2 5-a-day
885 Cals | 41g Prot | 54g Fat | 24g SatFat | 8g Fibre

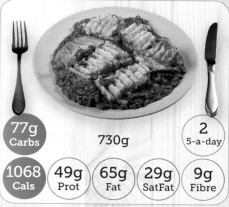

77g Carbs
730g
2 5-a-day
1068 Cals | 49g Prot | 65g Fat | 29g SatFat | 9g Fibre

Spaghetti Bolognese

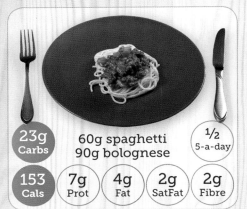

23g Carbs — 60g spaghetti / 90g bolognese — **½** 5-a-day

153 Cals | **7g** Prot | **4g** Fat | **2g** SatFat | **2g** Fibre

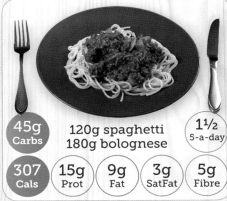

45g Carbs — 120g spaghetti / 180g bolognese — **1½** 5-a-day

307 Cals | **15g** Prot | **9g** Fat | **3g** SatFat | **5g** Fibre

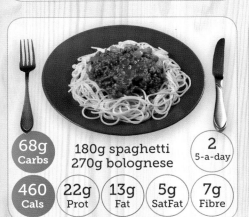

68g Carbs — 180g spaghetti / 270g bolognese — **2** 5-a-day

460 Cals | **22g** Prot | **13g** Fat | **5g** SatFat | **7g** Fibre

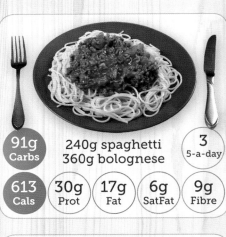

91g Carbs — 240g spaghetti / 360g bolognese — **3** 5-a-day

613 Cals | **30g** Prot | **17g** Fat | **6g** SatFat | **9g** Fibre

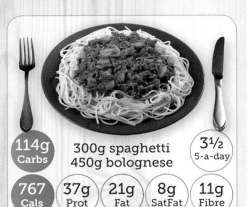

114g Carbs — 300g spaghetti / 450g bolognese — **3½** 5-a-day

767 Cals | **37g** Prot | **21g** Fat | **8g** SatFat | **11g** Fibre

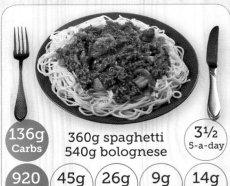

136g Carbs — 360g spaghetti / 540g bolognese — **3½** 5-a-day

920 Cals | **45g** Prot | **26g** Fat | **9g** SatFat | **14g** Fibre

Spaghetti Carbonara

Stir-fry
(cashew, without noodles)

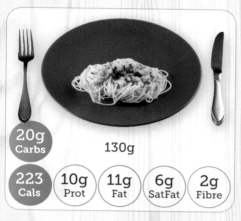

20g Carbs — 130g

223 Cals | **10g** Prot | **11g** Fat | **6g** SatFat | **2g** Fibre

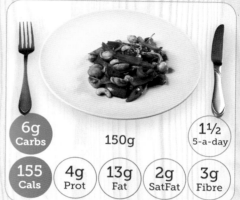

6g Carbs — 150g — **1½** 5-a-day

155 Cals | **4g** Prot | **13g** Fat | **2g** SatFat | **3g** Fibre

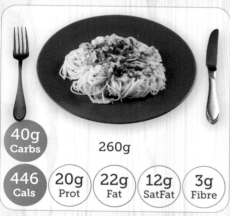

40g Carbs — 260g

446 Cals | **20g** Prot | **22g** Fat | **12g** SatFat | **3g** Fibre

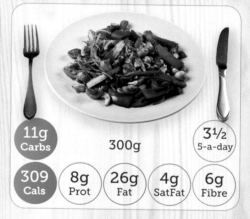

11g Carbs — 300g — **3½** 5-a-day

309 Cals | **8g** Prot | **26g** Fat | **4g** SatFat | **6g** Fibre

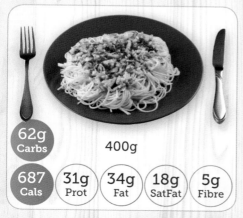

62g Carbs — 400g

687 Cals | **31g** Prot | **34g** Fat | **18g** SatFat | **5g** Fibre

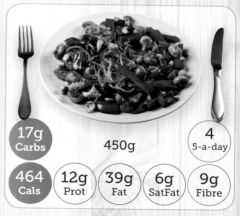

17g Carbs — 450g — **4** 5-a-day

464 Cals | **12g** Prot | **39g** Fat | **6g** SatFat | **9g** Fibre

Stir-fry
(chicken & noodles)

Toad in the Hole

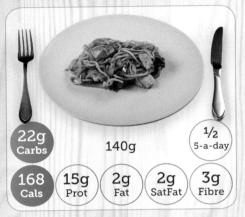

22g Carbs — 140g — **½** 5-a-day

168 Cals | **15g** Prot | **2g** Fat | **2g** SatFat | **3g** Fibre

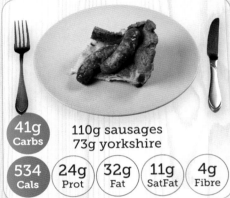

41g Carbs — 110g sausages / 73g yorkshire

534 Cals | **24g** Prot | **32g** Fat | **11g** SatFat | **4g** Fibre

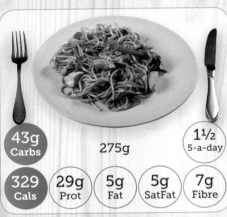

43g Carbs — 275g — **1½** 5-a-day

329 Cals | **29g** Prot | **5g** Fat | **5g** SatFat | **7g** Fibre

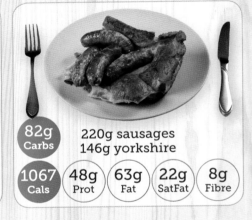

82g Carbs — 220g sausages / 146g yorkshire

1067 Cals | **48g** Prot | **63g** Fat | **22g** SatFat | **8g** Fibre

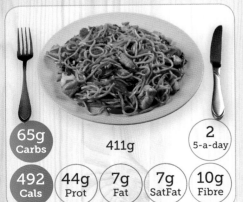

65g Carbs — 411g — **2** 5-a-day

492 Cals | **44g** Prot | **7g** Fat | **7g** SatFat | **10g** Fibre

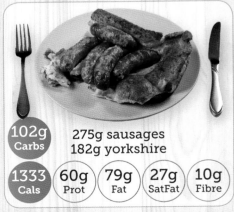

102g Carbs — 275g sausages / 182g yorkshire

1333 Cals | **60g** Prot | **79g** Fat | **27g** SatFat | **10g** Fibre

Coleslaw

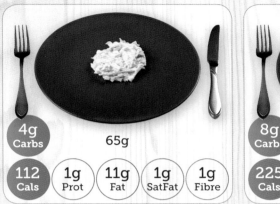

4g Carbs
65g

112 Cals | **1g** Prot | **11g** Fat | **1g** SatFat | **1g** Fibre

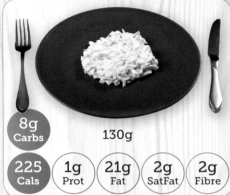

8g Carbs
130g

225 Cals | **1g** Prot | **21g** Fat | **2g** SatFat | **2g** Fibre

Gherkins

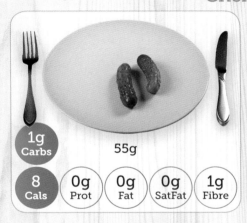

1g Carbs
55g

8 Cals | **0g** Prot | **0g** Fat | **0g** SatFat | **1g** Fibre

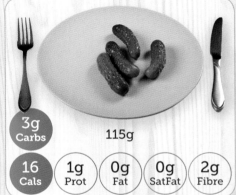

3g Carbs
115g

16 Cals | **1g** Prot | **0g** Fat | **0g** SatFat | **2g** Fibre

Olives (pitted in brine)

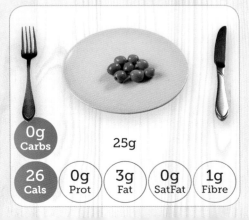

0g Carbs
25g

26 Cals | **0g** Prot | **3g** Fat | **0g** SatFat | **1g** Fibre

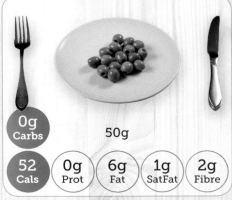

0g Carbs
50g

52 Cals | **0g** Prot | **6g** Fat | **1g** SatFat | **2g** Fibre

Onion Rings (battered)

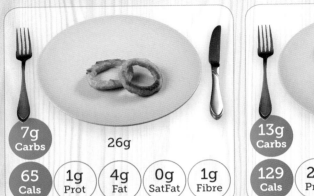

7g Carbs
26g
65 Cals | **1g** Prot | **4g** Fat | **0g** SatFat | **1g** Fibre

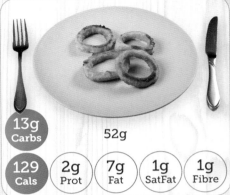

13g Carbs
52g
129 Cals | **2g** Prot | **7g** Fat | **1g** SatFat | **1g** Fibre

Pickled Onions

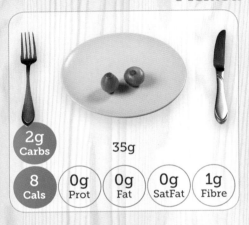

2g Carbs
35g
8 Cals | **0g** Prot | **0g** Fat | **0g** SatFat | **1g** Fibre

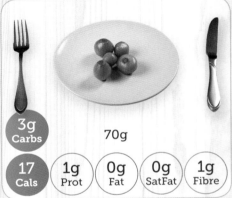

3g Carbs
70g
17 Cals | **1g** Prot | **0g** Fat | **0g** SatFat | **1g** Fibre

Sun-dried Tomatoes (in oil, drained)

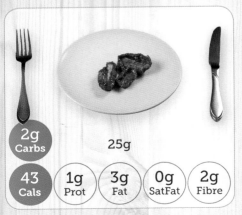

2g Carbs
25g
43 Cals | **1g** Prot | **3g** Fat | **0g** SatFat | **2g** Fibre

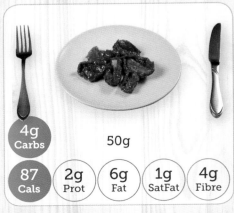

4g Carbs
50g
87 Cals | **2g** Prot | **6g** Fat | **1g** SatFat | **4g** Fibre

Stuffing (packet mix)

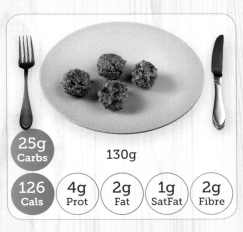

13g Carbs — 65g

63 Cals | **2g** Prot | **1g** Fat | **1g** SatFat | **1g** Fibre

25g Carbs — 130g

126 Cals | **4g** Prot | **2g** Fat | **1g** SatFat | **2g** Fibre

38g Carbs — 195g

189 Cals | **5g** Prot | **3g** Fat | **2g** SatFat | **3g** Fibre

Yorkshire Pudding

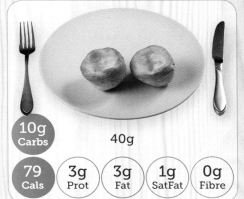

10g Carbs — 40g

79 Cals | **3g** Prot | **3g** Fat | **1g** SatFat | **0g** Fibre

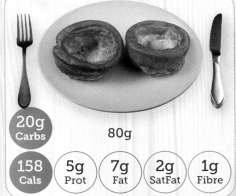

20g Carbs — 80g

158 Cals | **5g** Prot | **7g** Fat | **2g** SatFat | **1g** Fibre

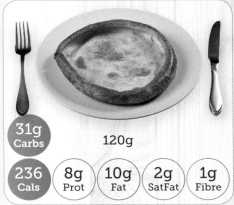

31g Carbs — 120g

236 Cals | **8g** Prot | **10g** Fat | **2g** SatFat | **1g** Fibre

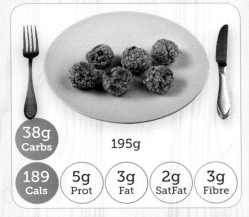

20cm Side Plate

Cornish Pasty

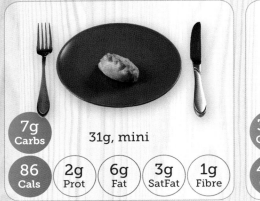

7g Carbs

31g, mini

86 Cals | **2g Prot** | **6g Fat** | **3g SatFat** | **1g Fibre**

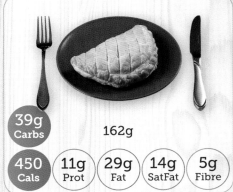

39g Carbs

162g

450 Cals | **11g Prot** | **29g Fat** | **14g SatFat** | **5g Fibre**

Pork Pie

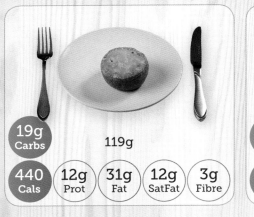

19g Carbs

119g

440 Cals | **12g Prot** | **31g Fat** | **12g SatFat** | **3g Fibre**

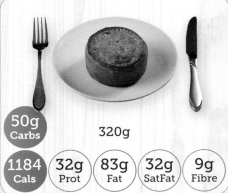

50g Carbs

320g

1184 Cals | **32g Prot** | **83g Fat** | **32g SatFat** | **9g Fibre**

Sausage Roll

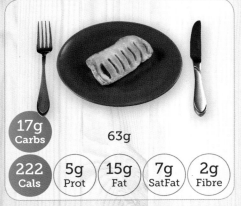

17g Carbs

63g

222 Cals | **5g Prot** | **15g Fat** | **7g SatFat** | **2g Fibre**

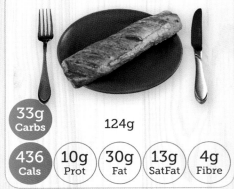

33g Carbs

124g

436 Cals | **10g Prot** | **30g Fat** | **13g SatFat** | **4g Fibre**

Sausages & Beans (tinned)

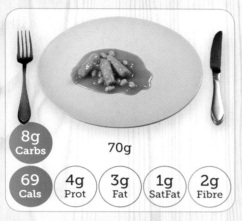

8g Carbs — 70g

69 Cals | **4g** Prot | **3g** Fat | **1g** SatFat | **2g** Fibre

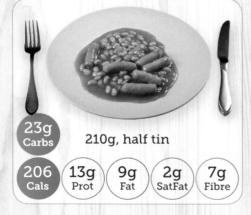

23g Carbs — 210g, half tin

206 Cals | **13g** Prot | **9g** Fat | **2g** SatFat | **7g** Fibre

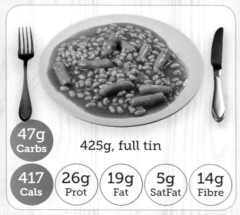

47g Carbs — 425g, full tin

417 Cals | **26g** Prot | **19g** Fat | **5g** SatFat | **14g** Fibre

Haggis

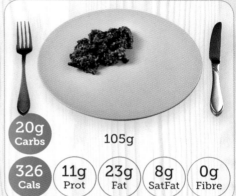

20g Carbs — 105g

326 Cals | **11g** Prot | **23g** Fat | **8g** SatFat | **0g** Fibre

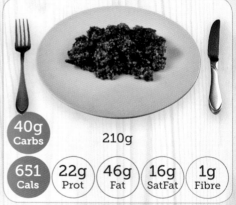

40g Carbs — 210g

651 Cals | **22g** Prot | **46g** Fat | **16g** SatFat | **1g** Fibre

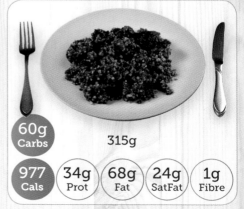

60g Carbs — 315g

977 Cals | **34g** Prot | **68g** Fat | **24g** SatFat | **1g** Fibre

26cm Dinner Plate

Black Pudding (dry fried)

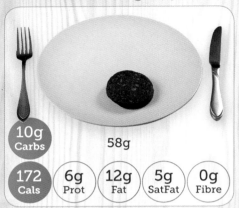

10g Carbs

58g

172 Cals | **6g** Prot | **12g** Fat | **5g** SatFat | **0g** Fibre

Chicken Goujon (baked)

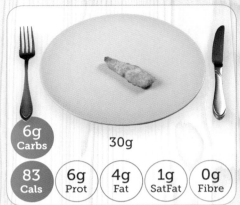

6g Carbs

30g

83 Cals | **6g** Prot | **4g** Fat | **1g** SatFat | **0g** Fibre

Brussels Pâté

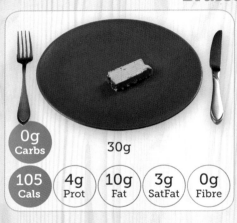

0g Carbs

30g

105 Cals | **4g** Prot | **10g** Fat | **3g** SatFat | **0g** Fibre

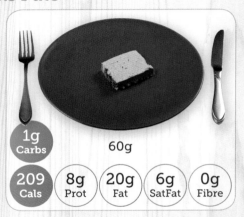

1g Carbs

60g

209 Cals | **8g** Prot | **20g** Fat | **6g** SatFat | **0g** Fibre

BBQ Ribs

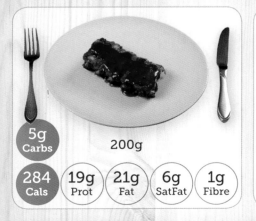

5g Carbs

200g

284 Cals | **19g** Prot | **21g** Fat | **6g** SatFat | **1g** Fibre

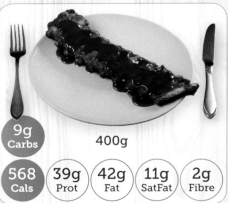

9g Carbs

400g

568 Cals | **39g** Prot | **42g** Fat | **11g** SatFat | **2g** Fibre

Gammon (grilled)

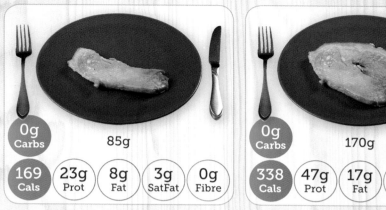

0g Carbs — 85g
169 Cals | **23g** Prot | **8g** Fat | **3g** SatFat | **0g** Fibre

0g Carbs — 170g
338 Cals | **47g** Prot | **17g** Fat | **6g** SatFat | **0g** Fibre

Pork Chop (grilled)

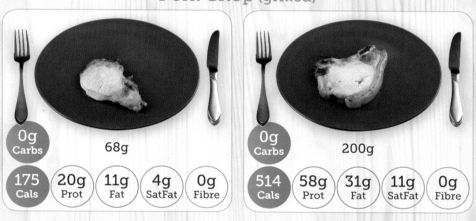

0g Carbs — 68g
175 Cals | **20g** Prot | **11g** Fat | **4g** SatFat | **0g** Fibre

0g Carbs — 200g
514 Cals | **58g** Prot | **31g** Fat | **11g** SatFat | **0g** Fibre

Roast Pork

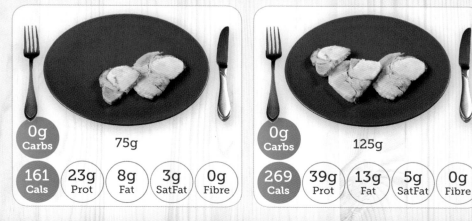

0g Carbs — 75g
161 Cals | **23g** Prot | **8g** Fat | **3g** SatFat | **0g** Fibre

0g Carbs — 125g
269 Cals | **39g** Prot | **13g** Fat | **5g** SatFat | **0g** Fibre

26cm Dinner Plate

Back Bacon (fried)

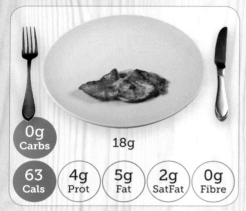

0g Carbs

18g

63 Cals | 4g Prot | 5g Fat | 2g SatFat | 0g Fibre

Back Bacon (grilled)

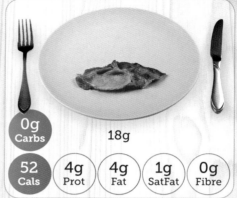

0g Carbs

18g

52 Cals | 4g Prot | 4g Fat | 1g SatFat | 0g Fibre

Streaky Bacon (fried)

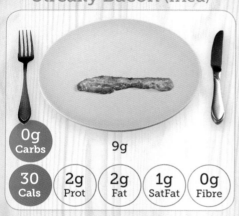

0g Carbs

9g

30 Cals | 2g Prot | 2g Fat | 1g SatFat | 0g Fibre

Streaky Bacon (grilled)

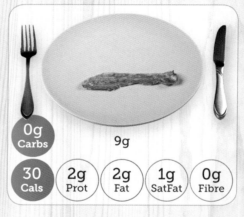

0g Carbs

9g

30 Cals | 2g Prot | 2g Fat | 1g SatFat | 0g Fibre

Sausage (grilled)

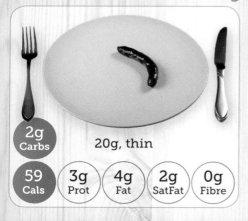

2g Carbs

20g, thin

59 Cals | 3g Prot | 4g Fat | 2g SatFat | 0g Fibre

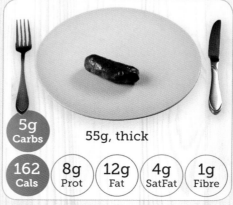

5g Carbs

55g, thick

162 Cals | 8g Prot | 12g Fat | 4g SatFat | 1g Fibre

Chorizo

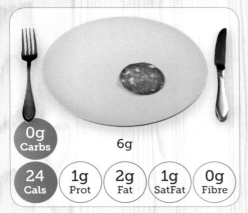

0g Carbs

6g

24 Cals | 1g Prot | 2g Fat | 1g SatFat | 0g Fibre

Pancetta (dry fried)

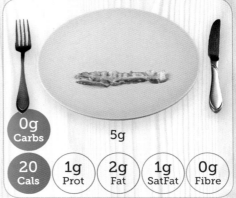

0g Carbs

5g

20 Cals | 1g Prot | 2g Fat | 1g SatFat | 0g Fibre

Parma Ham

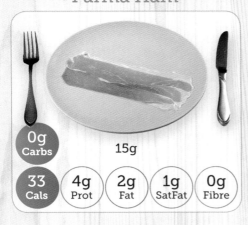

0g Carbs

15g

33 Cals | 4g Prot | 2g Fat | 1g SatFat | 0g Fibre

Prosciutto

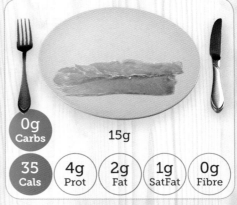

0g Carbs

15g

35 Cals | 4g Prot | 2g Fat | 1g SatFat | 0g Fibre

Salami

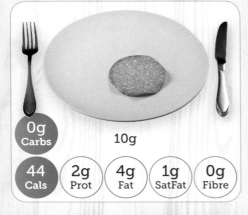

0g Carbs

10g

44 Cals | 2g Prot | 4g Fat | 1g SatFat | 0g Fibre

Wafer-thin Chicken

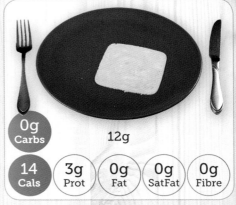

0g Carbs

12g

14 Cals | 3g Prot | 0g Fat | 0g SatFat | 0g Fibre

26cm Dinner Plate

Beef Slice

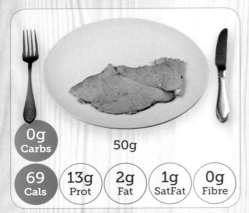

0g
Carbs

50g

69 Cals | 13g Prot | 2g Fat | 1g SatFat | 0g Fibre

Wafer-thin Beef

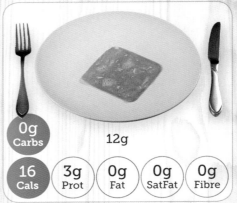

0g
Carbs

12g

16 Cals | 3g Prot | 0g Fat | 0g SatFat | 0g Fibre

Ham Slice

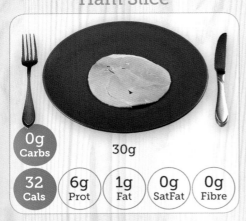

0g
Carbs

30g

32 Cals | 6g Prot | 1g Fat | 0g SatFat | 0g Fibre

Wafer-thin Ham

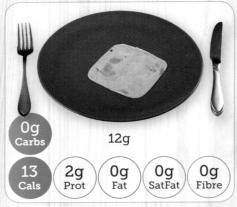

0g
Carbs

12g

13 Cals | 2g Prot | 0g Fat | 0g SatFat | 0g Fibre

Turkey Slice

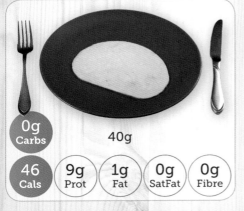

0g
Carbs

40g

46 Cals | 9g Prot | 1g Fat | 0g SatFat | 0g Fibre

Wafer-thin Turkey

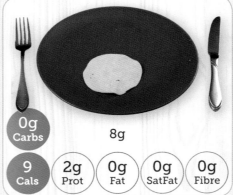

0g
Carbs

8g

9 Cals | 2g Prot | 0g Fat | 0g SatFat | 0g Fibre

Beef Burger (fried)

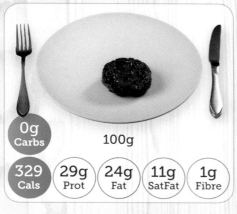

0g Carbs

100g

329 Cals | **29g Prot** | **24g Fat** | **11g SatFat** | **1g Fibre**

Beef Burger (grilled)

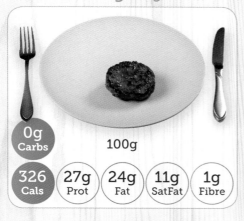

0g Carbs

100g

326 Cals | **27g Prot** | **24g Fat** | **11g SatFat** | **1g Fibre**

Corned Beef

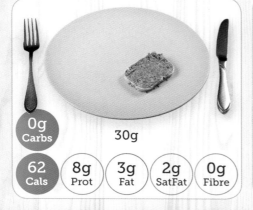

0g Carbs

30g

62 Cals | **8g Prot** | **3g Fat** | **2g SatFat** | **0g Fibre**

Roast Beef

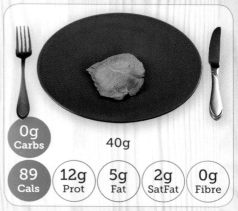

0g Carbs

40g

89 Cals | **12g Prot** | **5g Fat** | **2g SatFat** | **0g Fibre**

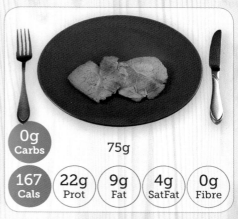

0g Carbs

75g

167 Cals | **22g Prot** | **9g Fat** | **4g SatFat** | **0g Fibre**

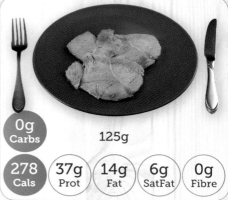

0g Carbs

125g

278 Cals | **37g Prot** | **14g Fat** | **6g SatFat** | **0g Fibre**

Rump Steak (fried)

Sirloin Steak (fried)

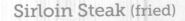

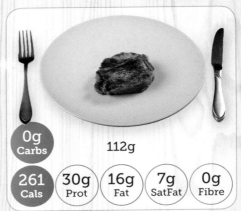

0g Carbs
68g
155 Cals | **19g** Prot | **9g** Fat | **3g** SatFat | **0g** Fibre

0g Carbs
112g
261 Cals | **30g** Prot | **16g** Fat | **7g** SatFat | **0g** Fibre

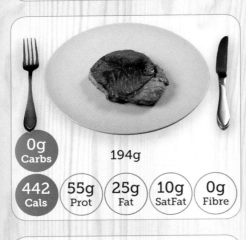

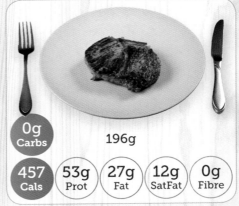

0g Carbs
194g
442 Cals | **55g** Prot | **25g** Fat | **10g** SatFat | **0g** Fibre

0g Carbs
196g
457 Cals | **53g** Prot | **27g** Fat | **12g** SatFat | **0g** Fibre

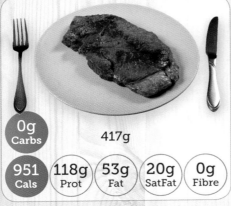

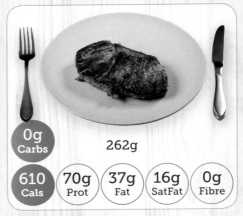

0g Carbs
417g
951 Cals | **118g** Prot | **53g** Fat | **20g** SatFat | **0g** Fibre

0g Carbs
262g
610 Cals | **70g** Prot | **37g** Fat | **16g** SatFat | **0g** Fibre

Lamb Chop (grilled)

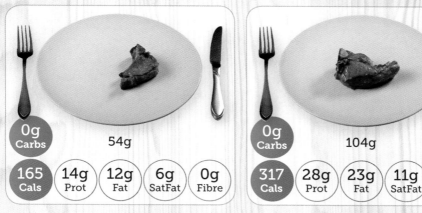

0g Carbs — 54g
165 Cals | **14g** Prot | **12g** Fat | **6g** SatFat | **0g** Fibre

0g Carbs — 104g
317 Cals | **28g** Prot | **23g** Fat | **11g** SatFat | **0g** Fibre

Lamb Steak (grilled)

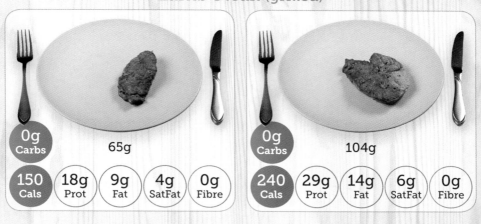

0g Carbs — 65g
150 Cals | **18g** Prot | **9g** Fat | **4g** SatFat | **0g** Fibre

0g Carbs — 104g
240 Cals | **29g** Prot | **14g** Fat | **6g** SatFat | **0g** Fibre

Roast Lamb

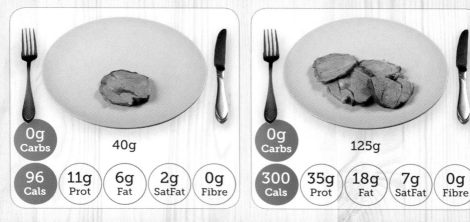

0g Carbs — 40g
96 Cals | **11g** Prot | **6g** Fat | **2g** SatFat | **0g** Fibre

0g Carbs — 125g
300 Cals | **35g** Prot | **18g** Fat | **7g** SatFat | **0g** Fibre

BBQ Chicken Wings

Chicken Drumsticks
(roasted)

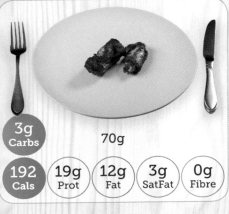

3g Carbs

70g

192 Cals | **19g** Prot | **12g** Fat | **3g** SatFat | **0g** Fibre

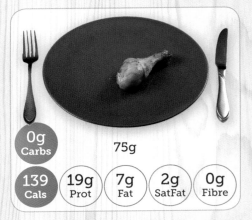

0g Carbs

75g

139 Cals | **19g** Prot | **7g** Fat | **2g** SatFat | **0g** Fibre

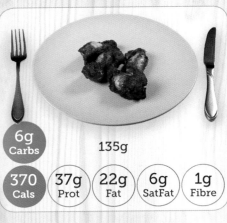

6g Carbs

135g

370 Cals | **37g** Prot | **22g** Fat | **6g** SatFat | **1g** Fibre

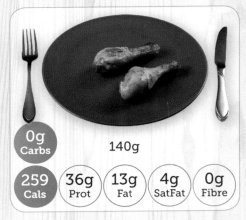

0g Carbs

140g

259 Cals | **36g** Prot | **13g** Fat | **4g** SatFat | **0g** Fibre

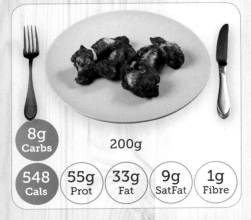

8g Carbs

200g

548 Cals | **55g** Prot | **33g** Fat | **9g** SatFat | **1g** Fibre

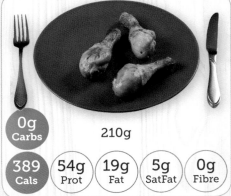

0g Carbs

210g

389 Cals | **54g** Prot | **19g** Fat | **5g** SatFat | **0g** Fibre

Chicken Breast (grilled, without skin)

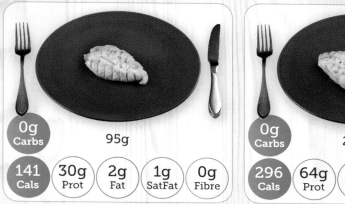

0g
Carbs

95g

141
Cals

30g
Prot

2g
Fat

1g
SatFat

0g
Fibre

0g
Carbs

200g

296
Cals

64g
Prot

4g
Fat

1g
SatFat

0g
Fibre

Chicken Breast (grilled, with skin)

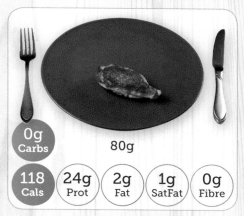
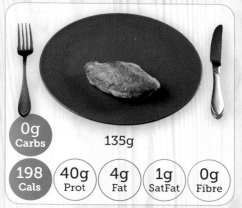

0g
Carbs

80g

118
Cals

24g
Prot

2g
Fat

1g
SatFat

0g
Fibre

0g
Carbs

135g

198
Cals

40g
Prot

4g
Fat

1g
SatFat

0g
Fibre

Roast Chicken (with skin)

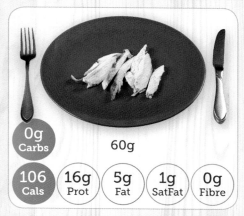
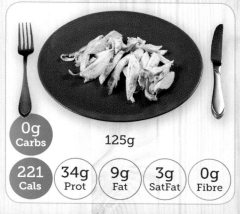

0g
Carbs

60g

106
Cals

16g
Prot

5g
Fat

1g
SatFat

0g
Fibre

0g
Carbs

125g

221
Cals

34g
Prot

9g
Fat

3g
SatFat

0g
Fibre

26cm Dinner Plate

Chicken Kiev

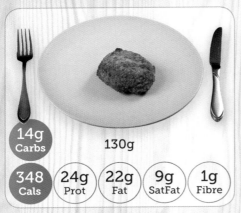

14g Carbs

130g

348 Cals | **24g** Prot | **22g** Fat | **9g** SatFat | **1g** Fibre

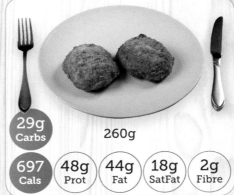

29g Carbs

260g

697 Cals | **48g** Prot | **44g** Fat | **18g** SatFat | **2g** Fibre

Roast Turkey (with skin)

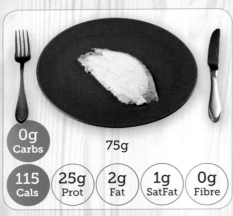

0g Carbs

75g

115 Cals | **25g** Prot | **2g** Fat | **1g** SatFat | **0g** Fibre

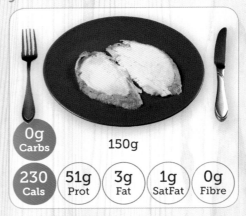

0g Carbs

150g

230 Cals | **51g** Prot | **3g** Fat | **1g** SatFat | **0g** Fibre

Turkey Breast (grilled)

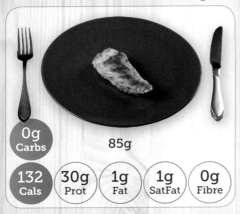

0g Carbs

85g

132 Cals | **30g** Prot | **1g** Fat | **1g** SatFat | **0g** Fibre

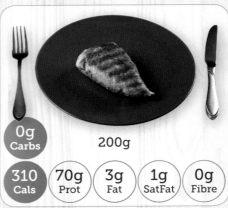

0g Carbs

200g

310 Cals | **70g** Prot | **3g** Fat | **1g** SatFat | **0g** Fibre

Fish (battered, baked)

Fish (breaded, baked)

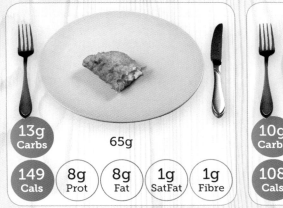

13g Carbs

65g

149 Cals | **8g** Prot | **8g** Fat | **1g** SatFat | **1g** Fibre

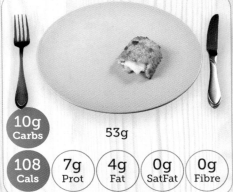

10g Carbs

53g

108 Cals | **7g** Prot | **4g** Fat | **0g** SatFat | **0g** Fibre

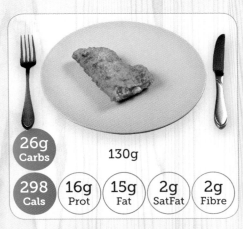

26g Carbs

130g

298 Cals | **16g** Prot | **15g** Fat | **2g** SatFat | **2g** Fibre

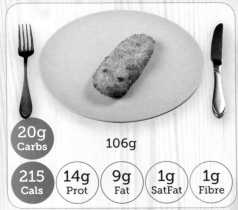

20g Carbs

106g

215 Cals | **14g** Prot | **9g** Fat | **1g** SatFat | **1g** Fibre

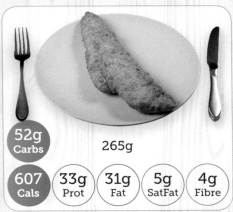

52g Carbs

265g

607 Cals | **33g** Prot | **31g** Fat | **5g** SatFat | **4g** Fibre

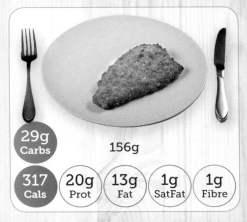

29g Carbs

156g

317 Cals | **20g** Prot | **13g** Fat | **1g** SatFat | **1g** Fibre

26cm Dinner Plate

Fish Cake (baked)

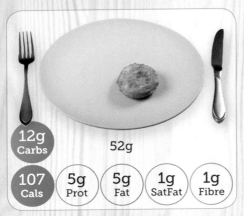

12g Carbs

52g

107 Cals | 5g Prot | 5g Fat | 1g SatFat | 1g Fibre

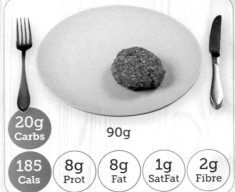

20g Carbs

90g

185 Cals | 8g Prot | 8g Fat | 1g SatFat | 2g Fibre

Fish Finger (baked)

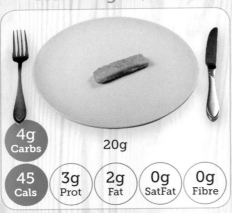

4g Carbs

20g

45 Cals | 3g Prot | 2g Fat | 0g SatFat | 0g Fibre

Fish Goujon (baked)

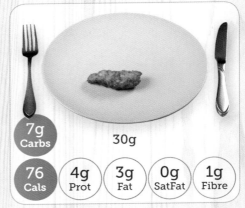

7g Carbs

30g

76 Cals | 4g Prot | 3g Fat | 0g SatFat | 1g Fibre

Scampi (fried)

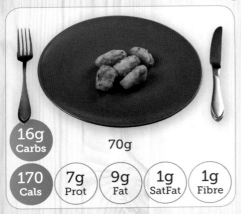

16g Carbs

70g

170 Cals | 7g Prot | 9g Fat | 1g SatFat | 1g Fibre

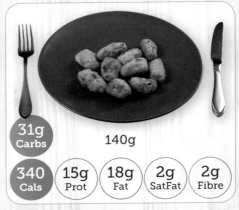

31g Carbs

140g

340 Cals | 15g Prot | 18g Fat | 2g SatFat | 2g Fibre

Prawns (boiled)

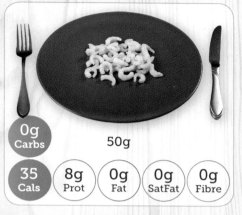

0g Carbs
50g
35 Cals | **8g** Prot | **0g** Fat | **0g** SatFat | **0g** Fibre

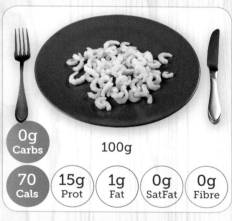

0g Carbs
100g
70 Cals | **15g** Prot | **1g** Fat | **0g** SatFat | **0g** Fibre

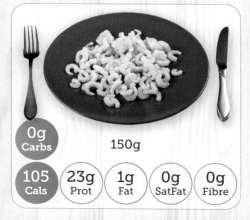

0g Carbs
150g
105 Cals | **23g** Prot | **1g** Fat | **0g** SatFat | **0g** Fibre

King Prawns (boiled)

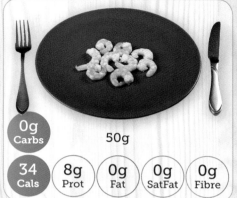

0g Carbs
50g
34 Cals | **8g** Prot | **0g** Fat | **0g** SatFat | **0g** Fibre

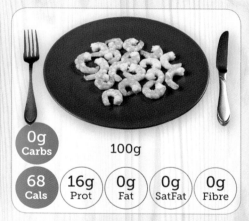

0g Carbs
100g
68 Cals | **16g** Prot | **0g** Fat | **0g** SatFat | **0g** Fibre

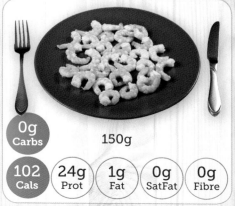

0g Carbs
150g
102 Cals | **24g** Prot | **1g** Fat | **0g** SatFat | **0g** Fibre

Salmon (tinned in brine)

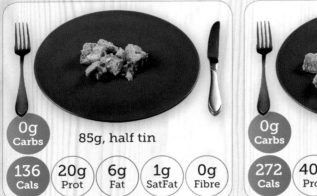

0g
Carbs

85g, half tin

136
Cals

20g
Prot

6g
Fat

1g
SatFat

0g
Fibre

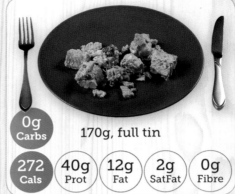

0g
Carbs

170g, full tin

272
Cals

40g
Prot

12g
Fat

2g
SatFat

0g
Fibre

Tuna (tinned in brine)

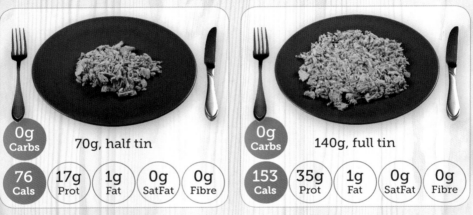

0g
Carbs

70g, half tin

76
Cals

17g
Prot

1g
Fat

0g
SatFat

0g
Fibre

0g
Carbs

140g, full tin

153
Cals

35g
Prot

1g
Fat

0g
SatFat

0g
Fibre

Tuna (tinned in oil)

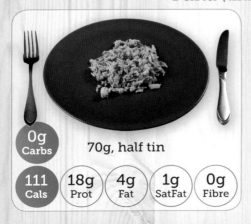

0g
Carbs

70g, half tin

111
Cals

18g
Prot

4g
Fat

1g
SatFat

0g
Fibre

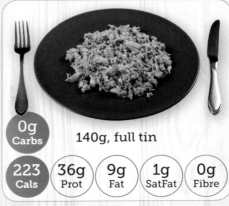

0g
Carbs

140g, full tin

223
Cals

36g
Prot

9g
Fat

1g
SatFat

0g
Fibre

Sardines (tinned in brine)

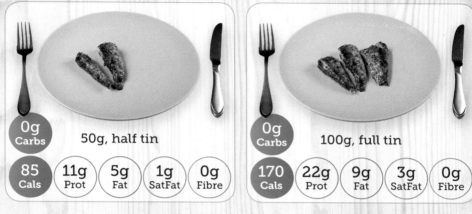

0g Carbs — 50g, half tin

85 Cals | **11g** Prot | **5g** Fat | **1g** SatFat | **0g** Fibre

0g Carbs — 100g, full tin

170 Cals | **22g** Prot | **9g** Fat | **3g** SatFat | **0g** Fibre

Sardines (tinned in oil)

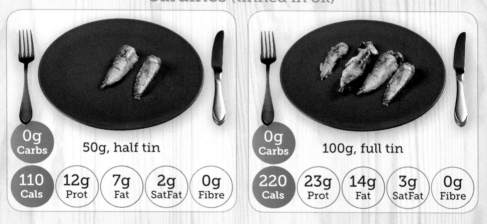

0g Carbs — 50g, half tin

110 Cals | **12g** Prot | **7g** Fat | **2g** SatFat | **0g** Fibre

0g Carbs — 100g, full tin

220 Cals | **23g** Prot | **14g** Fat | **3g** SatFat | **0g** Fibre

Sardines (tinned in tomato sauce)

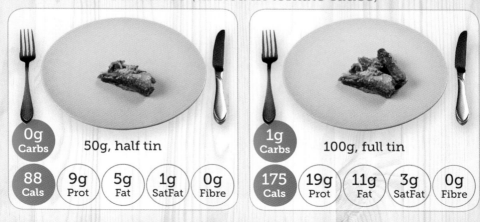

0g Carbs — 50g, half tin

88 Cals | **9g** Prot | **5g** Fat | **1g** SatFat | **0g** Fibre

1g Carbs — 100g, full tin

175 Cals | **19g** Prot | **11g** Fat | **3g** SatFat | **0g** Fibre

26cm Dinner Plate

Smoked Mackerel

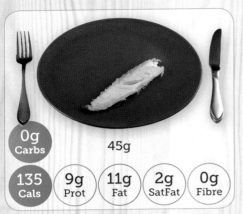

0g Carbs

45g

135 Cals | **9g** Prot | **11g** Fat | **2g** SatFat | **0g** Fibre

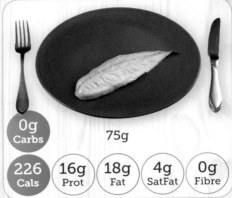

0g Carbs

75g

226 Cals | **16g** Prot | **18g** Fat | **4g** SatFat | **0g** Fibre

Smoked Salmon

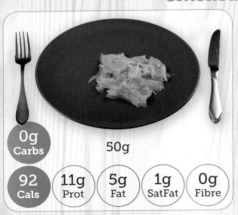

0g Carbs

50g

92 Cals | **11g** Prot | **5g** Fat | **1g** SatFat | **0g** Fibre

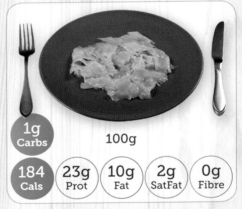

1g Carbs

100g

184 Cals | **23g** Prot | **10g** Fat | **2g** SatFat | **0g** Fibre

Saltfish (boiled)

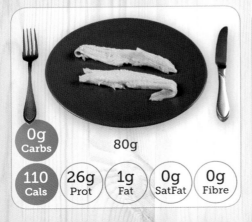

0g Carbs

80g

110 Cals | **26g** Prot | **1g** Fat | **0g** SatFat | **0g** Fibre

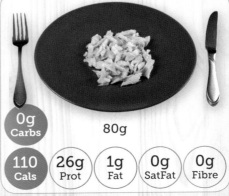

0g Carbs

80g

110 Cals | **26g** Prot | **1g** Fat | **0g** SatFat | **0g** Fibre

Cod / Haddock (baked)

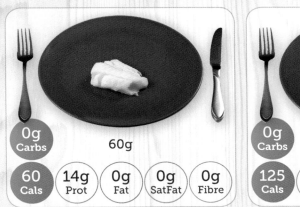

0g Carbs
60g
60 Cals | **14g** Prot | **0g** Fat | **0g** SatFat | **0g** Fibre

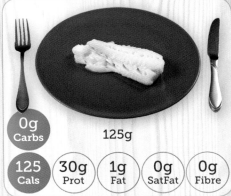

0g Carbs
125g
125 Cals | **30g** Prot | **1g** Fat | **0g** SatFat | **0g** Fibre

Plaice (grilled)

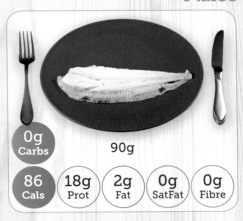

0g Carbs
90g
86 Cals | **18g** Prot | **2g** Fat | **0g** SatFat | **0g** Fibre

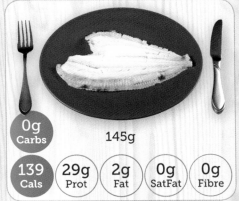

0g Carbs
145g
139 Cals | **29g** Prot | **2g** Fat | **0g** SatFat | **0g** Fibre

Scallops (fried)

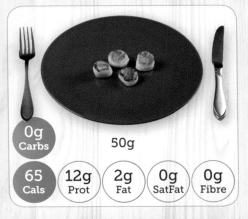

0g Carbs
50g
65 Cals | **12g** Prot | **2g** Fat | **0g** SatFat | **0g** Fibre

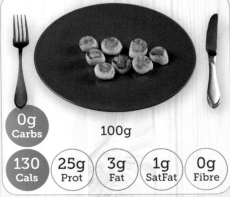

0g Carbs
100g
130 Cals | **25g** Prot | **3g** Fat | **1g** SatFat | **0g** Fibre

26cm Dinner Plate

Salmon Steak (grilled)

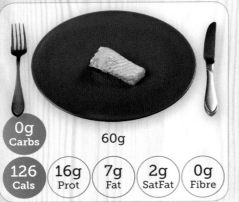

0g Carbs

60g

126 Cals | 16g Prot | 7g Fat | 2g SatFat | 0g Fibre

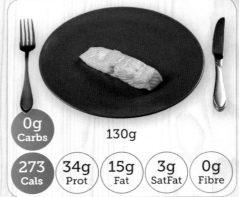

0g Carbs

130g

273 Cals | 34g Prot | 15g Fat | 3g SatFat | 0g Fibre

Trout Fillet (baked)

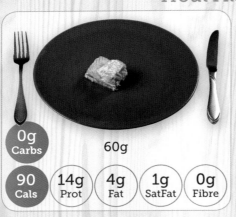

0g Carbs

60g

90 Cals | 14g Prot | 4g Fat | 1g SatFat | 0g Fibre

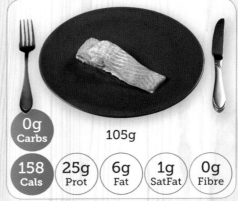

0g Carbs

105g

158 Cals | 25g Prot | 6g Fat | 1g SatFat | 0g Fibre

Tuna Steak (grilled)

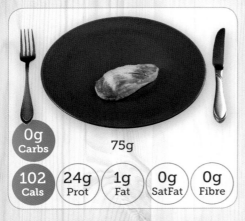

0g Carbs

75g

102 Cals | 24g Prot | 1g Fat | 0g SatFat | 0g Fibre

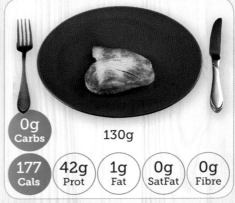

0g Carbs

130g

177 Cals | 42g Prot | 1g Fat | 0g SatFat | 0g Fibre

Crab Meat (tinned)

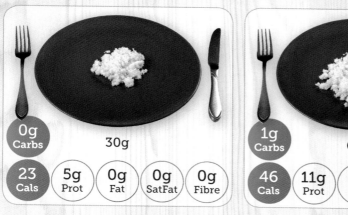

0g
Carbs

30g

23
Cals

5g Prot

0g Fat

0g SatFat

0g Fibre

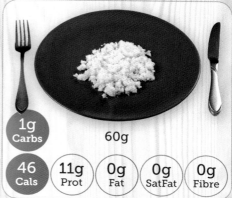

1g
Carbs

60g

46
Cals

11g Prot

0g Fat

0g SatFat

0g Fibre

Seafood Sticks

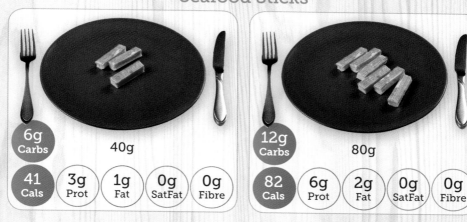

6g
Carbs

40g

41
Cals

3g Prot

1g Fat

0g SatFat

0g Fibre

12g
Carbs

80g

82
Cals

6g Prot

2g Fat

0g SatFat

0g Fibre

Calamari (fried)

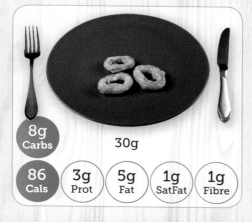

8g
Carbs

30g

86
Cals

3g Prot

5g Fat

1g SatFat

1g Fibre

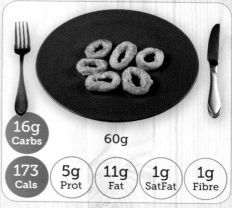

16g
Carbs

60g

173
Cals

5g Prot

11g Fat

1g SatFat

1g Fibre

Beef RAW (per 100g weight)

	Carbs	Cals	Prot	Fat	SatFat	Fibre
Beef Sausage	8g	258	13g	20g	8g	2g
Braising Steak	0g	160	21g	9g	4g	0g
Fillet Steak	0g	140	21g	6g	3g	0g
Mince	0g	225	20g	16g	7g	0g
Rump Steak	0g	174	21g	10g	4g	0g
Sirloin Steak	0g	201	22g	13g	6g	0g
Stewing Steak	0g	146	22g	6g	3g	0g

Beef COOKED (per 100g weight)

	Carbs	Cals	Prot	Fat	SatFat	Fibre
Beef Sausage (grilled)	11g	265	17g	17g	8g	2g
Braising Steak (braised)	0g	246	33g	13g	5g	0g
Fillet Steak (fried)	0g	184	28g	8g	3g	0g
Mince (stewed)	0g	209	22g	14g	6g	0g
Rump Steak (fried)	0g	228	28g	13g	5g	0g
Sirloin Steak (fried)	0g	233	27g	14g	6g	0g
Stewing Steak (stewed)	0g	203	29g	10g	4g	0g

Game COOKED (per 100g weight)

	Carbs	Cals	Prot	Fat	SatFat	Fibre
Partridge (roasted, meat only)	0g	212	37g	7g	2g	0g
Pheasant (roasted, meat only)	0g	220	28g	12g	4g	0g
Rabbit (stewed, meat only)	0g	114	21g	3g	2g	0g
Venison (roasted)	0g	165	36g	3g	1g	0g

Lamb RAW (per 100g weight)

	Carbs	Cals	Prot	Fat	SatFat	Fibre
Chop	0g	277	18g	23g	11g	0g
Leg	0g	187	19g	12g	5g	0g
Mince	0g	196	19g	13g	6g	0g
Neck Fillet	0g	232	18g	18g	8g	0g
Rack of Lamb	0g	283	17g	24g	12g	0g
Shoulder	0g	235	18g	18g	9g	0g

Lamb COOKED (per 100g weight)

	Carbs	Cals	Prot	Fat	SatFat	Fibre
Chop (grilled)	0g	305	27g	22g	11g	0g
Leg (roasted)	0g	240	28g	14g	6g	0g
Mince (stewed)	0g	208	24g	12g	6g	0g
Neck Fillet (grilled)	0g	302	26g	22g	10g	0g
Rack of Lamb (roasted)	0g	363	23g	30g	15g	0g
Shoulder (roasted)	0g	298	25g	22g	10g	0g

Poultry RAW (per 100g weight)

	Carbs	Cals	Prot	Fat	SatFat	Fibre
Chicken (dark meat)	0g	109	21g	3g	1g	0g
Chicken (light meat)	0g	106	24g	1g	0g	0g
Duck (meat only)	0g	137	20g	7g	2g	0g
Goose (meat & skin)	0g	361	17g	33g	10g	0g
Turkey (dark meat)	0g	104	20g	3g	1g	0g
Turkey (light meat)	0g	105	24g	1g	0g	0g

Poultry COOKED (per 100g weight)

	Carbs	Cals	Prot	Fat	SatFat	Fibre
Chicken (dark meat, roasted)	0g	196	24g	11g	3g	0g
Chicken (light meat, roasted)	0g	153	30g	4g	1g	0g
Duck (meat only, roasted)	0g	195	25g	10g	3g	0g
Goose (meat & skin, roasted)	0g	301	28g	21g	7g	0g
Turkey (dark meat, roasted)	0g	177	29g	7g	2g	0g
Turkey (light meat, roasted)	0g	153	34g	2g	1g	0g

Pork RAW (per 100g weight)

	Carbs	Cals	Prot	Fat	SatFat	Fibre
Bacon (back)	0g	215	17g	17g	6g	0g
Bacon (streaky)	0g	276	16g	24g	8g	0g
Belly	0g	258	19g	20g	7g	0g
Chop	0g	270	19g	22g	8g	0g
Mince	0g	164	19g	10g	4g	0g
Steak (lean)	0g	123	22g	4g	1g	0g

Pork COOKED (per 100g weight)

	Carbs	Cals	Prot	Fat	SatFat	Fibre
Bacon (back, grilled)	0g	287	23g	22g	8g	0g
Bacon (streaky, grilled)	0g	337	24g	27g	10g	0g
Belly (roasted)	0g	293	25g	21g	7g	0g
Chop (grilled)	0g	257	29g	16g	6g	0g
Mince (stewed)	0g	191	24g	10g	4g	0g
Sausage (grilled)	10g	294	15g	22g	8g	2g
Steak (lean, grilled)	0g	169	34g	4g	1g	0g

Seafood RAW (per 100g weight)

	Carbs	Cals	Prot	Fat	SatFat	Fibre
Cod / Haddock	0g	75	18g	1g	0g	0g
Coley	0g	82	18g	1g	0g	0g
Mussels	3g	74	12g	2g	0g	0g
Pollock	0g	72	16g	1g	0g	0g
Prawns	0g	77	18g	1g	0g	0g
Rainbow Trout	0g	127	20g	5g	1g	0g
Salmon	0g	179	22g	10g	2g	0g
Sardines	0g	134	20g	6g	2g	0g
Scallops	2g	96	18g	2g	0g	0g
Sea Bream	0g	96	18g	3g	0g	0g
Tuna Steak	0g	107	25g	1g	0g	0g

Seafood COOKED (per 100g weight)

	Carbs	Cals	Prot	Fat	SatFat	Fibre
Cod / Haddock (baked)	0g	100	24g	1g	0g	0g
Coley (baked)	0g	111	24g	2g	0g	0g
Kipper (grilled)	0g	245	22g	18g	4g	0g
Mackerel (smoked)	0g	301	21g	24g	5g	0g
Prawns (cooked)	0g	70	15g	1g	0g	0g
Salmon (baked)	0g	215	27g	12g	3g	0g
Sardines (grilled)	0g	172	25g	8g	2g	0g
Tuna Steak (baked)	0g	136	32g	1g	0g	0g

Almond Milk

5g Carbs

150ml

36 Cals | **1g** Prot | **2g** Fat | **0g** SatFat | **0g** Fibre

Coconut Milk

7g Carbs

150ml
(drink, not tinned)

33 Cals | **0g** Prot | **0g** Fat | **0g** SatFat | **0g** Fibre

Goat's Milk

7g Carbs

150ml

93 Cals | **5g** Prot | **6g** Fat | **4g** SatFat | **0g** Fibre

Hemp Milk

5g Carbs

150ml

59 Cals | **1g** Prot | **4g** Fat | **0g** SatFat | **0g** Fibre

Oat Milk

11g Carbs

150ml

69 Cals | **1g** Prot | **2g** Fat | **0g** SatFat | **1g** Fibre

Rice Milk

15g Carbs

150ml

73 Cals | **0g** Prot | **2g** Fat | **0g** SatFat | **0g** Fibre

Milk (whole)

7g Carbs
150ml
95 Cals | **5g** Prot | **5g** Fat | **3g** SatFat | **0g** Fibre

13g Carbs
284ml, half pint
179 Cals | **10g** Prot | **10g** Fat | **7g** SatFat | **0g** Fibre

26g Carbs
568ml, pint
358 Cals | **19g** Prot | **20g** Fat | **13g** SatFat | **0g** Fibre

Milk (semi-skimmed)

7g Carbs
150ml
69 Cals | **5g** Prot | **3g** Fat | **2g** SatFat | **0g** Fibre

13g Carbs
284ml, half pint
131 Cals | **10g** Prot | **5g** Fat | **3g** SatFat | **0g** Fibre

27g Carbs
568ml, pint
261 Cals | **20g** Prot | **10g** Fat | **6g** SatFat | **0g** Fibre

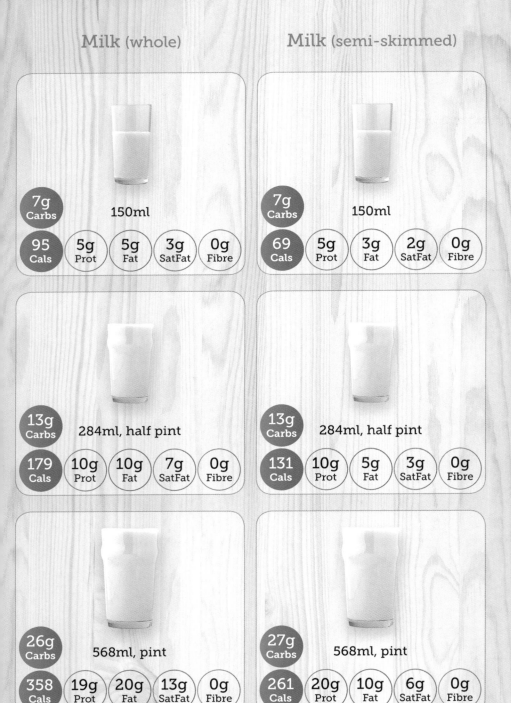

Milk (1%)

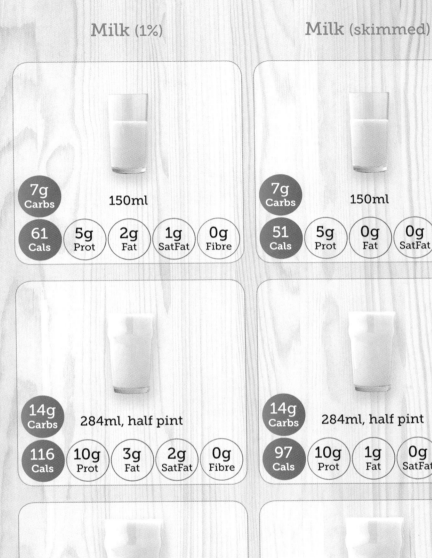

7g Carbs

150ml

61 Cals | **5g** Prot | **2g** Fat | **1g** SatFat | **0g** Fibre

14g Carbs

284ml, half pint

116 Cals | **10g** Prot | **3g** Fat | **2g** SatFat | **0g** Fibre

27g Carbs

568ml, pint

232 Cals | **20g** Prot | **6g** Fat | **3g** SatFat | **0g** Fibre

Milk (skimmed)

7g Carbs

150ml

51 Cals | **5g** Prot | **0g** Fat | **0g** SatFat | **0g** Fibre

14g Carbs

284ml, half pint

97 Cals | **10g** Prot | **1g** Fat | **0g** SatFat | **0g** Fibre

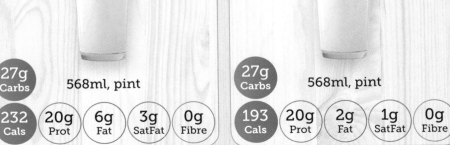

27g Carbs

568ml, pint

193 Cals | **20g** Prot | **2g** Fat | **1g** SatFat | **0g** Fibre

Soya Milk (sweetened)

4g Carbs

150ml

65 Cals | **5g** Prot | **4g** Fat | **1g** SatFat | **1g** Fibre

Soya Milk (unsweetened)

1g Carbs

150ml

39 Cals | **4g** Prot | **2g** Fat | **0g** SatFat | **1g** Fibre

Milkshake (powder & semi-skimmed milk)

33g Carbs

284ml, half pint (chocolate)

203 Cals | **9g** Prot | **4g** Fat | **3g** SatFat | **0g** Fibre

29g Carbs

284ml, half pint (strawberry)

196 Cals | **9g** Prot | **5g** Fat | **3g** SatFat | **0g** Fibre

Milk (per 100ml)

	Carbs	Cals	Prot	Fat	SatFat	Fibre
Milk (whole)	5g	63	3g	4g	2g	0g
Milk (semi-skimmed)	5g	46	4g	2g	1g	0g
Milk (1%)	5g	41	4g	1g	1g	0g
Milk (skimmed)	5g	34	4g	0g	0g	0g
Almond Milk	3g	24	1g	1g	0g	0g
Coconut Milk (drink, not tinned)	5g	22	0g	0g	0g	0g
Soya Milk (sweetened)	3g	43	3g	2g	0g	1g
Soya Milk (unsweetened)	1g	26	2g	2g	0g	0g

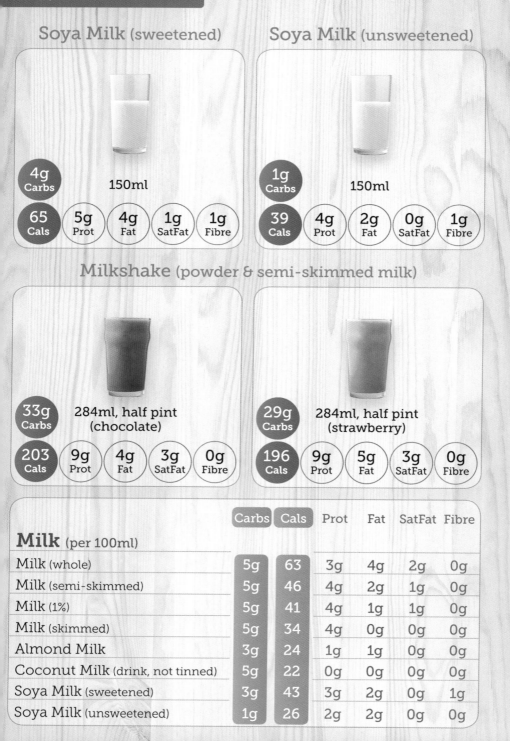

Single Cream

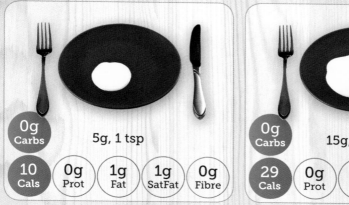

0g Carbs

5g, 1 tsp

10 Cals | **0g** Prot | **1g** Fat | **1g** SatFat | **0g** Fibre

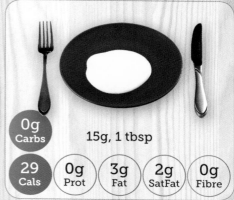

0g Carbs

15g, 1 tbsp

29 Cals | **0g** Prot | **3g** Fat | **2g** SatFat | **0g** Fibre

Double Cream

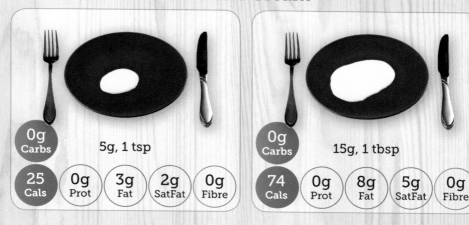

0g Carbs

5g, 1 tsp

25 Cals | **0g** Prot | **3g** Fat | **2g** SatFat | **0g** Fibre

0g Carbs

15g, 1 tbsp

74 Cals | **0g** Prot | **8g** Fat | **5g** SatFat | **0g** Fibre

Clotted Cream

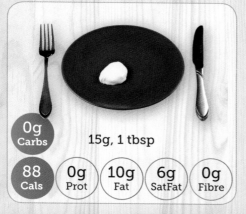

0g Carbs

15g, 1 tbsp

88 Cals | **0g** Prot | **10g** Fat | **6g** SatFat | **0g** Fibre

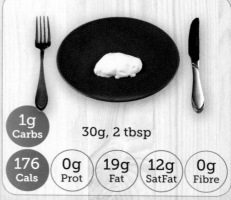

1g Carbs

30g, 2 tbsp

176 Cals | **0g** Prot | **19g** Fat | **12g** SatFat | **0g** Fibre

20cm Side Plate

Crème Fraîche

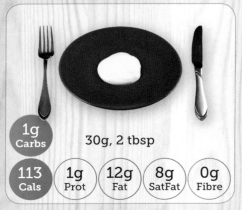

1g Carbs

30g, 2 tbsp

113 Cals | **1g** Prot | **12g** Fat | **8g** SatFat | **0g** Fibre

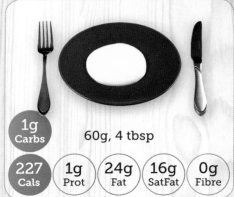

1g Carbs

60g, 4 tbsp

227 Cals | **1g** Prot | **24g** Fat | **16g** SatFat | **0g** Fibre

Soured Cream

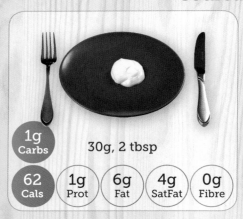

1g Carbs

30g, 2 tbsp

62 Cals | **1g** Prot | **6g** Fat | **4g** SatFat | **0g** Fibre

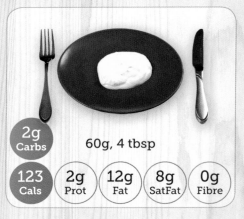

2g Carbs

60g, 4 tbsp

123 Cals | **2g** Prot | **12g** Fat | **8g** SatFat | **0g** Fibre

Whipped Cream

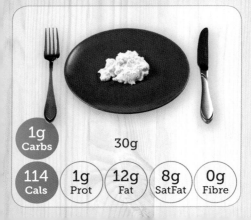

1g Carbs

30g

114 Cals | **1g** Prot | **12g** Fat | **8g** SatFat | **0g** Fibre

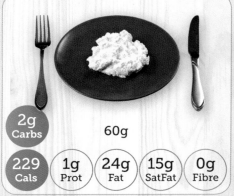

2g Carbs

60g

229 Cals | **1g** Prot | **24g** Fat | **15g** SatFat | **0g** Fibre

Almonds

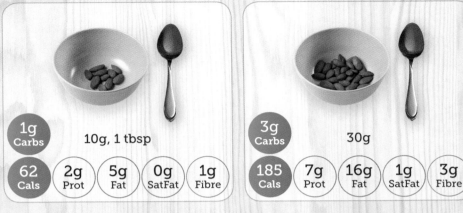

1g Carbs
10g, 1 tbsp
62 Cals | 2g Prot | 5g Fat | 0g SatFat | 1g Fibre

3g Carbs
30g
185 Cals | 7g Prot | 16g Fat | 1g SatFat | 3g Fibre

Brazil Nuts

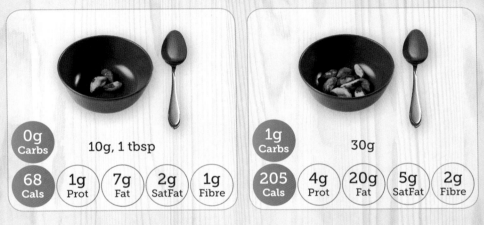

0g Carbs
10g, 1 tbsp
68 Cals | 1g Prot | 7g Fat | 2g SatFat | 1g Fibre

1g Carbs
30g
205 Cals | 4g Prot | 20g Fat | 5g SatFat | 2g Fibre

Cashews

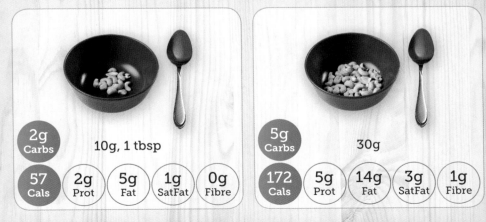

2g Carbs
10g, 1 tbsp
57 Cals | 2g Prot | 5g Fat | 1g SatFat | 0g Fibre

5g Carbs
30g
172 Cals | 5g Prot | 14g Fat | 3g SatFat | 1g Fibre

14cm Cereal Bowl

Dried Fruit & Nuts

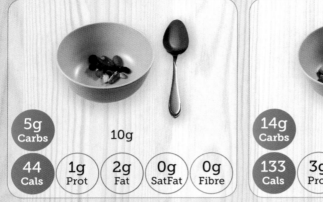

5g Carbs
10g

44 Cals | **1g** Prot | **2g** Fat | **0g** SatFat | **0g** Fibre

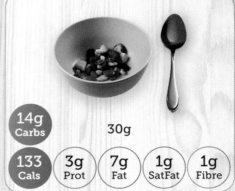

14g Carbs
30g

133 Cals | **3g** Prot | **7g** Fat | **1g** SatFat | **1g** Fibre

Hazelnuts

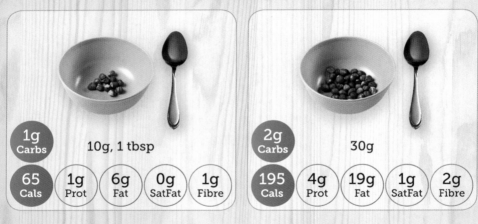

1g Carbs
10g, 1 tbsp

65 Cals | **1g** Prot | **6g** Fat | **0g** SatFat | **1g** Fibre

2g Carbs
30g

195 Cals | **4g** Prot | **19g** Fat | **1g** SatFat | **2g** Fibre

Macadamia Nuts

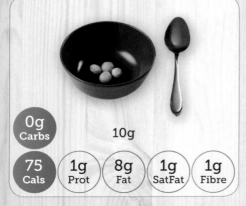

0g Carbs
10g

75 Cals | **1g** Prot | **8g** Fat | **1g** SatFat | **1g** Fibre

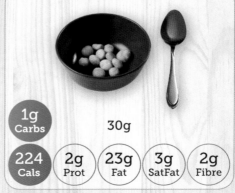

1g Carbs
30g

224 Cals | **2g** Prot | **23g** Fat | **3g** SatFat | **2g** Fibre

Peanuts (roasted)

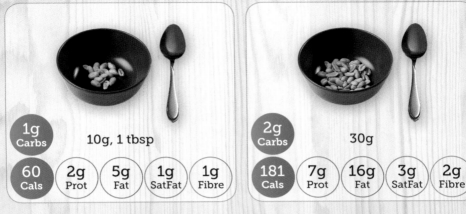

1g Carbs   10g, 1 tbsp

60 Cals | **2g** Prot | **5g** Fat | **1g** SatFat | **1g** Fibre

2g Carbs   30g

181 Cals | **7g** Prot | **16g** Fat | **3g** SatFat | **2g** Fibre

Pecans

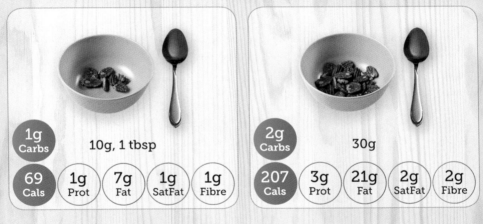

1g Carbs   10g, 1 tbsp

69 Cals | **1g** Prot | **7g** Fat | **1g** SatFat | **1g** Fibre

2g Carbs   30g

207 Cals | **3g** Prot | **21g** Fat | **2g** SatFat | **2g** Fibre

Pine Nuts

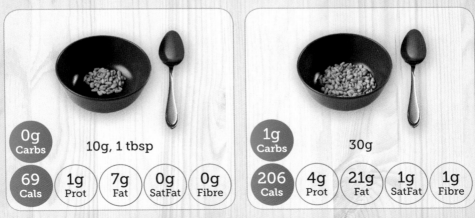

0g Carbs   10g, 1 tbsp

69 Cals | **1g** Prot | **7g** Fat | **0g** SatFat | **0g** Fibre

1g Carbs   30g

206 Cals | **4g** Prot | **21g** Fat | **1g** SatFat | **1g** Fibre

14cm Cereal Bowl

Pistachios

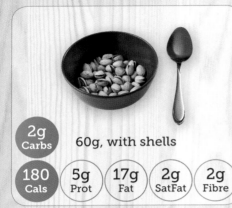

2g Carbs

60g, with shells

180 Cals | **5g** Prot | **17g** Fat | **2g** SatFat | **2g** Fibre

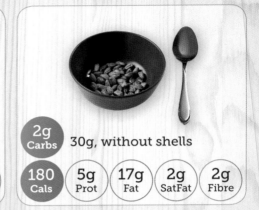

2g Carbs

30g, without shells

180 Cals | **5g** Prot | **17g** Fat | **2g** SatFat | **2g** Fibre

Soya Nuts

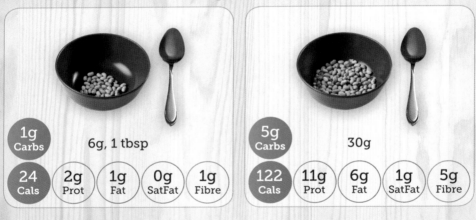

1g Carbs

6g, 1 tbsp

24 Cals | **2g** Prot | **1g** Fat | **0g** SatFat | **1g** Fibre

5g Carbs

30g

122 Cals | **11g** Prot | **6g** Fat | **1g** SatFat | **5g** Fibre

Walnuts

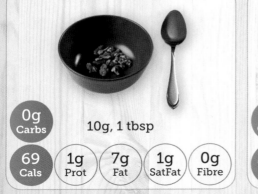

0g Carbs

10g, 1 tbsp

69 Cals | **1g** Prot | **7g** Fat | **1g** SatFat | **0g** Fibre

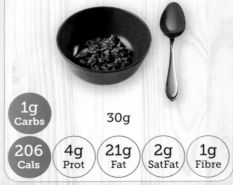

1g Carbs

30g

206 Cals | **4g** Prot | **21g** Fat | **2g** SatFat | **1g** Fibre

Linseeds / Flaxseeds

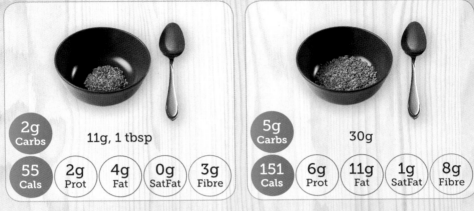

2g Carbs
11g, 1 tbsp
55 Cals | **2g** Prot | **4g** Fat | **0g** SatFat | **3g** Fibre

5g Carbs
30g
151 Cals | **6g** Prot | **11g** Fat | **1g** SatFat | **8g** Fibre

Pumpkin Seeds

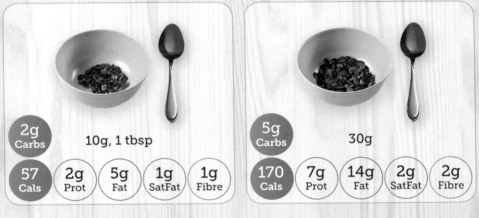

2g Carbs
10g, 1 tbsp
57 Cals | **2g** Prot | **5g** Fat | **1g** SatFat | **1g** Fibre

5g Carbs
30g
170 Cals | **7g** Prot | **14g** Fat | **2g** SatFat | **2g** Fibre

Sunflower Seeds

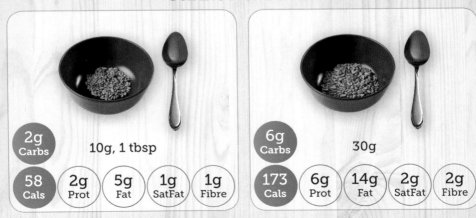

2g Carbs
10g, 1 tbsp
58 Cals | **2g** Prot | **5g** Fat | **1g** SatFat | **1g** Fibre

6g Carbs
30g
173 Cals | **6g** Prot | **14g** Fat | **2g** SatFat | **2g** Fibre

Macaroni

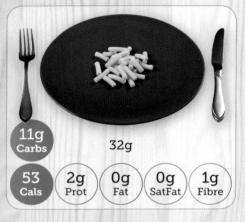

11g Carbs — 32g

53 Cals | **2g** Prot | **0g** Fat | **0g** SatFat | **1g** Fibre

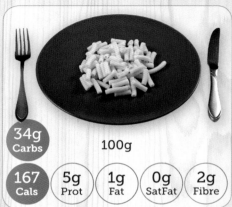

34g Carbs — 100g

167 Cals | **5g** Prot | **1g** Fat | **0g** SatFat | **2g** Fibre

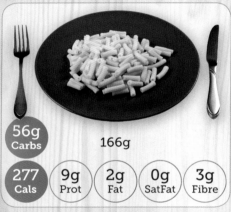

56g Carbs — 166g

277 Cals | **9g** Prot | **2g** Fat | **0g** SatFat | **3g** Fibre

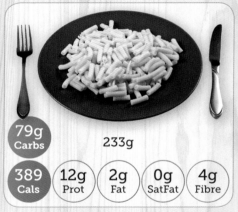

79g Carbs — 233g

389 Cals | **12g** Prot | **2g** Fat | **0g** SatFat | **4g** Fibre

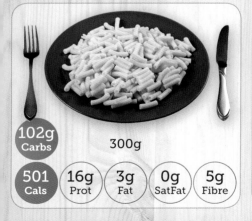

102g Carbs — 300g

501 Cals | **16g** Prot | **3g** Fat | **0g** SatFat | **5g** Fibre

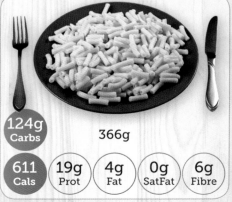

124g Carbs — 366g

611 Cals | **19g** Prot | **4g** Fat | **0g** SatFat | **6g** Fibre

Pasta Bows

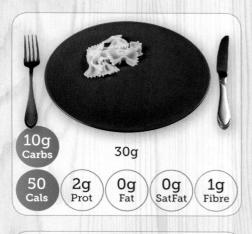

10g Carbs — 30g

50 Cals	2g Prot	0g Fat	0g SatFat	1g Fibre

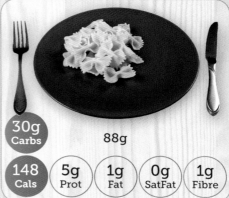

30g Carbs — 88g

148 Cals	5g Prot	1g Fat	0g SatFat	1g Fibre

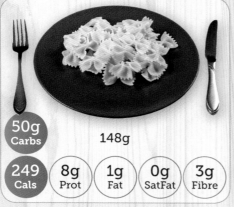

50g Carbs — 148g

249 Cals	8g Prot	1g Fat	0g SatFat	3g Fibre

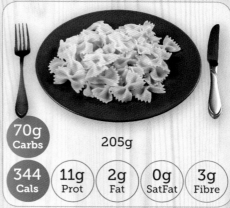

70g Carbs — 205g

344 Cals	11g Prot	2g Fat	0g SatFat	3g Fibre

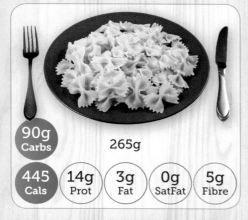

90g Carbs — 265g

445 Cals	14g Prot	3g Fat	0g SatFat	5g Fibre

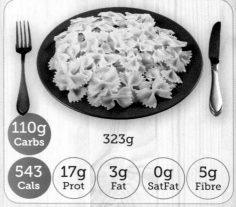

110g Carbs — 323g

543 Cals	17g Prot	3g Fat	0g SatFat	5g Fibre

26cm Dinner Plate

Pasta Shells

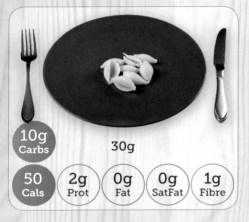

10g Carbs
30g

50 Cals | **2g** Prot | **0g** Fat | **0g** SatFat | **1g** Fibre

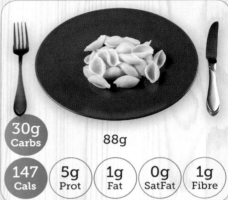

30g Carbs
88g

147 Cals | **5g** Prot | **1g** Fat | **0g** SatFat | **1g** Fibre

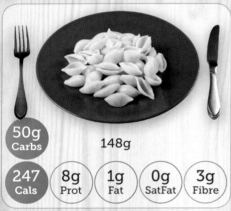

50g Carbs
148g

247 Cals | **8g** Prot | **1g** Fat | **0g** SatFat | **3g** Fibre

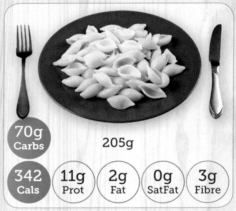

70g Carbs
205g

342 Cals | **11g** Prot | **2g** Fat | **0g** SatFat | **3g** Fibre

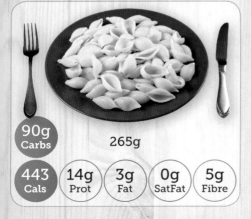

90g Carbs
265g

443 Cals | **14g** Prot | **3g** Fat | **0g** SatFat | **5g** Fibre

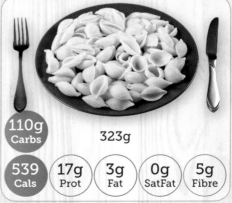

110g Carbs
323g

539 Cals | **17g** Prot | **3g** Fat | **0g** SatFat | **5g** Fibre

Pasta Twists

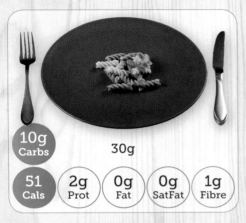

10g Carbs
30g

51 Cals | **2g** Prot | **0g** Fat | **0g** SatFat | **1g** Fibre

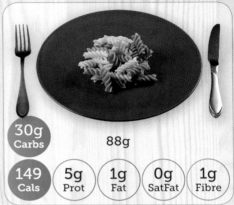

30g Carbs
88g

149 Cals | **5g** Prot | **1g** Fat | **0g** SatFat | **1g** Fibre

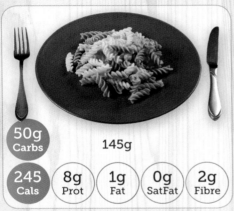

50g Carbs
145g

245 Cals | **8g** Prot | **1g** Fat | **0g** SatFat | **2g** Fibre

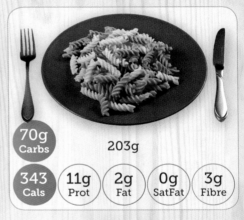

70g Carbs
203g

343 Cals | **11g** Prot | **2g** Fat | **0g** SatFat | **3g** Fibre

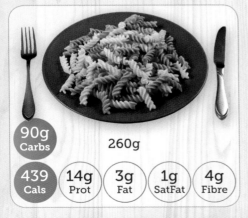

90g Carbs
260g

439 Cals | **14g** Prot | **3g** Fat | **1g** SatFat | **4g** Fibre

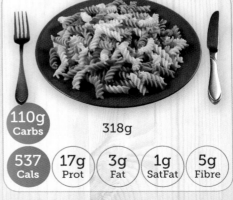

110g Carbs
318g

537 Cals | **17g** Prot | **3g** Fat | **1g** SatFat | **5g** Fibre

26cm Dinner Plate

Penne

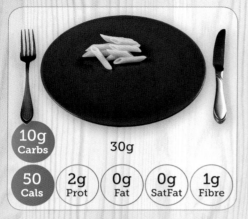

10g Carbs

30g

50 Cals | **2g** Prot | **0g** Fat | **0g** SatFat | **1g** Fibre

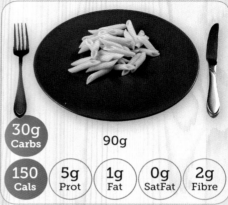

30g Carbs

90g

150 Cals | **5g** Prot | **1g** Fat | **0g** SatFat | **2g** Fibre

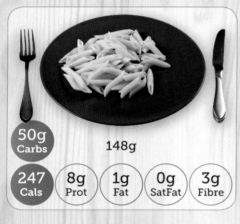

50g Carbs

148g

247 Cals | **8g** Prot | **1g** Fat | **0g** SatFat | **3g** Fibre

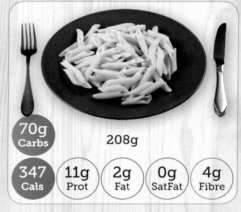

70g Carbs

208g

347 Cals | **11g** Prot | **2g** Fat | **0g** SatFat | **4g** Fibre

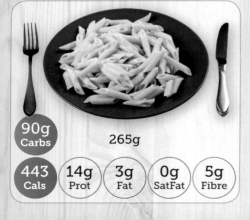

90g Carbs

265g

443 Cals | **14g** Prot | **3g** Fat | **0g** SatFat | **5g** Fibre

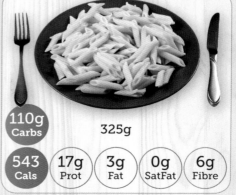

110g Carbs

325g

543 Cals | **17g** Prot | **3g** Fat | **0g** SatFat | **6g** Fibre

Ravioli (fresh, meat-filled)

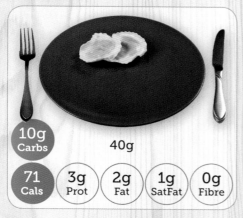

10g Carbs — 40g

71 Cals | **3g** Prot | **2g** Fat | **1g** SatFat | **0g** Fibre

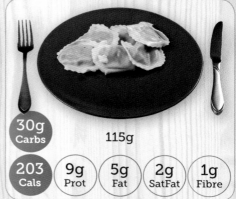

30g Carbs — 115g

203 Cals | **9g** Prot | **5g** Fat | **2g** SatFat | **1g** Fibre

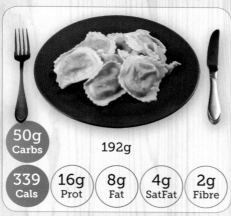

50g Carbs — 192g

339 Cals | **16g** Prot | **8g** Fat | **4g** SatFat | **2g** Fibre

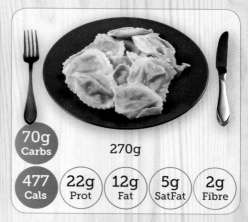

70g Carbs — 270g

477 Cals | **22g** Prot | **12g** Fat | **5g** SatFat | **2g** Fibre

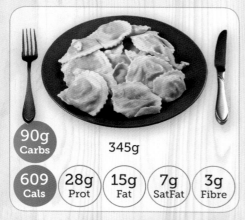

90g Carbs — 345g

609 Cals | **28g** Prot | **15g** Fat | **7g** SatFat | **3g** Fibre

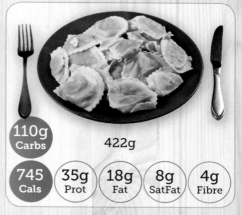

110g Carbs — 422g

745 Cals | **35g** Prot | **18g** Fat | **8g** SatFat | **4g** Fibre

26cm Dinner Plate

Spaghetti (white)

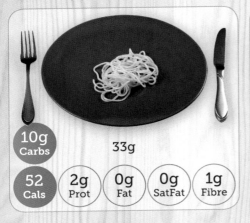

10g Carbs — 33g

52 Cals | **2g Prot** | **0g Fat** | **0g SatFat** | **1g Fibre**

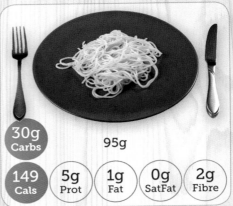

30g Carbs — 95g

149 Cals | **5g Prot** | **1g Fat** | **0g SatFat** | **2g Fibre**

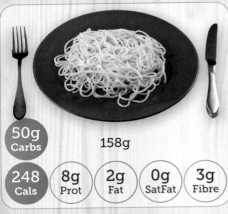

50g Carbs — 158g

248 Cals | **8g Prot** | **2g Fat** | **0g SatFat** | **3g Fibre**

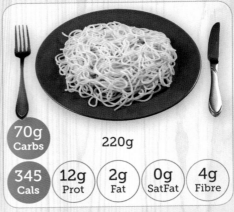

70g Carbs — 220g

345 Cals | **12g Prot** | **2g Fat** | **0g SatFat** | **4g Fibre**

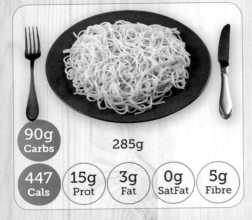

90g Carbs — 285g

447 Cals | **15g Prot** | **3g Fat** | **0g SatFat** | **5g Fibre**

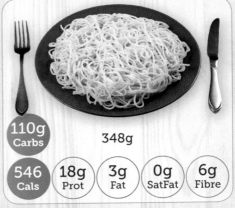

110g Carbs — 348g

546 Cals | **18g Prot** | **3g Fat** | **0g SatFat** | **6g Fibre**

Spaghetti (whole wheat)

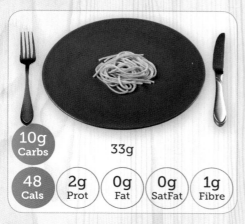

10g Carbs

33g

48 Cals | **2g Prot** | **0g Fat** | **0g SatFat** | **1g Fibre**

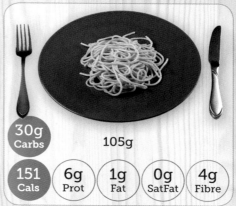

30g Carbs

105g

151 Cals | **6g Prot** | **1g Fat** | **0g SatFat** | **4g Fibre**

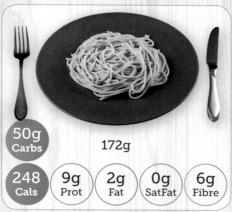

50g Carbs

172g

248 Cals | **9g Prot** | **2g Fat** | **0g SatFat** | **6g Fibre**

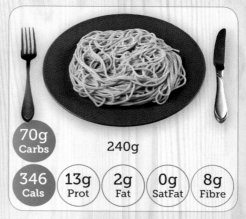

70g Carbs

240g

346 Cals | **13g Prot** | **2g Fat** | **0g SatFat** | **8g Fibre**

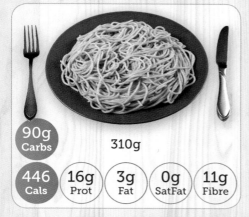

90g Carbs

310g

446 Cals | **16g Prot** | **3g Fat** | **0g SatFat** | **11g Fibre**

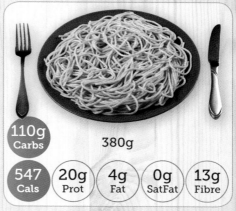

110g Carbs

380g

547 Cals | **20g Prot** | **4g Fat** | **0g SatFat** | **13g Fibre**

Tagliatelle

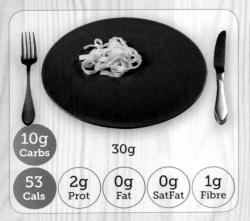

10g Carbs — 30g

53 Cals	2g Prot	0g Fat	0g SatFat	1g Fibre

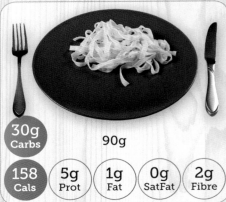

30g Carbs — 90g

158 Cals	5g Prot	1g Fat	0g SatFat	2g Fibre

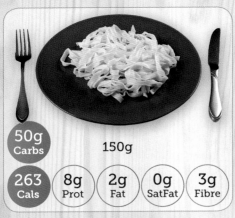

50g Carbs — 150g

263 Cals	8g Prot	2g Fat	0g SatFat	3g Fibre

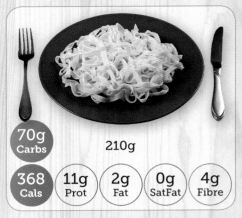

70g Carbs — 210g

368 Cals	11g Prot	2g Fat	0g SatFat	4g Fibre

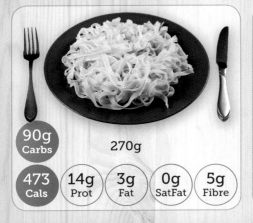

90g Carbs — 270g

473 Cals	14g Prot	3g Fat	0g SatFat	5g Fibre

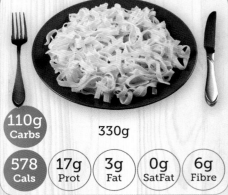

110g Carbs — 330g

578 Cals	17g Prot	3g Fat	0g SatFat	6g Fibre

Tortellini (fresh, cheese-filled)

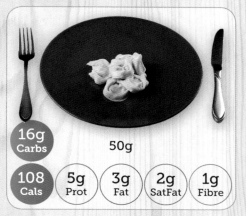

16g Carbs

50g

108 Cals | **5g** Prot | **3g** Fat | **2g** SatFat | **1g** Fibre

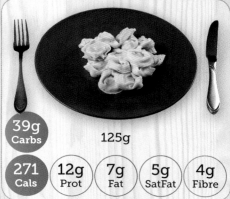

39g Carbs

125g

271 Cals | **12g** Prot | **7g** Fat | **5g** SatFat | **4g** Fibre

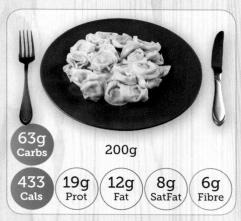

63g Carbs

200g

433 Cals | **19g** Prot | **12g** Fat | **8g** SatFat | **6g** Fibre

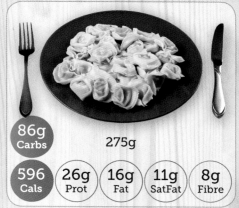

86g Carbs

275g

596 Cals | **26g** Prot | **16g** Fat | **11g** SatFat | **8g** Fibre

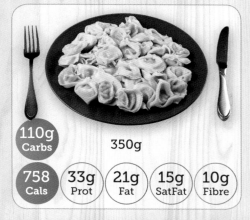

110g Carbs

350g

758 Cals | **33g** Prot | **21g** Fat | **15g** SatFat | **10g** Fibre

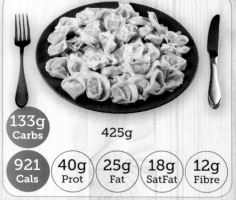

133g Carbs

425g

921 Cals | **40g** Prot | **25g** Fat | **18g** SatFat | **12g** Fibre

26cm Dinner Plate

Vermicelli

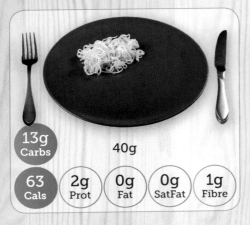

13g Carbs — 40g

63 Cals | **2g** Prot | **0g** Fat | **0g** SatFat | **1g** Fibre

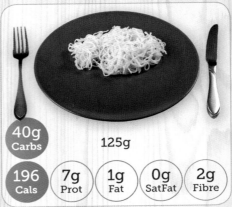

40g Carbs — 125g

196 Cals | **7g** Prot | **1g** Fat | **0g** SatFat | **2g** Fibre

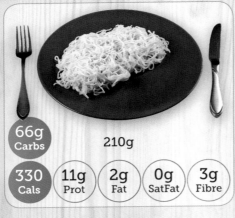

66g Carbs — 210g

330 Cals | **11g** Prot | **2g** Fat | **0g** SatFat | **3g** Fibre

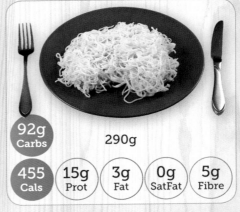

92g Carbs — 290g

455 Cals | **15g** Prot | **3g** Fat | **0g** SatFat | **5g** Fibre

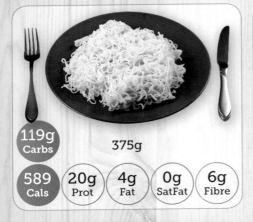

119g Carbs — 375g

589 Cals | **20g** Prot | **4g** Fat | **0g** SatFat | **6g** Fibre

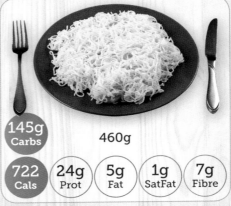

145g Carbs — 460g

722 Cals | **24g** Prot | **5g** Fat | **1g** SatFat | **7g** Fibre

Noodles (egg)

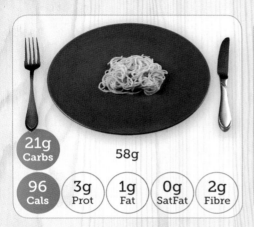

21g Carbs

58g

96 Cals | **3g** Prot | **1g** Fat | **0g** SatFat | **2g** Fibre

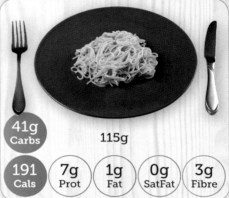

41g Carbs

115g

191 Cals | **7g** Prot | **1g** Fat | **0g** SatFat | **3g** Fibre

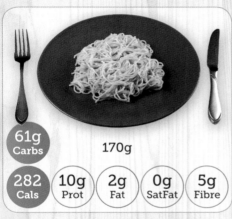

61g Carbs

170g

282 Cals | **10g** Prot | **2g** Fat | **0g** SatFat | **5g** Fibre

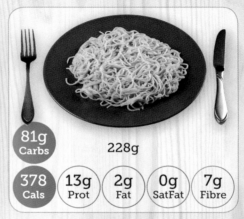

81g Carbs

228g

378 Cals | **13g** Prot | **2g** Fat | **0g** SatFat | **7g** Fibre

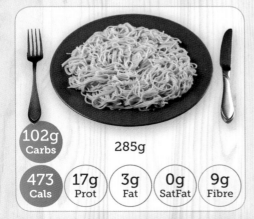

102g Carbs

285g

473 Cals | **17g** Prot | **3g** Fat | **0g** SatFat | **9g** Fibre

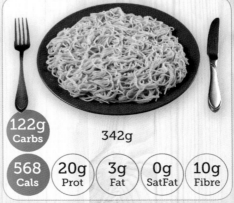

122g Carbs

342g

568 Cals | **20g** Prot | **3g** Fat | **0g** SatFat | **10g** Fibre

Noodles (rice)

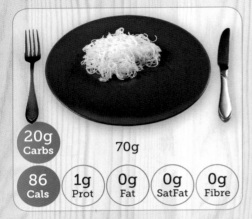

20g Carbs — 70g

86 Cals | **1g** Prot | **0g** Fat | **0g** SatFat | **0g** Fibre

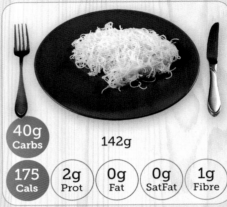

40g Carbs — 142g

175 Cals | **2g** Prot | **0g** Fat | **0g** SatFat | **1g** Fibre

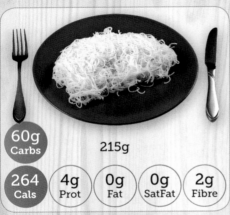

60g Carbs — 215g

264 Cals | **4g** Prot | **0g** Fat | **0g** SatFat | **2g** Fibre

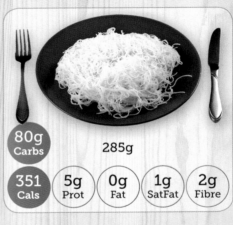

80g Carbs — 285g

351 Cals | **5g** Prot | **0g** Fat | **1g** SatFat | **2g** Fibre

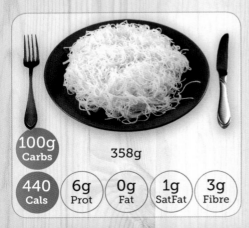

100g Carbs — 358g

440 Cals | **6g** Prot | **0g** Fat | **1g** SatFat | **3g** Fibre

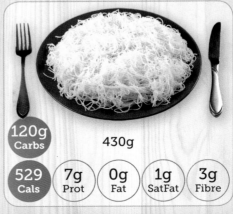

120g Carbs — 430g

529 Cals | **7g** Prot | **0g** Fat | **1g** SatFat | **3g** Fibre

Pasta Shapes (tinned)

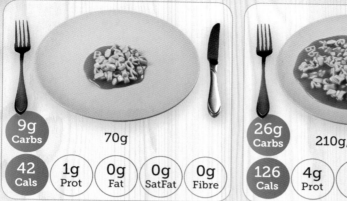

9g Carbs

70g

42 Cals | 1g Prot | 0g Fat | 0g SatFat | 0g Fibre

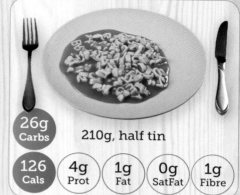

26g Carbs

210g, half tin

126 Cals | 4g Prot | 1g Fat | 0g SatFat | 1g Fibre

Ravioli (tinned)

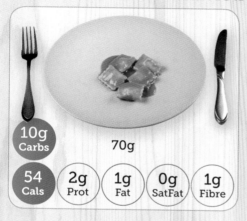

10g Carbs

70g

54 Cals | 2g Prot | 1g Fat | 0g SatFat | 1g Fibre

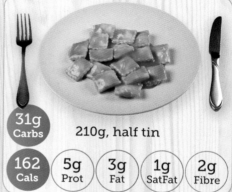

31g Carbs

210g, half tin

162 Cals | 5g Prot | 3g Fat | 1g SatFat | 2g Fibre

Spaghetti (tinned)

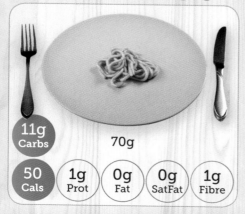

11g Carbs

70g

50 Cals | 1g Prot | 0g Fat | 0g SatFat | 1g Fibre

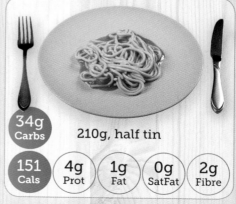

34g Carbs

210g, half tin

151 Cals | 4g Prot | 1g Fat | 0g SatFat | 2g Fibre

Spaghetti Hoops (tinned)

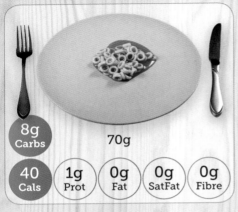

8g Carbs — 70g

40 Cals | **1g** Prot | **0g** Fat | **0g** SatFat | **0g** Fibre

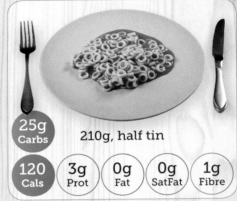

25g Carbs — 210g, half tin

120 Cals | **3g** Prot | **0g** Fat | **0g** SatFat | **1g** Fibre

Pasta & Noodles UNCOOKED (per 100g weight)

	Carbs	Cals	Prot	Fat	SatFat	Fibre
Egg Noodles	73g	338	12g	2g	0g	5g
Gluten Free Pasta	78g	355	7g	1g	0g	2g
Pasta	76g	343	11g	2g	0g	5g
Pasta (fresh)	57g	282	11g	3g	1g	3g
Rice Noodles	79g	353	7g	1g	1g	2g
Spaghetti	73g	360	13g	1g	0g	3g
Vermicelli Pasta	76g	343	11g	2g	0g	5g
Whole Wheat Spaghetti	68g	329	13g	3g	0g	12g

Pasta & Noodles COOKED (per 100g weight)

	Carbs	Cals	Prot	Fat	SatFat	Fibre
Egg Noodles	36g	166	6g	1g	0g	3g
Gluten Free Pasta	35g	156	3g	0g	0g	1g
Pasta	34g	167	5g	1g	0g	2g
Pasta (fresh)	32g	159	7g	2g	0g	3g
Rice Noodles	28g	123	2g	0g	0g	1g
Spaghetti	32g	157	5g	1g	0g	2g
Vermicelli Pasta	34g	167	5g	1g	0g	2g
Whole Wheat Spaghetti	29g	144	5g	1g	0g	4g

Chips (deep fried)

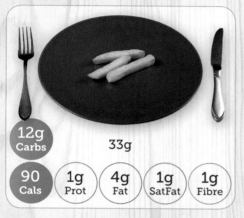

12g Carbs — 33g

90 Cals | 1g Prot | 4g Fat | 1g SatFat | 1g Fibre

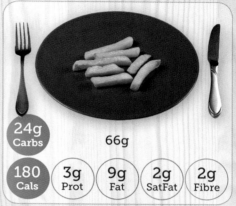

24g Carbs — 66g

180 Cals | 3g Prot | 9g Fat | 2g SatFat | 2g Fibre

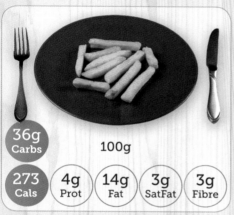

36g Carbs — 100g

273 Cals | 4g Prot | 14g Fat | 3g SatFat | 3g Fibre

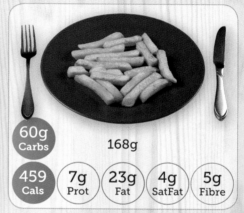

60g Carbs — 168g

459 Cals | 7g Prot | 23g Fat | 4g SatFat | 5g Fibre

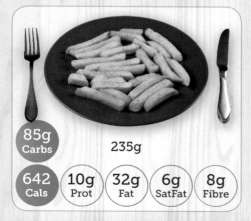

85g Carbs — 235g

642 Cals | 10g Prot | 32g Fat | 6g SatFat | 8g Fibre

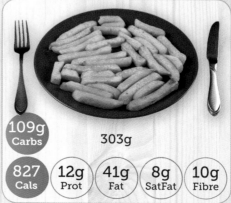

109g Carbs — 303g

827 Cals | 12g Prot | 41g Fat | 8g SatFat | 10g Fibre

Chips (oven)

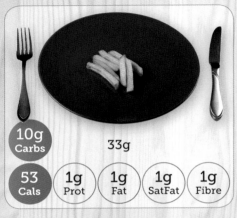

10g Carbs — 33g

53 Cals | **1g** Prot | **1g** Fat | **1g** SatFat | **1g** Fibre

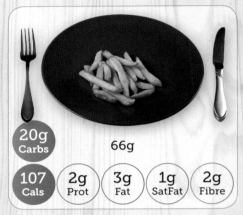

20g Carbs — 66g

107 Cals | **2g** Prot | **3g** Fat | **1g** SatFat | **2g** Fibre

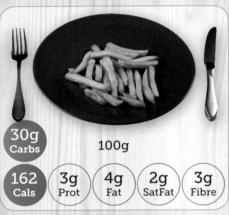

30g Carbs — 100g

162 Cals | **3g** Prot | **4g** Fat | **2g** SatFat | **3g** Fibre

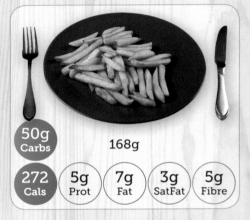

50g Carbs — 168g

272 Cals | **5g** Prot | **7g** Fat | **3g** SatFat | **5g** Fibre

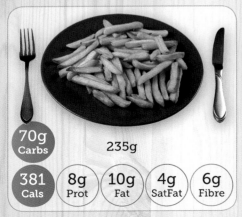

70g Carbs — 235g

381 Cals | **8g** Prot | **10g** Fat | **4g** SatFat | **6g** Fibre

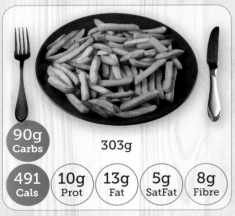

90g Carbs — 303g

491 Cals | **10g** Prot | **13g** Fat | **5g** SatFat | **8g** Fibre

Dauphinoise Potatoes

Gnocchi

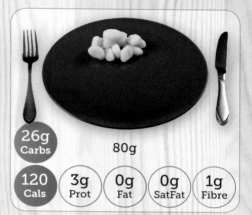

Dauphinoise Potatoes

11g Carbs	72g			
181 Cals	2g Prot	15g Fat	9g SatFat	1g Fibre

Gnocchi

26g Carbs	80g			
120 Cals	3g Prot	0g Fat	0g SatFat	1g Fibre

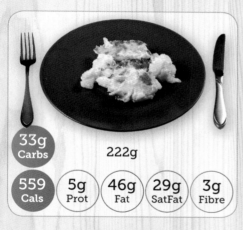

33g Carbs	222g			
559 Cals	5g Prot	46g Fat	29g SatFat	3g Fibre

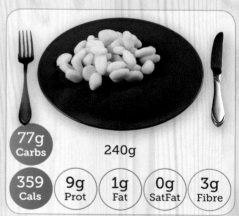

77g Carbs	240g			
359 Cals	9g Prot	1g Fat	0g SatFat	3g Fibre

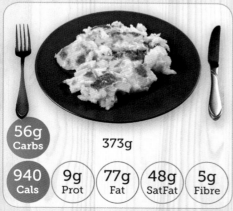

56g Carbs	373g			
940 Cals	9g Prot	77g Fat	48g SatFat	5g Fibre

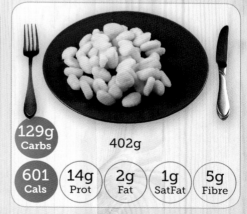

129g Carbs	402g			
601 Cals	14g Prot	2g Fat	1g SatFat	5g Fibre

Jacket Potato (baked)   New Potatoes (boiled)

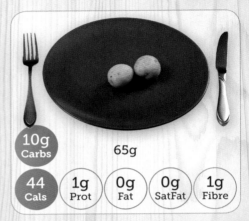

20g Carbs   95g
87 Cals   **2g** Prot   **0g** Fat   **0g** SatFat   **2g** Fibre

10g Carbs   65g
44 Cals   **1g** Prot   **0g** Fat   **0g** SatFat   **1g** Fibre

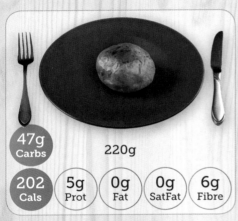
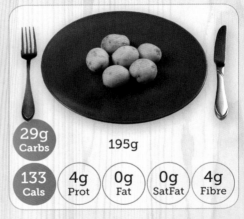

47g Carbs   220g
202 Cals   **5g** Prot   **0g** Fat   **0g** SatFat   **6g** Fibre

29g Carbs   195g
133 Cals   **4g** Prot   **0g** Fat   **0g** SatFat   **4g** Fibre

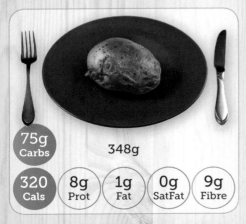
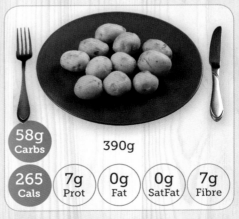

75g Carbs   348g
320 Cals   **8g** Prot   **1g** Fat   **0g** SatFat   **9g** Fibre

58g Carbs   390g
265 Cals   **7g** Prot   **0g** Fat   **0g** SatFat   **7g** Fibre

Mashed Potato
(with butter)

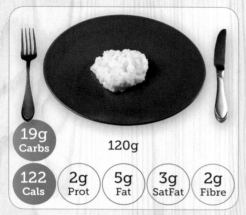

19g Carbs

120g

122 Cals | **2g** Prot | **5g** Fat | **3g** SatFat | **2g** Fibre

Mashed Potato
(with semi-skimmed milk)

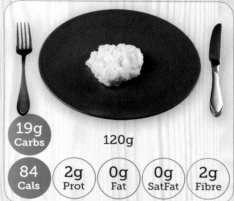

19g Carbs

120g

84 Cals | **2g** Prot | **0g** Fat | **0g** SatFat | **2g** Fibre

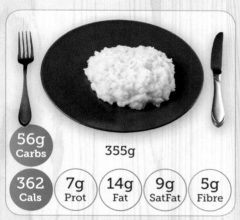

56g Carbs

355g

362 Cals | **7g** Prot | **14g** Fat | **9g** SatFat | **5g** Fibre

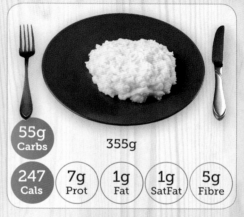

55g Carbs

355g

247 Cals | **7g** Prot | **1g** Fat | **1g** SatFat | **5g** Fibre

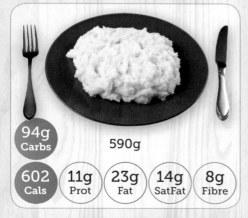

94g Carbs

590g

602 Cals | **11g** Prot | **23g** Fat | **14g** SatFat | **8g** Fibre

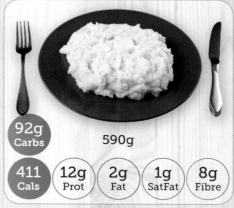

92g Carbs

590g

411 Cals | **12g** Prot | **2g** Fat | **1g** SatFat | **8g** Fibre

Potato Slices (baked)

Roast Potatoes (in oil)

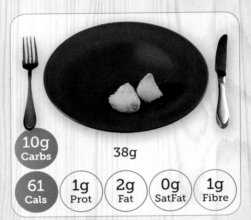

8g Carbs — 28g

52 Cals | 1g Prot | 2g Fat | 0g SatFat | 1g Fibre

10g Carbs — 38g

61 Cals | 1g Prot | 2g Fat | 0g SatFat | 1g Fibre

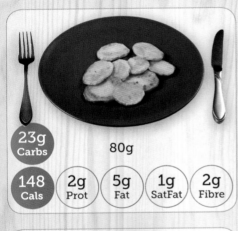
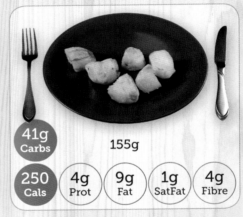

23g Carbs — 80g

148 Cals | 2g Prot | 5g Fat | 1g SatFat | 2g Fibre

41g Carbs — 155g

250 Cals | 4g Prot | 9g Fat | 1g SatFat | 4g Fibre

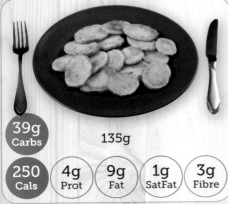
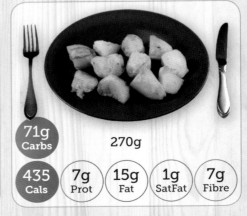

39g Carbs — 135g

250 Cals | 4g Prot | 9g Fat | 1g SatFat | 3g Fibre

71g Carbs — 270g

435 Cals | 7g Prot | 15g Fat | 1g SatFat | 7g Fibre

Sweet Potatoes (baked)

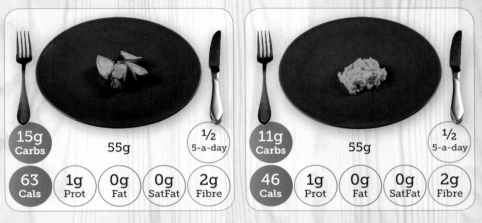

15g Carbs · 55g · ½ 5-a-day
63 Cals · 1g Prot · 0g Fat · 0g SatFat · 2g Fibre

45g Carbs · 160g · 1 5-a-day
184 Cals · 3g Prot · 1g Fat · 0g SatFat · 7g Fibre

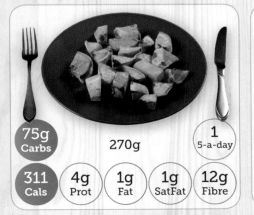

75g Carbs · 270g · 1 5-a-day
311 Cals · 4g Prot · 1g Fat · 1g SatFat · 12g Fibre

Mashed Sweet Potato

11g Carbs · 55g · ½ 5-a-day
46 Cals · 1g Prot · 0g Fat · 0g SatFat · 2g Fibre

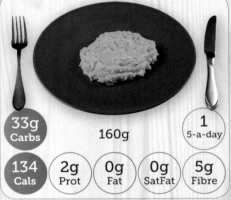

33g Carbs · 160g · 1 5-a-day
134 Cals · 2g Prot · 0g Fat · 0g SatFat · 5g Fibre

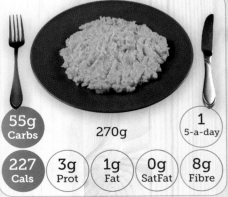

55g Carbs · 270g · 1 5-a-day
227 Cals · 3g Prot · 1g Fat · 0g SatFat · 8g Fibre

Potato Salad
(with mayonnaise)

Wedges (baked)

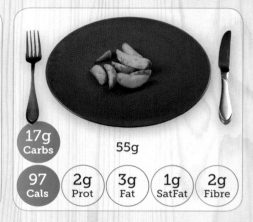

Potato Salad — 60g

7g Carbs | 95 Cals | 1g Prot | 7g Fat | 1g SatFat | 1g Fibre

Wedges — 55g

17g Carbs | 97 Cals | 2g Prot | 3g Fat | 1g SatFat | 2g Fibre

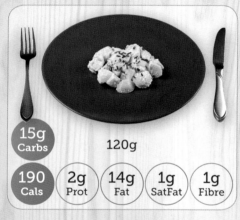

Potato Salad — 120g

15g Carbs | 190 Cals | 2g Prot | 14g Fat | 1g SatFat | 1g Fibre

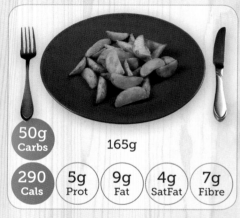

Wedges — 165g

50g Carbs | 290 Cals | 5g Prot | 9g Fat | 4g SatFat | 7g Fibre

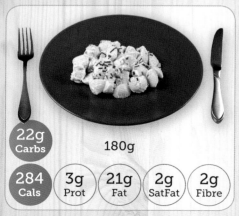

Potato Salad — 180g

22g Carbs | 284 Cals | 3g Prot | 21g Fat | 2g SatFat | 2g Fibre

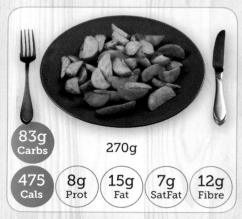

Wedges — 270g

83g Carbs | 475 Cals | 8g Prot | 15g Fat | 7g SatFat | 12g Fibre

26cm Dinner Plate

Hash Brown (baked)

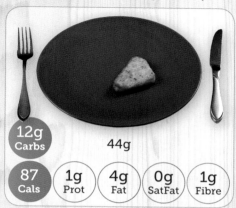

12g Carbs — 44g — 87 Cals — 1g Prot — 4g Fat — 0g SatFat — 1g Fibre

Potato Croquette (fried)

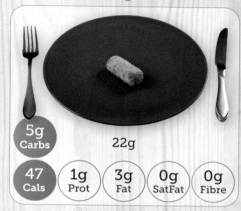

5g Carbs — 22g — 47 Cals — 1g Prot — 3g Fat — 0g SatFat — 0g Fibre

Potato Rosti (grilled)

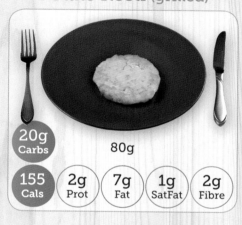

20g Carbs — 80g — 155 Cals — 2g Prot — 7g Fat — 1g SatFat — 2g Fibre

Potato Waffle (baked)

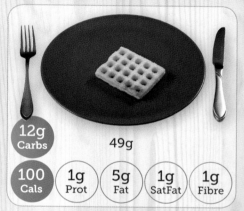

12g Carbs — 49g — 100 Cals — 1g Prot — 5g Fat — 1g SatFat — 1g Fibre

Potato Smiles (baked)

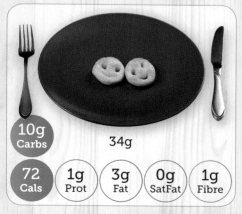

10g Carbs — 34g — 72 Cals — 1g Prot — 3g Fat — 0g SatFat — 1g Fibre

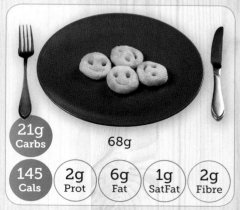

21g Carbs — 68g — 145 Cals — 2g Prot — 6g Fat — 1g SatFat — 2g Fibre

Cassava Chips (baked)

Eba / Gari

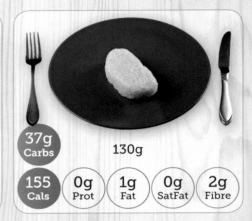

Cassava Chips (baked)

23g Carbs — 45g
122 Cals | 0g Prot | 3g Fat | 1g SatFat | 1g Fibre

Eba / Gari

37g Carbs — 130g
155 Cals | 0g Prot | 1g Fat | 0g SatFat | 2g Fibre

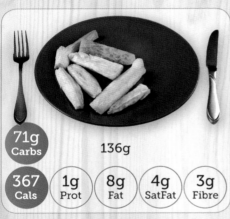

71g Carbs — 136g
367 Cals | 1g Prot | 8g Fat | 4g SatFat | 3g Fibre

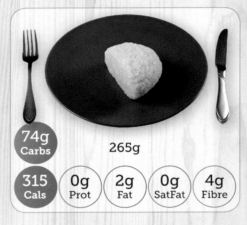

74g Carbs — 265g
315 Cals | 0g Prot | 2g Fat | 0g SatFat | 4g Fibre

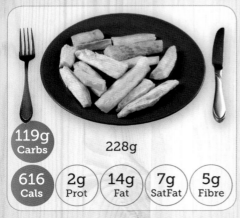

119g Carbs — 228g
616 Cals | 2g Prot | 14g Fat | 7g SatFat | 5g Fibre

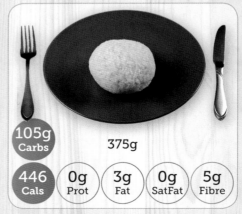

105g Carbs — 375g
446 Cals | 0g Prot | 3g Fat | 0g SatFat | 5g Fibre

Fufu (plantain)

Yam (boiled)

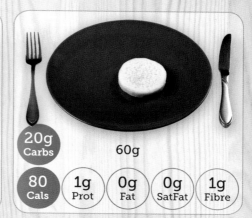

Fufu (plantain) — 130g
- 40g Carbs
- 174 Cals
- 2g Prot
- 0g Fat
- 0g SatFat
- 1g Fibre

Yam (boiled) — 60g
- 20g Carbs
- 80 Cals
- 1g Prot
- 0g Fat
- 0g SatFat
- 1g Fibre

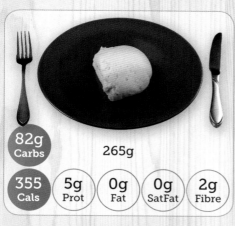
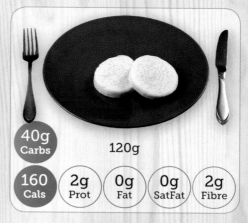

Fufu (plantain) — 265g
- 82g Carbs
- 355 Cals
- 5g Prot
- 0g Fat
- 0g SatFat
- 2g Fibre

Yam (boiled) — 120g
- 40g Carbs
- 160 Cals
- 2g Prot
- 0g Fat
- 0g SatFat
- 2g Fibre

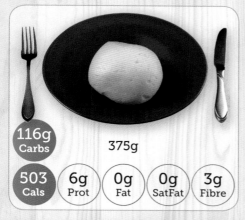
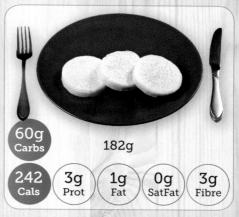

Fufu (plantain) — 375g
- 116g Carbs
- 503 Cals
- 6g Prot
- 0g Fat
- 0g SatFat
- 3g Fibre

Yam (boiled) — 182g
- 60g Carbs
- 242 Cals
- 3g Prot
- 1g Fat
- 0g SatFat
- 3g Fibre

	Carbs	Cals	Prot	Fat	SatFat	Fibre
Potatoes & Tubers RAW (per 100g weight)						
Cassava	37g	142	1g	0g	0g	2g
New Potatoes	16g	68	2g	0g	0g	2g
Potato	20g	82	2g	0g	0g	2g
Sweet Potato	21g	87	1g	0g	0g	3g
Yam	28g	114	2g	0g	0g	2g
Potatoes & Tubers COOKED (per 100g weight)						
Chips (deep fried)	33g	214	4g	8g	4g	3g
Chips (oven)	35g	189	3g	5g	1g	4g
Dauphinoise Potatoes	15g	252	2g	21g	13g	1g
Gnocchi	32g	150	4g	1g	0g	1g
Hash Brown (baked)	28g	197	2g	9g	1g	2g
Jacket Potato (baked)	23g	97	3g	0g	0g	3g
Mashed Potato (with butter)	16g	102	2g	4g	2g	1g
Mashed Potato (with semi-skim milk)	16g	70	2g	0g	0g	1g
New Potatoes (boiled)	15g	68	2g	0g	0g	2g
Potato Croquette (fried)	22g	214	4g	13g	2g	2g
Potato Rosti (grilled)	25g	194	3g	9g	1g	2g
Potato Salad (with mayonnaise)	13g	239	2g	21g	2g	1g
Potato Slices (baked)	29g	185	3g	7g	1g	2g
Potato Smiles (baked)	31g	213	3g	9g	1g	2g
Potato Waffle (baked)	24g	204	2g	11g	1g	2g
Roast Potatoes (in oil)	26g	161	3g	6g	1g	3g
Sweet Potato (baked)	28g	115	2g	0g	0g	4g
Sweet Potato Mash	21g	84	1g	0g	0g	3g
Wedges (baked)	31g	176	3g	6g	3g	4g
Cassava Chips (baked)	91g	353	2g	0g	0g	5g
Eba / Gari	28g	119	0g	1g	0g	1g
Fufu (plantain)	31g	134	2g	0g	0g	1g
Yam (boiled)	33g	133	2g	0g	0g	2g

Basmati Rice

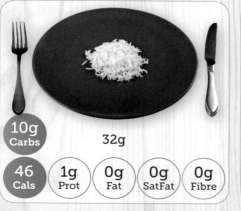

10g Carbs

32g

46 Cals | **1g** Prot | **0g** Fat | **0g** SatFat | **0g** Fibre

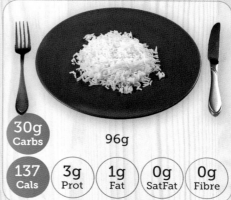

30g Carbs

96g

137 Cals | **3g** Prot | **1g** Fat | **0g** SatFat | **0g** Fibre

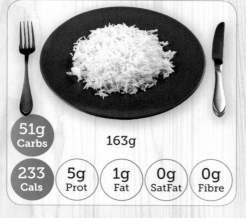

51g Carbs

163g

233 Cals | **5g** Prot | **1g** Fat | **0g** SatFat | **0g** Fibre

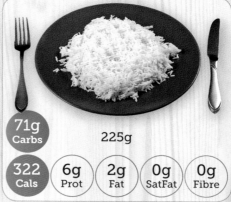

71g Carbs

225g

322 Cals | **6g** Prot | **2g** Fat | **0g** SatFat | **0g** Fibre

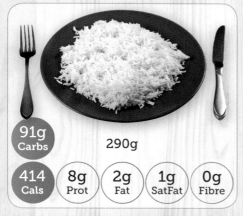

91g Carbs

290g

414 Cals | **8g** Prot | **2g** Fat | **1g** SatFat | **0g** Fibre

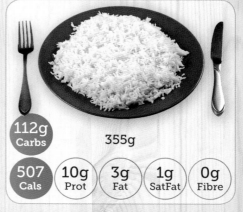

112g Carbs

355g

507 Cals | **10g** Prot | **3g** Fat | **1g** SatFat | **0g** Fibre

26cm Dinner Plate

Brown Rice (wholegrain)

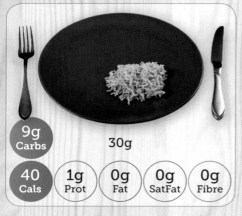

9g Carbs

30g

40 Cals | **1g** Prot | **0g** Fat | **0g** SatFat | **0g** Fibre

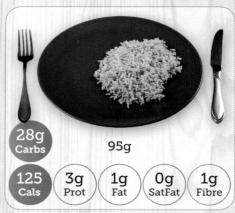

28g Carbs

95g

125 Cals | **3g** Prot | **1g** Fat | **0g** SatFat | **1g** Fibre

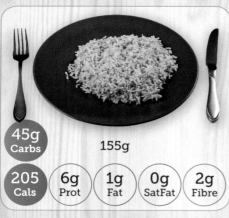

45g Carbs

155g

205 Cals | **6g** Prot | **1g** Fat | **0g** SatFat | **2g** Fibre

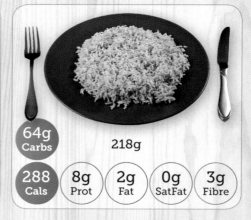

64g Carbs

218g

288 Cals | **8g** Prot | **2g** Fat | **0g** SatFat | **3g** Fibre

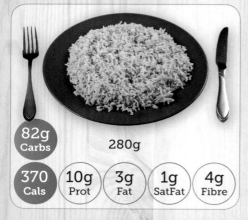

82g Carbs

280g

370 Cals | **10g** Prot | **3g** Fat | **1g** SatFat | **4g** Fibre

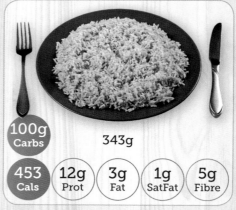

100g Carbs

343g

453 Cals | **12g** Prot | **3g** Fat | **1g** SatFat | **5g** Fibre

White Rice (long grain)

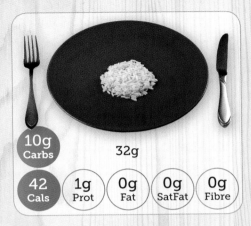

10g Carbs
32g
42 Cals | 1g Prot | 0g Fat | 0g SatFat | 0g Fibre

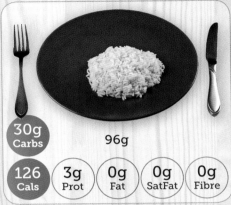

30g Carbs
96g
126 Cals | 3g Prot | 0g Fat | 0g SatFat | 0g Fibre

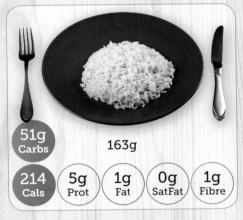

51g Carbs
163g
214 Cals | 5g Prot | 1g Fat | 0g SatFat | 1g Fibre

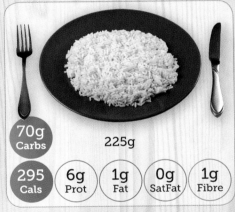

70g Carbs
225g
295 Cals | 6g Prot | 1g Fat | 0g SatFat | 1g Fibre

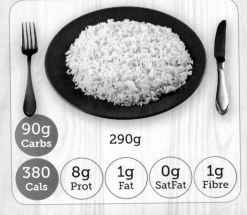

90g Carbs
290g
380 Cals | 8g Prot | 1g Fat | 0g SatFat | 1g Fibre

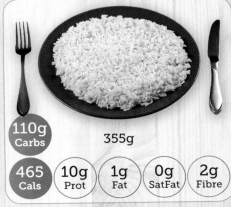

110g Carbs
355g
465 Cals | 10g Prot | 1g Fat | 0g SatFat | 2g Fibre

26cm Dinner Plate

Egg Fried Rice

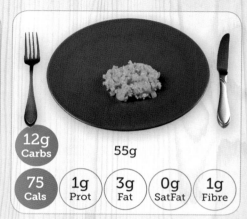

18g Carbs   55g

102 Cals | **2g** Prot | **3g** Fat | **0g** SatFat | **1g** Fibre

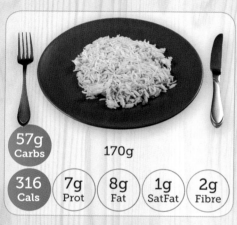

57g Carbs   170g

316 Cals | **7g** Prot | **8g** Fat | **1g** SatFat | **2g** Fibre

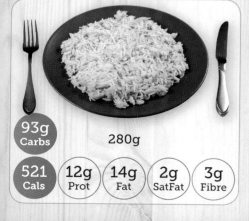

93g Carbs   280g

521 Cals | **12g** Prot | **14g** Fat | **2g** SatFat | **3g** Fibre

Jollof Rice

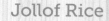

12g Carbs   55g

75 Cals | **1g** Prot | **3g** Fat | **0g** SatFat | **1g** Fibre

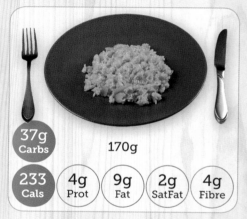

37g Carbs   170g

233 Cals | **4g** Prot | **9g** Fat | **2g** SatFat | **4g** Fibre

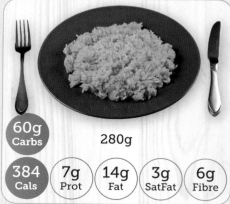

60g Carbs   280g

384 Cals | **7g** Prot | **14g** Fat | **3g** SatFat | **6g** Fibre

Mexican Rice

Pilau Rice

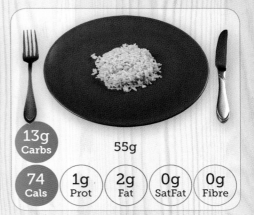

Mexican Rice

17g Carbs · 55g · 86 Cals · 2g Prot · 1g Fat · 0g SatFat · 0g Fibre

Pilau Rice

13g Carbs · 55g · 74 Cals · 1g Prot · 2g Fat · 0g SatFat · 0g Fibre

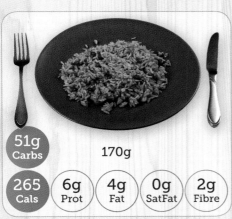
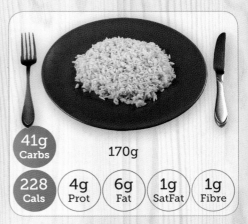

Mexican Rice

51g Carbs · 170g · 265 Cals · 6g Prot · 4g Fat · 0g SatFat · 2g Fibre

Pilau Rice

41g Carbs · 170g · 228 Cals · 4g Prot · 6g Fat · 1g SatFat · 1g Fibre

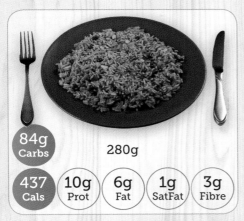
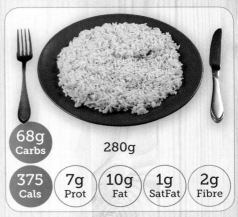

Mexican Rice

84g Carbs · 280g · 437 Cals · 10g Prot · 6g Fat · 1g SatFat · 3g Fibre

Pilau Rice

68g Carbs · 280g · 375 Cals · 7g Prot · 10g Fat · 1g SatFat · 2g Fibre

Rice & Peas

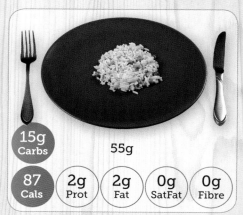

14g Carbs

55g

85 Cals | 3g Prot | 2g Fat | 2g SatFat | 1g Fibre

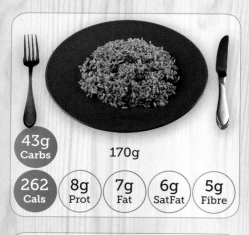

43g Carbs

170g

262 Cals | 8g Prot | 7g Fat | 6g SatFat | 5g Fibre

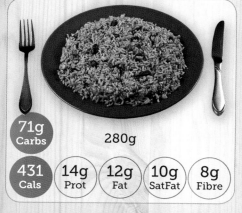

71g Carbs

280g

431 Cals | 14g Prot | 12g Fat | 10g SatFat | 8g Fibre

Special Fried Rice

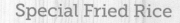

15g Carbs

55g

87 Cals | 2g Prot | 2g Fat | 0g SatFat | 0g Fibre

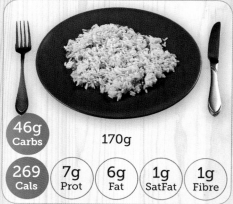

46g Carbs

170g

269 Cals | 7g Prot | 6g Fat | 1g SatFat | 1g Fibre

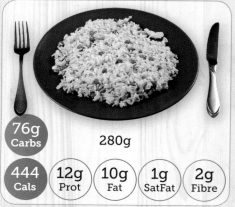

76g Carbs

280g

444 Cals | 12g Prot | 10g Fat | 1g SatFat | 2g Fibre

26cm Dinner Plate

Sticky White Rice

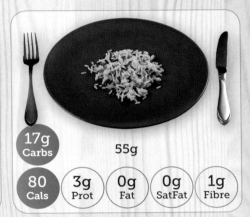

19g Carbs

70g

100 Cals | **2g** Prot | **2g** Fat | **0g** SatFat | **0g** Fibre

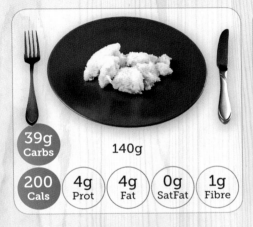

39g Carbs

140g

200 Cals | **4g** Prot | **4g** Fat | **0g** SatFat | **1g** Fibre

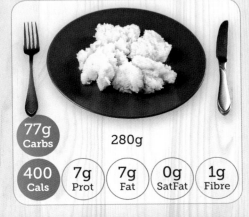

77g Carbs

280g

400 Cals | **7g** Prot | **7g** Fat | **0g** SatFat | **1g** Fibre

Wild Rice

17g Carbs

55g

80 Cals | **3g** Prot | **0g** Fat | **0g** SatFat | **1g** Fibre

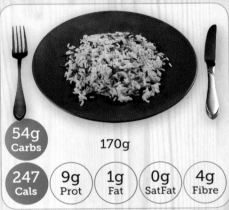

54g Carbs

170g

247 Cals | **9g** Prot | **1g** Fat | **0g** SatFat | **4g** Fibre

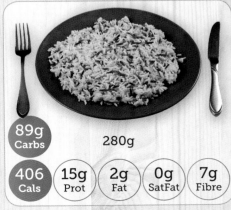

89g Carbs

280g

406 Cals | **15g** Prot | **2g** Fat | **0g** SatFat | **7g** Fibre

26cm Dinner Plate

Bulgur Wheat

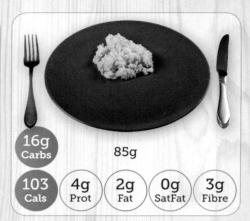

16g Carbs — 100g

89 Cals | **3g** Prot | **1g** Fat | **0g** SatFat | **3g** Fibre

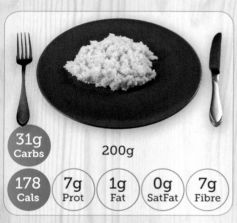

31g Carbs — 200g

178 Cals | **7g** Prot | **1g** Fat | **0g** SatFat | **7g** Fibre

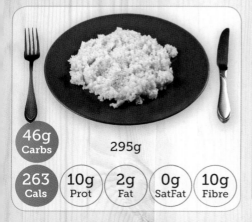

46g Carbs — 295g

263 Cals | **10g** Prot | **2g** Fat | **0g** SatFat | **10g** Fibre

Quinoa

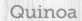

16g Carbs — 85g

103 Cals | **4g** Prot | **2g** Fat | **0g** SatFat | **3g** Fibre

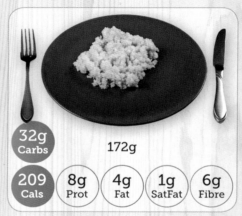

32g Carbs — 172g

209 Cals | **8g** Prot | **4g** Fat | **1g** SatFat | **6g** Fibre

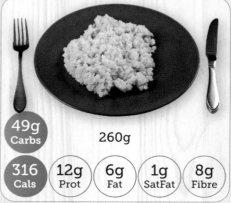

49g Carbs — 260g

316 Cals | **12g** Prot | **6g** Fat | **1g** SatFat | **8g** Fibre

Couscous

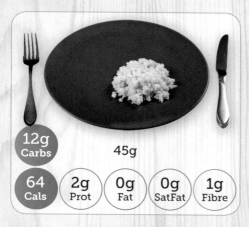

12g Carbs

45g

64 Cals | **2g** Prot | **0g** Fat | **0g** SatFat | **1g** Fibre

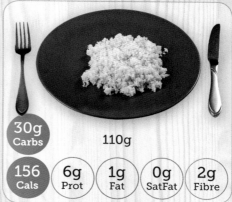

30g Carbs

110g

156 Cals | **6g** Prot | **1g** Fat | **0g** SatFat | **2g** Fibre

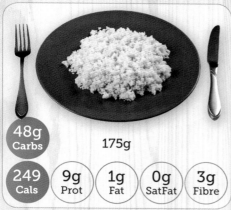

48g Carbs

175g

249 Cals | **9g** Prot | **1g** Fat | **0g** SatFat | **3g** Fibre

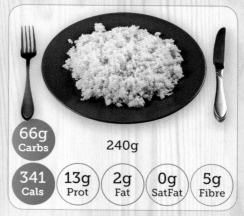

66g Carbs

240g

341 Cals | **13g** Prot | **2g** Fat | **0g** SatFat | **5g** Fibre

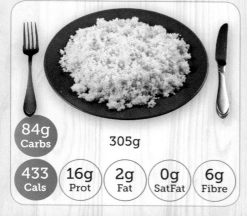

84g Carbs

305g

433 Cals | **16g** Prot | **2g** Fat | **0g** SatFat | **6g** Fibre

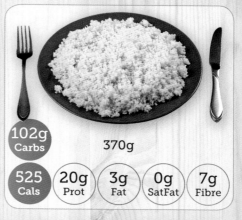

102g Carbs

370g

525 Cals | **20g** Prot | **3g** Fat | **0g** SatFat | **7g** Fibre

Polenta

Polenta (sliced)

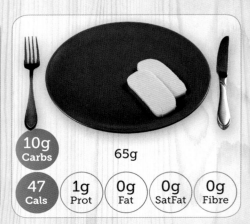

10g Carbs — 65g
47 Cals | **1g** Prot | **0g** Fat | **0g** SatFat | **0g** Fibre

10g Carbs — 65g
47 Cals | **1g** Prot | **0g** Fat | **0g** SatFat | **0g** Fibre

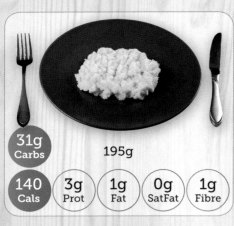
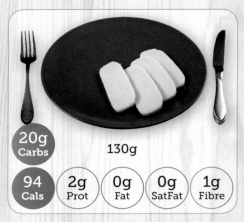

31g Carbs — 195g
140 Cals | **3g** Prot | **1g** Fat | **0g** SatFat | **1g** Fibre

20g Carbs — 130g
94 Cals | **2g** Prot | **0g** Fat | **0g** SatFat | **1g** Fibre

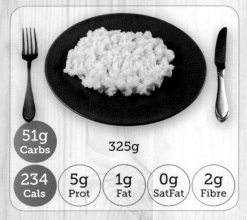
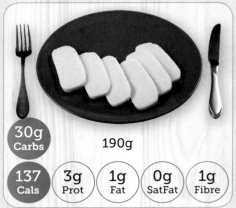

51g Carbs — 325g
234 Cals | **5g** Prot | **1g** Fat | **0g** SatFat | **2g** Fibre

30g Carbs — 190g
137 Cals | **3g** Prot | **1g** Fat | **0g** SatFat | **1g** Fibre

	Carbs	Cals	Prot	Fat	SatFat	Fibre
Rice & Grains UNCOOKED (per 100g weight)						
Basmati Rice	84g	351	8g	1g	0g	1g
Brown Rice (wholegrain)	77g	333	8g	2g	0g	3g
Easy Cook Rice (long grain)	82g	347	7g	1g	0g	2g
White Rice (long grain)	85g	355	7g	1g	0g	1g
Wild Rice	76g	343	12g	1g	0g	4g
Barley (wholegrain)	84g	360	8g	2g	0g	8g
Buckwheat	85g	364	8g	2g	1g	3g
Bulgur Wheat	78g	352	11g	2g	0g	7g
Couscous	79g	364	12g	2g	0g	4g
Pearl Barley	84g	360	8g	2g	0g	4g
Pearled Spelt	68g	314	12g	2g	1g	6g
Quinoa	56g	309	14g	5g	1g	7g
Rice & Grains COOKED (per 100g weight)						
Basmati Rice	32g	143	3g	1g	0g	0g
Brown Rice (wholegrain)	29g	132	4g	1g	0g	2g
Egg Fried Rice	33g	186	4g	5g	1g	1g
Jollof Rice	22g	137	2g	5g	1g	2g
Mexican Rice	30g	156	4g	2g	0g	1g
Pilau Rice	24g	134	3g	4g	0g	1g
Rice & Peas	25g	154	5g	4g	4g	3g
Special Fried Rice	27g	158	4g	3g	1g	1g
Sticky White Rice	28g	143	3g	3g	0g	0g
White Rice (long grain)	31g	131	3g	0g	0g	1g
Wild Rice	32g	145	5g	1g	0g	3g
Bulgur Wheat	16g	89	3g	1g	0g	3g
Couscous	28g	142	5g	1g	0g	2g
Pearl Barley	28g	120	3g	1g	0g	4g
Polenta	16g	72	2g	0g	0g	1g
Quinoa	19g	122	5g	2g	1g	3g

26cm Dinner Plate

BLT

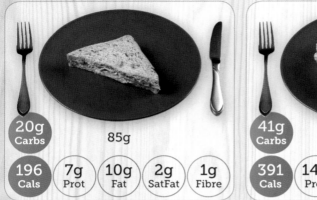

20g Carbs — 85g

196 Cals | **7g** Prot | **10g** Fat | **2g** SatFat | **1g** Fibre

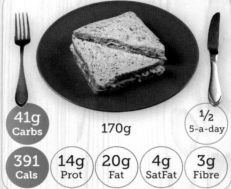

41g Carbs — 170g — ½ 5-a-day

391 Cals | **14g** Prot | **20g** Fat | **4g** SatFat | **3g** Fibre

Cheese & Pickle

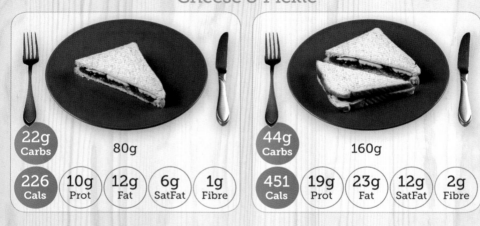

22g Carbs — 80g

226 Cals | **10g** Prot | **12g** Fat | **6g** SatFat | **1g** Fibre

44g Carbs — 160g

451 Cals | **19g** Prot | **23g** Fat | **12g** SatFat | **2g** Fibre

Chicken Salad

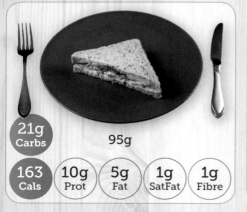

21g Carbs — 95g

163 Cals | **10g** Prot | **5g** Fat | **1g** SatFat | **1g** Fibre

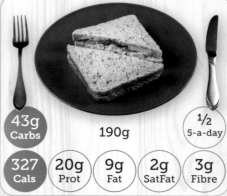

43g Carbs — 190g — ½ 5-a-day

327 Cals | **20g** Prot | **9g** Fat | **2g** SatFat | **3g** Fibre

Coronation Chicken

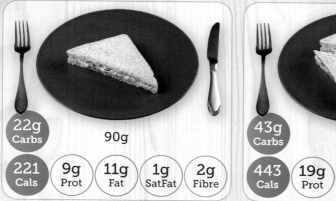

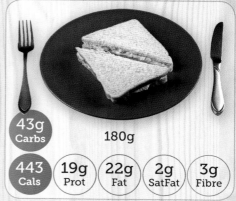

22g Carbs				
90g				
221 Cals	9g Prot	11g Fat	1g SatFat	2g Fibre

43g Carbs				
180g				
443 Cals	19g Prot	22g Fat	2g SatFat	3g Fibre

Egg Mayo

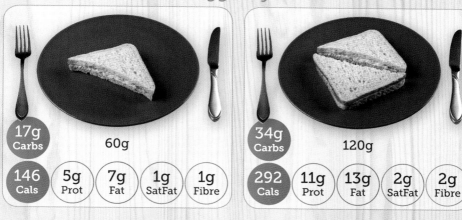

17g Carbs				
60g				
146 Cals	5g Prot	7g Fat	1g SatFat	1g Fibre

34g Carbs				
120g				
292 Cals	11g Prot	13g Fat	2g SatFat	2g Fibre

Grilled Cheese

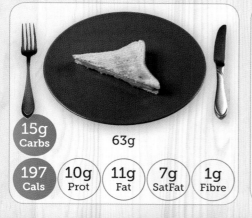

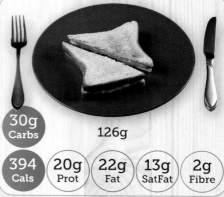

15g Carbs				
63g				
197 Cals	10g Prot	11g Fat	7g SatFat	1g Fibre

30g Carbs				
126g				
394 Cals	20g Prot	22g Fat	13g SatFat	2g Fibre

26cm Dinner Plate

Ham Salad

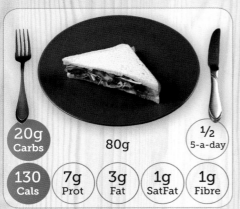

20g Carbs
80g
½ 5-a-day

130 Cals | **7g** Prot | **3g** Fat | **1g** SatFat | **1g** Fibre

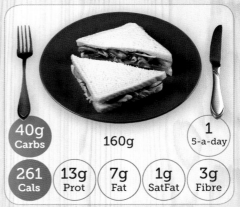

40g Carbs
160g
1 5-a-day

261 Cals | **13g** Prot | **7g** Fat | **1g** SatFat | **3g** Fibre

Prawn Mayo

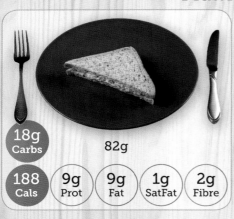

18g Carbs
82g

188 Cals | **9g** Prot | **9g** Fat | **1g** SatFat | **2g** Fibre

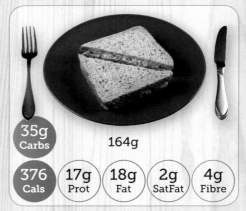

35g Carbs
164g

376 Cals | **17g** Prot | **18g** Fat | **2g** SatFat | **4g** Fibre

Tuna Mayo & Sweetcorn

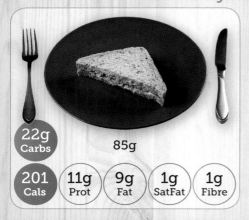

22g Carbs
85g

201 Cals | **11g** Prot | **9g** Fat | **1g** SatFat | **1g** Fibre

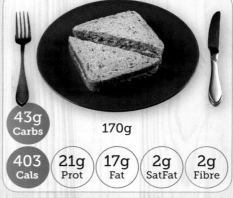

43g Carbs
170g

403 Cals | **21g** Prot | **17g** Fat | **2g** SatFat | **2g** Fibre

Bombay Mix

Crisps

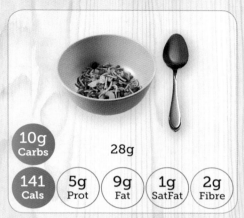

10g Carbs

28g

141 Cals | **5g** Prot | **9g** Fat | **1g** SatFat | **2g** Fibre

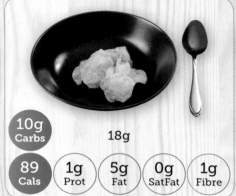

10g Carbs

18g

89 Cals | **1g** Prot | **5g** Fat | **0g** SatFat | **1g** Fibre

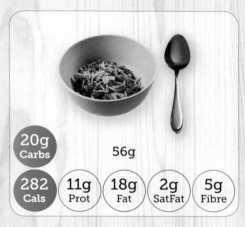

20g Carbs

56g

282 Cals | **11g** Prot | **18g** Fat | **2g** SatFat | **5g** Fibre

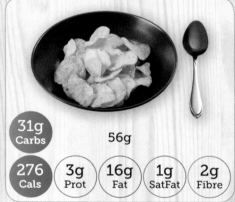

31g Carbs

56g

276 Cals | **3g** Prot | **16g** Fat | **1g** SatFat | **2g** Fibre

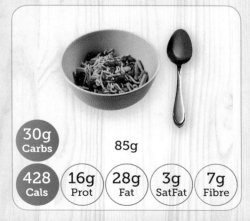

30g Carbs

85g

428 Cals | **16g** Prot | **28g** Fat | **3g** SatFat | **7g** Fibre

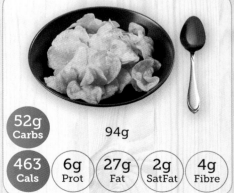

52g Carbs

94g

463 Cals | **6g** Prot | **27g** Fat | **2g** SatFat | **4g** Fibre

Popcorn (salted)   ## Popcorn (sweet)

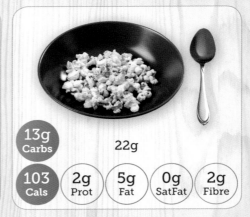

6g Carbs	10g			
47 Cals	**1g** Prot	**2g** Fat	**0g** SatFat	**1g** Fibre

13g Carbs	22g			
103 Cals	**2g** Prot	**5g** Fat	**0g** SatFat	**2g** Fibre

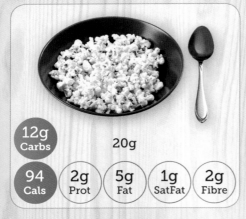

12g Carbs	20g			
94 Cals	**2g** Prot	**5g** Fat	**1g** SatFat	**2g** Fibre

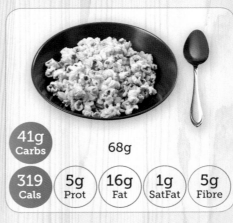

41g Carbs	68g			
319 Cals	**5g** Prot	**16g** Fat	**1g** SatFat	**5g** Fibre

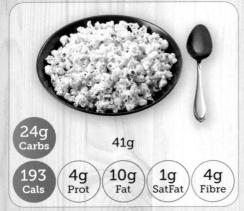

24g Carbs	41g			
193 Cals	**4g** Prot	**10g** Fat	**1g** SatFat	**4g** Fibre

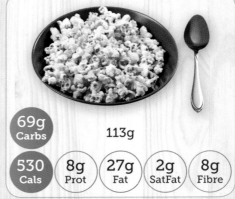

69g Carbs	113g			
530 Cals	**8g** Prot	**27g** Fat	**2g** SatFat	**8g** Fibre

Pretzels

Tortilla Chips

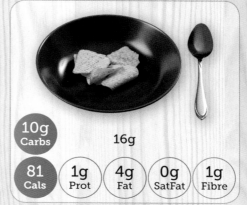

Pretzels

10g Carbs	13g

50 Cals	1g Prot	0g Fat	0g SatFat	0g Fibre

Tortilla Chips

10g Carbs	16g

81 Cals	1g Prot	4g Fat	0g SatFat	1g Fibre

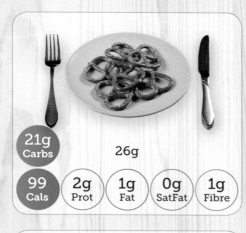
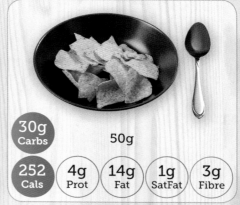

21g Carbs	26g

99 Cals	2g Prot	1g Fat	0g SatFat	1g Fibre

30g Carbs	50g

252 Cals	4g Prot	14g Fat	1g SatFat	3g Fibre

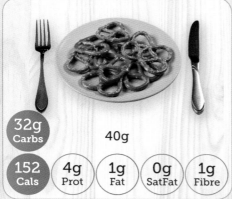
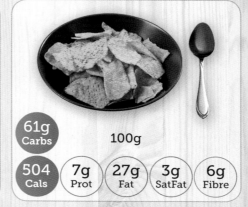

32g Carbs	40g

152 Cals	4g Prot	1g Fat	0g SatFat	1g Fibre

61g Carbs	100g

504 Cals	7g Prot	27g Fat	3g SatFat	6g Fibre

20cm Side Plate

Fudge

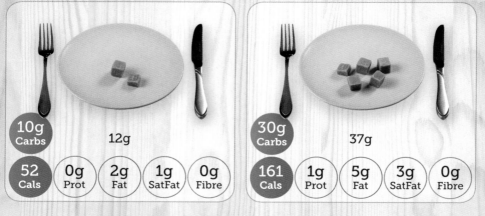

10g Carbs — 12g
52 Cals | **0g** Prot | **2g** Fat | **1g** SatFat | **0g** Fibre

30g Carbs — 37g
161 Cals | **1g** Prot | **5g** Fat | **3g** SatFat | **0g** Fibre

Marshmallows (small)

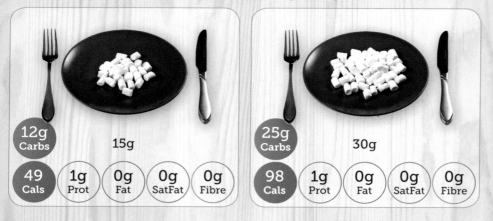

12g Carbs — 15g
49 Cals | **1g** Prot | **0g** Fat | **0g** SatFat | **0g** Fibre

25g Carbs — 30g
98 Cals | **1g** Prot | **0g** Fat | **0g** SatFat | **0g** Fibre

Marshmallows (large)

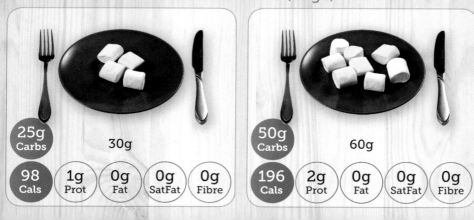

25g Carbs — 30g
98 Cals | **1g** Prot | **0g** Fat | **0g** SatFat | **0g** Fibre

50g Carbs — 60g
196 Cals | **2g** Prot | **0g** Fat | **0g** SatFat | **0g** Fibre

Chocolate (milk)

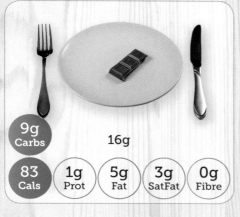

9g Carbs

16g

83 Cals | 1g Prot | 5g Fat | 3g SatFat | 0g Fibre

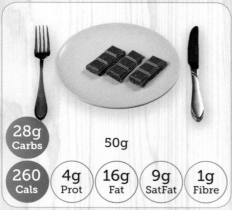

28g Carbs

50g

260 Cals | 4g Prot | 16g Fat | 9g SatFat | 1g Fibre

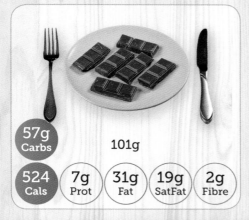

57g Carbs

101g

524 Cals | 7g Prot | 31g Fat | 19g SatFat | 2g Fibre

Chocolate (dark)

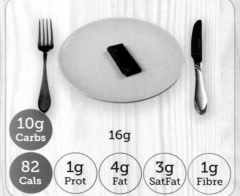

10g Carbs

16g

82 Cals | 1g Prot | 4g Fat | 3g SatFat | 1g Fibre

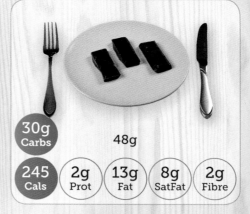

30g Carbs

48g

245 Cals | 2g Prot | 13g Fat | 8g SatFat | 2g Fibre

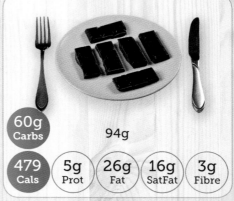

60g Carbs

94g

479 Cals | 5g Prot | 26g Fat | 16g SatFat | 3g Fibre

20cm Side Plate

Chocolate (white)

Chocolate (milk, with hazelnuts)

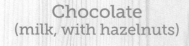

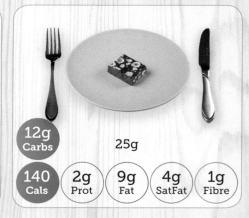

12g Carbs · 21g

111 Cals | **2g** Prot | **6g** Fat | **4g** SatFat | **0g** Fibre

12g Carbs · 25g

140 Cals | **2g** Prot | **9g** Fat | **4g** SatFat | **1g** Fibre

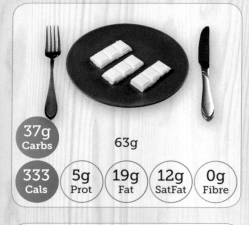

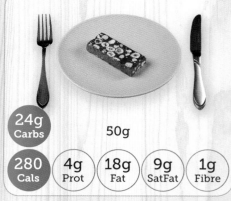

37g Carbs · 63g

333 Cals | **5g** Prot | **19g** Fat | **12g** SatFat | **0g** Fibre

24g Carbs · 50g

280 Cals | **4g** Prot | **18g** Fat | **9g** SatFat | **1g** Fibre

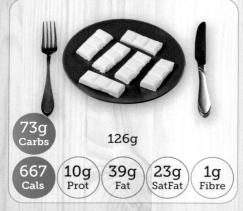

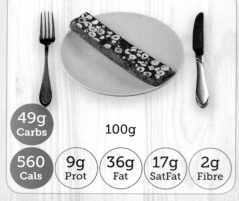

73g Carbs · 126g

667 Cals | **10g** Prot | **39g** Fat | **23g** SatFat | **1g** Fibre

49g Carbs · 100g

560 Cals | **9g** Prot | **36g** Fat | **17g** SatFat | **2g** Fibre

Chocolate Honeycomb Balls

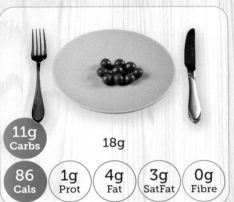

11g Carbs

18g

86 Cals | 1g Prot | 4g Fat | 3g SatFat | 0g Fibre

Individual Chocolate

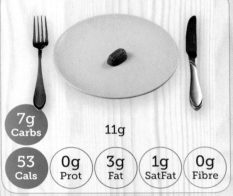

7g Carbs

11g

53 Cals | 0g Prot | 3g Fat | 1g SatFat | 0g Fibre

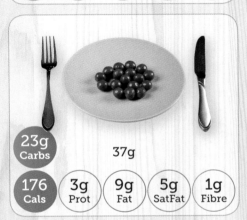

23g Carbs

37g

176 Cals | 3g Prot | 9g Fat | 5g SatFat | 1g Fibre

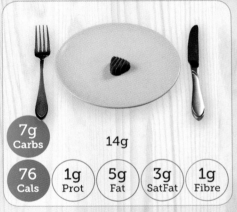

7g Carbs

14g

76 Cals | 1g Prot | 5g Fat | 3g SatFat | 1g Fibre

Chocolate Mint

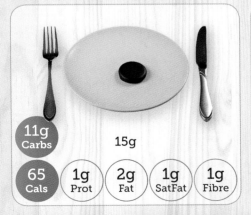

11g Carbs

15g

65 Cals | 1g Prot | 2g Fat | 1g SatFat | 1g Fibre

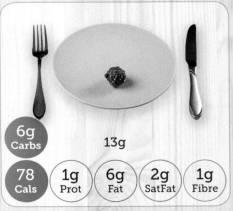

6g Carbs

13g

78 Cals | 1g Prot | 6g Fat | 2g SatFat | 1g Fibre

20cm Side Plate

Chocolate Bunny

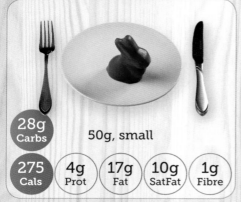

28g Carbs

50g, small

275 Cals | **4g** Prot | **17g** Fat | **10g** SatFat | **1g** Fibre

Easter Egg

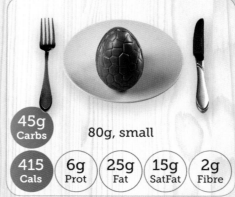

45g Carbs

80g, small

415 Cals | **6g** Prot | **25g** Fat | **15g** SatFat | **2g** Fibre

Chocolate Orange

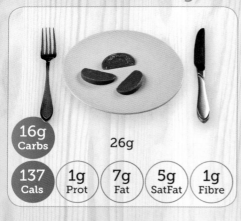

16g Carbs

26g

137 Cals | **1g** Prot | **7g** Fat | **5g** SatFat | **1g** Fibre

Easter Egg

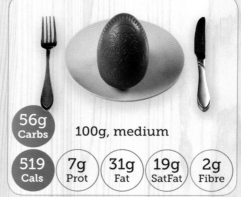

56g Carbs

100g, medium

519 Cals | **7g** Prot | **31g** Fat | **19g** SatFat | **2g** Fibre

Mini Eggs

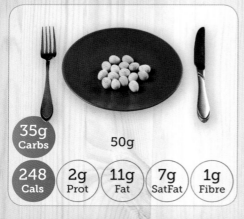

35g Carbs

50g

248 Cals | **2g** Prot | **11g** Fat | **7g** SatFat | **1g** Fibre

Easter Egg

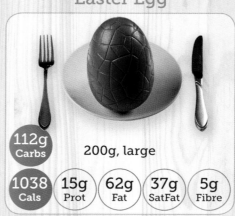

112g Carbs

200g, large

1038 Cals | **15g** Prot | **62g** Fat | **37g** SatFat | **5g** Fibre

Alpen Bar
(Fruit & Nut with Chocolate)

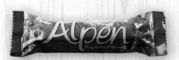

20g Carbs   28g

121 Cals | **2g** Prot | **4g** Fat | **1g** SatFat | **1g** Fibre

Nakd Bar (Berry Delight)

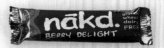

18g Carbs   35g   **1** 5-a-day

135 Cals | **3g** Prot | **5g** Fat | **1g** SatFat | **2g** Fibre

Alpen Bar
(Raspberry & Yogurt)

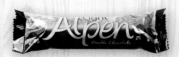

22g Carbs   29g

123 Cals | **1g** Prot | **3g** Fat | **2g** SatFat | **1g** Fibre

Nakd Bar (Cashew Cookie)

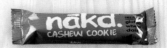

16g Carbs   35g   **1** 5-a-day

144 Cals | **4g** Prot | **8g** Fat | **2g** SatFat | **2g** Fibre

Alpen Bar Light
(Double Chocolate)

12g Carbs   21g

72 Cals | **1g** Prot | **1g** Fat | **1g** SatFat | **0g** Fibre

Nakd Bar (Cocoa Delight)

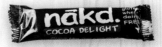

17g Carbs   35g   **1** 5-a-day

135 Cals | **3g** Prot | **5g** Fat | **1g** SatFat | **2g** Fibre

20cm Side Plate

Cola Bottles

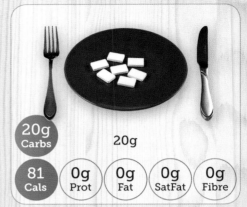

20g Carbs

27g

88 Cals | 2g Prot | 0g Fat | 0g SatFat | 0g Fibre

Dextrose Tablets

20g Carbs

20g

81 Cals | 0g Prot | 0g Fat | 0g SatFat | 0g Fibre

Jelly Babies

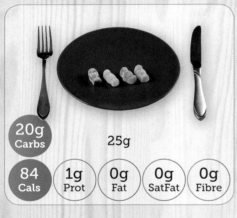

20g Carbs

25g

84 Cals | 1g Prot | 0g Fat | 0g SatFat | 0g Fibre

Jelly Beans

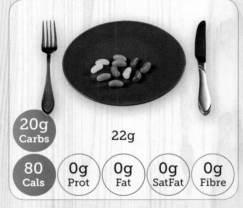

20g Carbs

22g

80 Cals | 0g Prot | 0g Fat | 0g SatFat | 0g Fibre

Licorice Allsorts

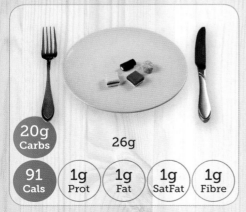

20g Carbs

26g

91 Cals | 1g Prot | 1g Fat | 1g SatFat | 1g Fibre

Wine Gums

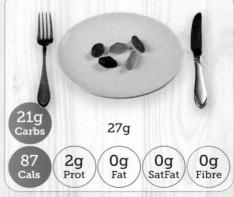

21g Carbs

27g

87 Cals | 2g Prot | 0g Fat | 0g SatFat | 0g Fibre

Broccoli & Stilton Soup

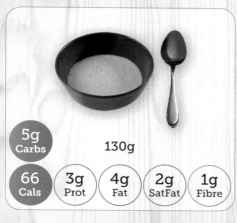

5g Carbs

130g

66 Cals | 3g Prot | 4g Fat | 2g SatFat | 1g Fibre

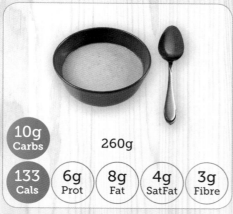

10g Carbs

260g

133 Cals | 6g Prot | 8g Fat | 4g SatFat | 3g Fibre

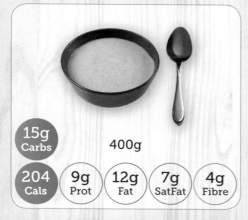

15g Carbs

400g

204 Cals | 9g Prot | 12g Fat | 7g SatFat | 4g Fibre

Chicken Noodle Soup

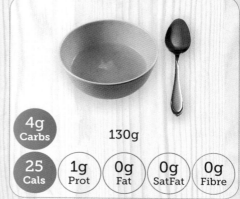

4g Carbs

130g

25 Cals | 1g Prot | 0g Fat | 0g SatFat | 0g Fibre

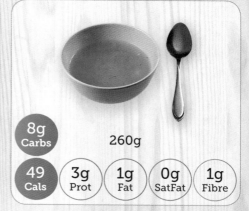

8g Carbs

260g

49 Cals | 3g Prot | 1g Fat | 0g SatFat | 1g Fibre

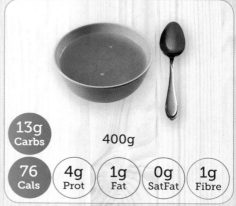

13g Carbs

400g

76 Cals | 4g Prot | 1g Fat | 0g SatFat | 1g Fibre

14cm Cereal Bowl

Chunky Veg Soup

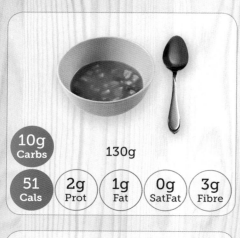

10g Carbs
130g

51 Cals | **2g** Prot | **1g** Fat | **0g** SatFat | **3g** Fibre

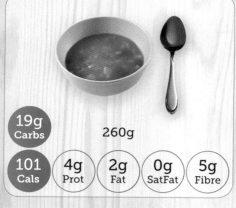

19g Carbs
260g

101 Cals | **4g** Prot | **2g** Fat | **0g** SatFat | **5g** Fibre

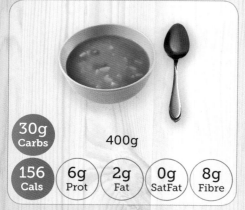

30g Carbs
400g

156 Cals | **6g** Prot | **2g** Fat | **0g** SatFat | **8g** Fibre

Mushroom Soup (cream of)

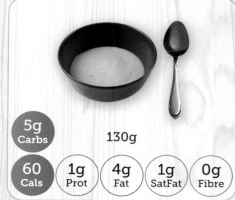

5g Carbs
130g

60 Cals | **1g** Prot | **4g** Fat | **1g** SatFat | **0g** Fibre

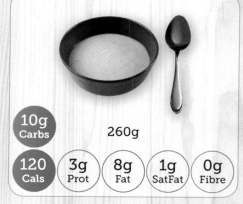

10g Carbs
260g

120 Cals | **3g** Prot | **8g** Fat | **1g** SatFat | **0g** Fibre

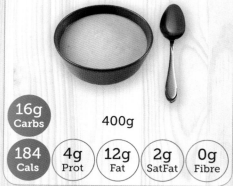

16g Carbs
400g

184 Cals | **4g** Prot | **12g** Fat | **2g** SatFat | **0g** Fibre

Onion Soup

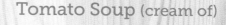

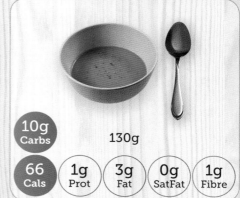

7g Carbs

130g

53 Cals | **1g Prot** | **3g Fat** | **0g SatFat** | **2g Fibre**

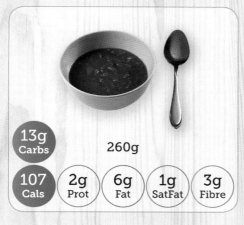

13g Carbs

260g

107 Cals | **2g Prot** | **6g Fat** | **1g SatFat** | **3g Fibre**

20g Carbs

400g

164 Cals | **4g Prot** | **9g Fat** | **1g SatFat** | **5g Fibre**

Tomato Soup (cream of)

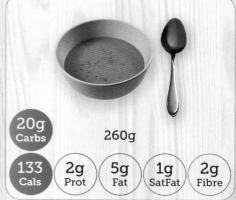

10g Carbs

130g

66 Cals | **1g Prot** | **3g Fat** | **0g SatFat** | **1g Fibre**

20g Carbs

260g

133 Cals | **2g Prot** | **5g Fat** | **1g SatFat** | **2g Fibre**

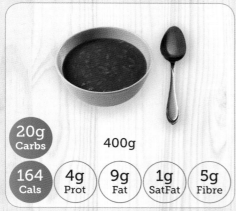

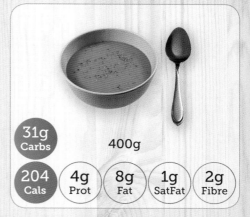

31g Carbs

400g

204 Cals | **4g Prot** | **8g Fat** | **1g SatFat** | **2g Fibre**

Butter

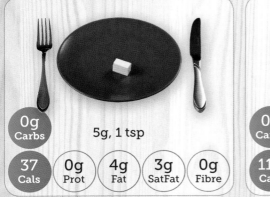

0g Carbs
5g, 1 tsp
37 Cals | **0g** Prot | **4g** Fat | **3g** SatFat | **0g** Fibre

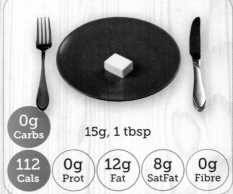

0g Carbs
15g, 1 tbsp
112 Cals | **0g** Prot | **12g** Fat | **8g** SatFat | **0g** Fibre

Margarine

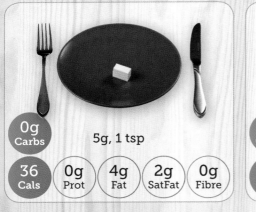

0g Carbs
5g, 1 tsp
36 Cals | **0g** Prot | **4g** Fat | **2g** SatFat | **0g** Fibre

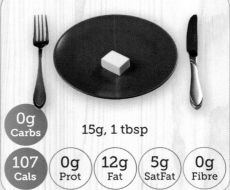

0g Carbs
15g, 1 tbsp
107 Cals | **0g** Prot | **12g** Fat | **5g** SatFat | **0g** Fibre

Margarine (light)

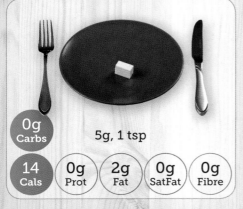

0g Carbs
5g, 1 tsp
14 Cals | **0g** Prot | **2g** Fat | **0g** SatFat | **0g** Fibre

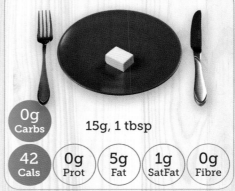

0g Carbs
15g, 1 tbsp
42 Cals | **0g** Prot | **5g** Fat | **1g** SatFat | **0g** Fibre

Olive Oil Spread

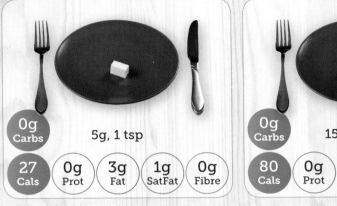

0g Carbs

5g, 1 tsp

27 Cals | **0g** Prot | **3g** Fat | **1g** SatFat | **0g** Fibre

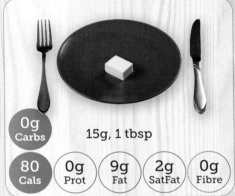

0g Carbs

15g, 1 tbsp

80 Cals | **0g** Prot | **9g** Fat | **2g** SatFat | **0g** Fibre

Lard

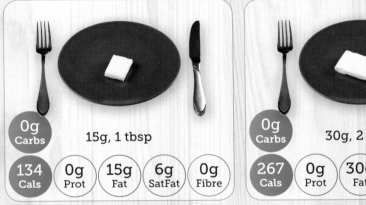

0g Carbs

15g, 1 tbsp

134 Cals | **0g** Prot | **15g** Fat | **6g** SatFat | **0g** Fibre

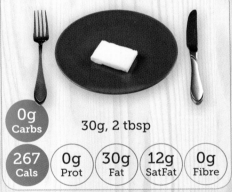

0g Carbs

30g, 2 tbsp

267 Cals | **0g** Prot | **30g** Fat | **12g** SatFat | **0g** Fibre

Ghee

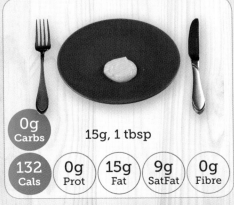

0g Carbs

15g, 1 tbsp

132 Cals | **0g** Prot | **15g** Fat | **9g** SatFat | **0g** Fibre

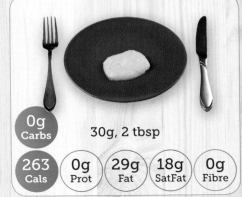

0g Carbs

30g, 2 tbsp

263 Cals | **0g** Prot | **29g** Fat | **18g** SatFat | **0g** Fibre

20cm Side Plate

Olive / Vegetable / Sesame Oil

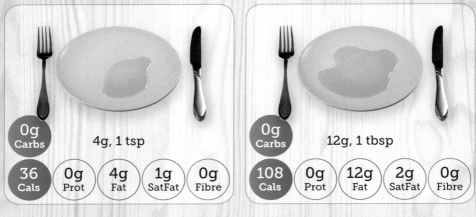

0g Carbs		4g, 1 tsp		
36 Cals	0g Prot	4g Fat	1g SatFat	0g Fibre

0g Carbs		12g, 1 tbsp		
108 Cals	0g Prot	12g Fat	2g SatFat	0g Fibre

Rapeseed Oil

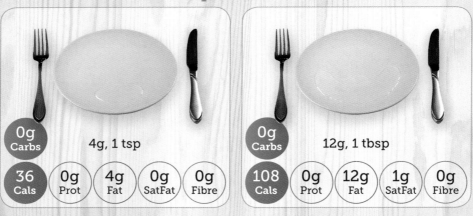

0g Carbs		4g, 1 tsp		
36 Cals	0g Prot	4g Fat	0g SatFat	0g Fibre

0g Carbs		12g, 1 tbsp		
108 Cals	0g Prot	12g Fat	1g SatFat	0g Fibre

Palm Oil

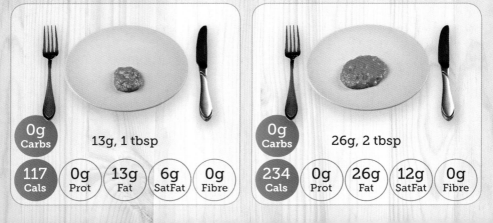

0g Carbs		13g, 1 tbsp		
117 Cals	0g Prot	13g Fat	6g SatFat	0g Fibre

0g Carbs		26g, 2 tbsp		
234 Cals	0g Prot	26g Fat	12g SatFat	0g Fibre

Chocolate Nut Spread

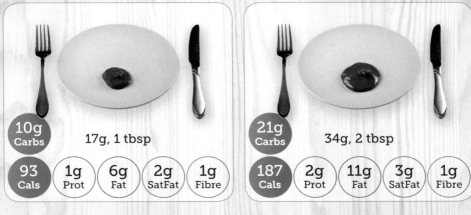

10g Carbs   17g, 1 tbsp

93 Cals | **1g** Prot | **6g** Fat | **2g** SatFat | **1g** Fibre

21g Carbs   34g, 2 tbsp

187 Cals | **2g** Prot | **11g** Fat | **3g** SatFat | **1g** Fibre

Honey

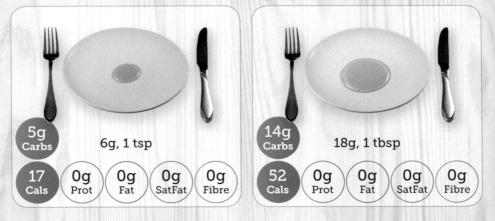

5g Carbs   6g, 1 tsp

17 Cals | **0g** Prot | **0g** Fat | **0g** SatFat | **0g** Fibre

14g Carbs   18g, 1 tbsp

52 Cals | **0g** Prot | **0g** Fat | **0g** SatFat | **0g** Fibre

Jam

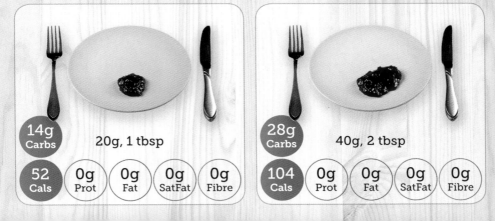

14g Carbs   20g, 1 tbsp

52 Cals | **0g** Prot | **0g** Fat | **0g** SatFat | **0g** Fibre

28g Carbs   40g, 2 tbsp

104 Cals | **0g** Prot | **0g** Fat | **0g** SatFat | **0g** Fibre

20cm Side Plate

Lemon Curd

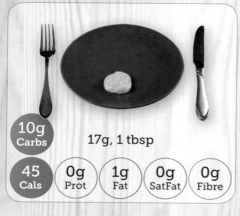

10g Carbs
45 Cals | 0g Prot | 1g Fat | 0g SatFat | 0g Fibre

17g, 1 tbsp

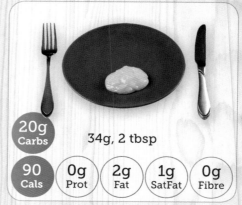

20g Carbs
90 Cals | 0g Prot | 2g Fat | 1g SatFat | 0g Fibre

34g, 2 tbsp

Maple Syrup

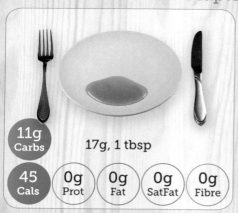

11g Carbs
45 Cals | 0g Prot | 0g Fat | 0g SatFat | 0g Fibre

17g, 1 tbsp

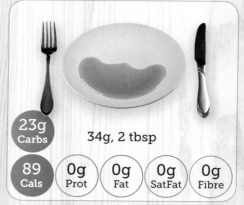

23g Carbs
89 Cals | 0g Prot | 0g Fat | 0g SatFat | 0g Fibre

34g, 2 tbsp

Marmalade

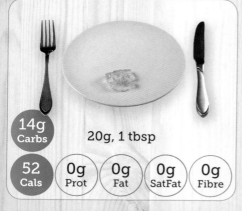

14g Carbs
52 Cals | 0g Prot | 0g Fat | 0g SatFat | 0g Fibre

20g, 1 tbsp

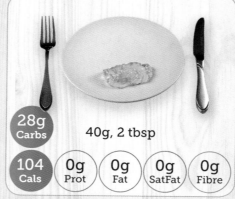

28g Carbs
104 Cals | 0g Prot | 0g Fat | 0g SatFat | 0g Fibre

40g, 2 tbsp

Marmite

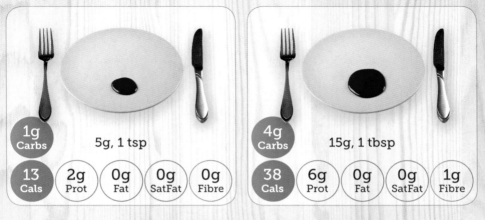

1g Carbs — 5g, 1 tsp

13 Cals | **2g** Prot | **0g** Fat | **0g** SatFat | **0g** Fibre

4g Carbs — 15g, 1 tbsp

38 Cals | **6g** Prot | **0g** Fat | **0g** SatFat | **1g** Fibre

Peanut Butter (crunchy)

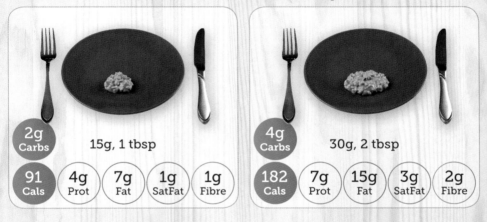

2g Carbs — 15g, 1 tbsp

91 Cals | **4g** Prot | **7g** Fat | **1g** SatFat | **1g** Fibre

4g Carbs — 30g, 2 tbsp

182 Cals | **7g** Prot | **15g** Fat | **3g** SatFat | **2g** Fibre

Peanut Butter (smooth)

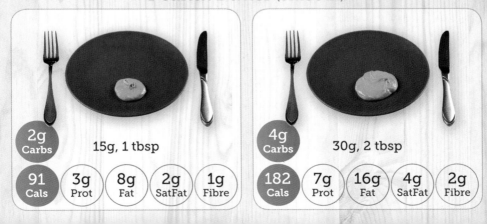

2g Carbs — 15g, 1 tbsp

91 Cals | **3g** Prot | **8g** Fat | **2g** SatFat | **1g** Fibre

4g Carbs — 30g, 2 tbsp

182 Cals | **7g** Prot | **16g** Fat | **4g** SatFat | **2g** Fibre

Sugar (white)

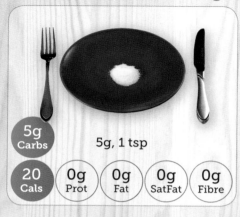

5g Carbs

5g, 1 tsp

20 Cals | **0g** Prot | **0g** Fat | **0g** SatFat | **0g** Fibre

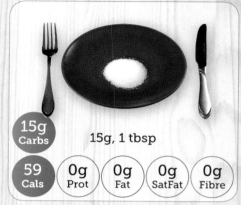

15g Carbs

15g, 1 tbsp

59 Cals | **0g** Prot | **0g** Fat | **0g** SatFat | **0g** Fibre

Sugar (brown)

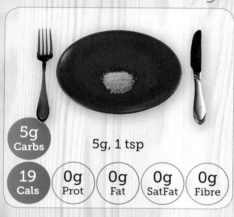

5g Carbs

5g, 1 tsp

19 Cals | **0g** Prot | **0g** Fat | **0g** SatFat | **0g** Fibre

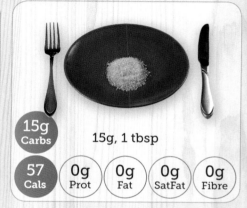

15g Carbs

15g, 1 tbsp

57 Cals | **0g** Prot | **0g** Fat | **0g** SatFat | **0g** Fibre

Sweetener

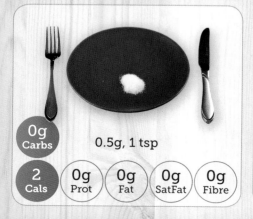

0g Carbs

0.5g, 1 tsp

2 Cals | **0g** Prot | **0g** Fat | **0g** SatFat | **0g** Fibre

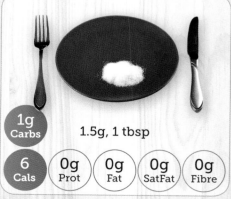

1g Carbs

1.5g, 1 tbsp

6 Cals | **0g** Prot | **0g** Fat | **0g** SatFat | **0g** Fibre

Apple Chutney

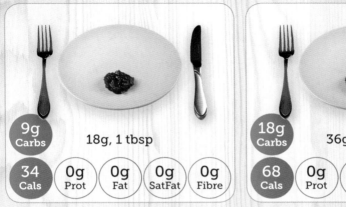

9g Carbs

18g, 1 tbsp

34 Cals | **0g** Prot | **0g** Fat | **0g** SatFat | **0g** Fibre

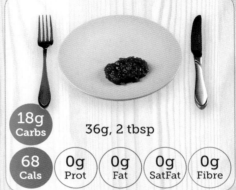

18g Carbs

36g, 2 tbsp

68 Cals | **0g** Prot | **0g** Fat | **0g** SatFat | **0g** Fibre

BBQ Sauce

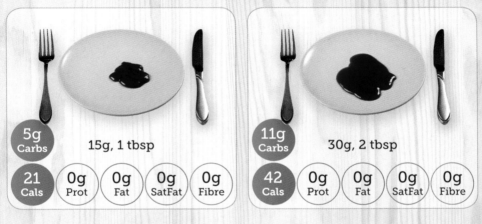

5g Carbs

15g, 1 tbsp

21 Cals | **0g** Prot | **0g** Fat | **0g** SatFat | **0g** Fibre

11g Carbs

30g, 2 tbsp

42 Cals | **0g** Prot | **0g** Fat | **0g** SatFat | **0g** Fibre

Béarnaise Sauce

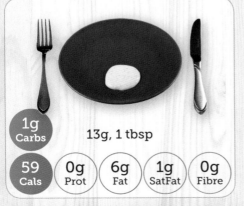

1g Carbs

13g, 1 tbsp

59 Cals | **0g** Prot | **6g** Fat | **1g** SatFat | **0g** Fibre

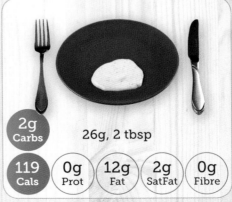

2g Carbs

26g, 2 tbsp

119 Cals | **0g** Prot | **12g** Fat | **2g** SatFat | **0g** Fibre

20cm Side Plate

Brown Sauce

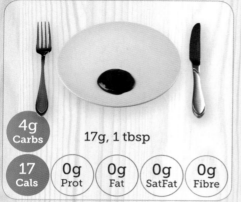

4g Carbs

17g, 1 tbsp

17 Cals | **0g** Prot | **0g** Fat | **0g** SatFat | **0g** Fibre

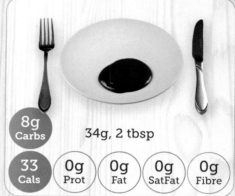

8g Carbs

34g, 2 tbsp

33 Cals | **0g** Prot | **0g** Fat | **0g** SatFat | **0g** Fibre

Caesar Dressing

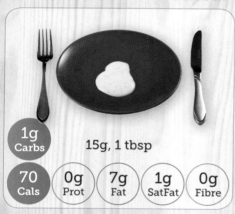

1g Carbs

15g, 1 tbsp

70 Cals | **0g** Prot | **7g** Fat | **1g** SatFat | **0g** Fibre

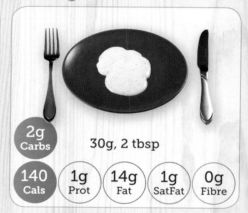

2g Carbs

30g, 2 tbsp

140 Cals | **1g** Prot | **14g** Fat | **1g** SatFat | **0g** Fibre

Chilli Sauce

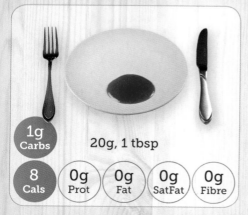

1g Carbs

20g, 1 tbsp

8 Cals | **0g** Prot | **0g** Fat | **0g** SatFat | **0g** Fibre

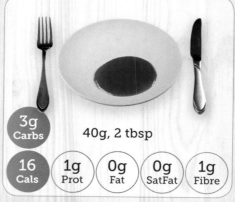

3g Carbs

40g, 2 tbsp

16 Cals | **1g** Prot | **0g** Fat | **0g** SatFat | **1g** Fibre

Cranberry Sauce

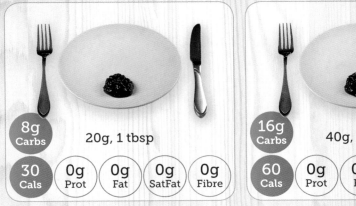

8g Carbs

20g, 1 tbsp

30 Cals | 0g Prot | 0g Fat | 0g SatFat | 0g Fibre

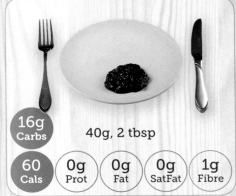

16g Carbs

40g, 2 tbsp

60 Cals | 0g Prot | 0g Fat | 0g SatFat | 1g Fibre

Gravy

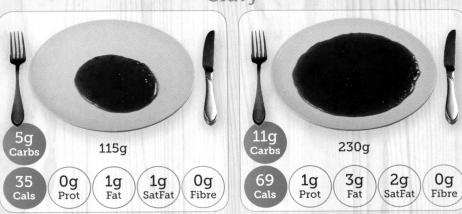

5g Carbs

115g

35 Cals | 0g Prot | 1g Fat | 1g SatFat | 0g Fibre

11g Carbs

230g

69 Cals | 1g Prot | 3g Fat | 2g SatFat | 0g Fibre

Guacamole

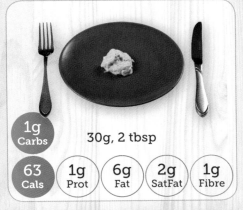

1g Carbs

30g, 2 tbsp

63 Cals | 1g Prot | 6g Fat | 2g SatFat | 1g Fibre

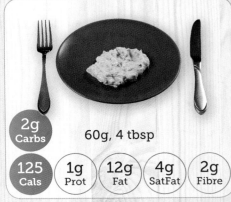

2g Carbs

60g, 4 tbsp

125 Cals | 1g Prot | 12g Fat | 4g SatFat | 2g Fibre

20cm Side Plate

Hollandaise Sauce

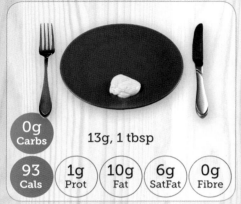

0g Carbs

13g, 1 tbsp

93 Cals | 1g Prot | 10g Fat | 6g SatFat | 0g Fibre

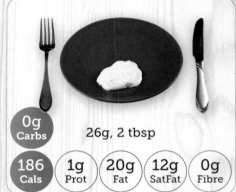

0g Carbs

26g, 2 tbsp

186 Cals | 1g Prot | 20g Fat | 12g SatFat | 0g Fibre

Horseradish Sauce

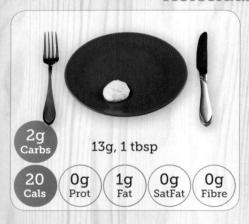

2g Carbs

13g, 1 tbsp

20 Cals | 0g Prot | 1g Fat | 0g SatFat | 0g Fibre

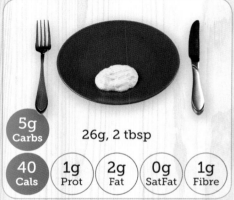

5g Carbs

26g, 2 tbsp

40 Cals | 1g Prot | 2g Fat | 0g SatFat | 1g Fibre

Houmous

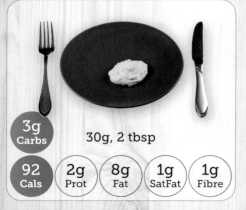

3g Carbs

30g, 2 tbsp

92 Cals | 2g Prot | 8g Fat | 1g SatFat | 1g Fibre

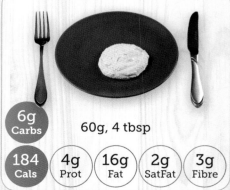

6g Carbs

60g, 4 tbsp

184 Cals | 4g Prot | 16g Fat | 2g SatFat | 3g Fibre

Ketchup

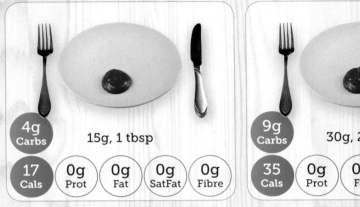

4g Carbs

15g, 1 tbsp

17 Cals | **0g** Prot | **0g** Fat | **0g** SatFat | **0g** Fibre

9g Carbs

30g, 2 tbsp

35 Cals | **0g** Prot | **0g** Fat | **0g** SatFat | **0g** Fibre

Lime Pickle

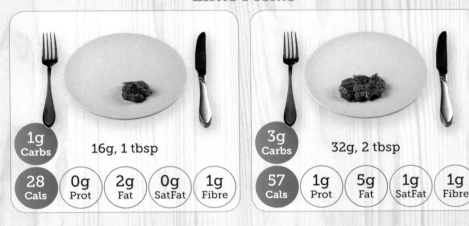

1g Carbs

16g, 1 tbsp

28 Cals | **0g** Prot | **2g** Fat | **0g** SatFat | **1g** Fibre

3g Carbs

32g, 2 tbsp

57 Cals | **1g** Prot | **5g** Fat | **1g** SatFat | **1g** Fibre

Mango Chutney

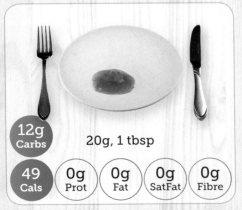
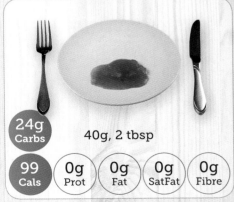

12g Carbs

20g, 1 tbsp

49 Cals | **0g** Prot | **0g** Fat | **0g** SatFat | **0g** Fibre

24g Carbs

40g, 2 tbsp

99 Cals | **0g** Prot | **0g** Fat | **0g** SatFat | **0g** Fibre

Mayonnaise

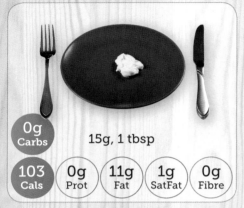

0g Carbs

15g, 1 tbsp

103 Cals | **0g** Prot | **11g** Fat | **1g** SatFat | **0g** Fibre

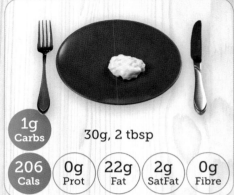

1g Carbs

30g, 2 tbsp

206 Cals | **0g** Prot | **22g** Fat | **2g** SatFat | **0g** Fibre

Mayonnaise (light)

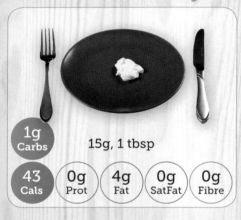

1g Carbs

15g, 1 tbsp

43 Cals | **0g** Prot | **4g** Fat | **0g** SatFat | **0g** Fibre

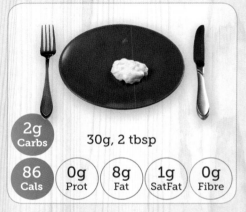

2g Carbs

30g, 2 tbsp

86 Cals | **0g** Prot | **8g** Fat | **1g** SatFat | **0g** Fibre

Mint Sauce

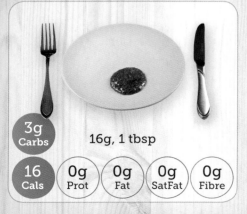

3g Carbs

16g, 1 tbsp

16 Cals | **0g** Prot | **0g** Fat | **0g** SatFat | **0g** Fibre

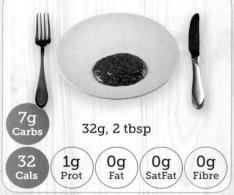

7g Carbs

32g, 2 tbsp

32 Cals | **1g** Prot | **0g** Fat | **0g** SatFat | **0g** Fibre

Mustard (English)

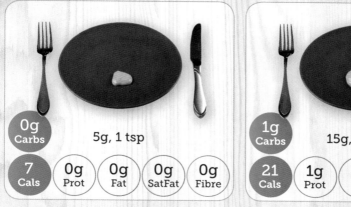

0g Carbs
5g, 1 tsp
7 Cals | **0g** Prot | **0g** Fat | **0g** SatFat | **0g** Fibre

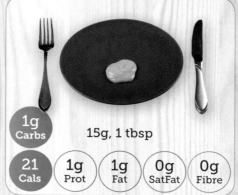

1g Carbs
15g, 1 tbsp
21 Cals | **1g** Prot | **1g** Fat | **0g** SatFat | **0g** Fibre

Mustard (wholegrain)

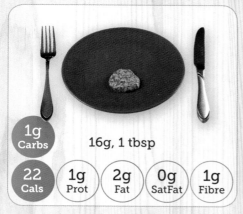

1g Carbs
16g, 1 tbsp
22 Cals | **1g** Prot | **2g** Fat | **0g** SatFat | **1g** Fibre

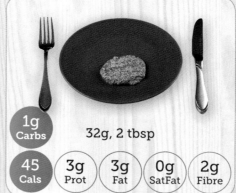

1g Carbs
32g, 2 tbsp
45 Cals | **3g** Prot | **3g** Fat | **0g** SatFat | **2g** Fibre

Parsley Sauce

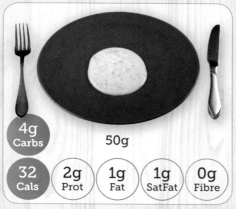

4g Carbs
50g
32 Cals | **2g** Prot | **1g** Fat | **1g** SatFat | **0g** Fibre

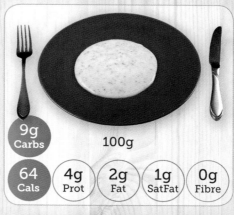

9g Carbs
100g
64 Cals | **4g** Prot | **2g** Fat | **1g** SatFat | **0g** Fibre

26cm Dinner Plate / 20cm Side Plate

Pesto

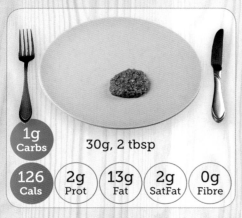

1g Carbs
30g, 2 tbsp

126 Cals | **2g** Prot | **13g** Fat | **2g** SatFat | **0g** Fibre

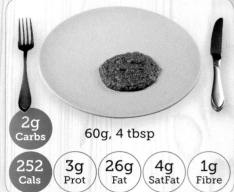

2g Carbs
60g, 4 tbsp

252 Cals | **3g** Prot | **26g** Fat | **4g** SatFat | **1g** Fibre

Piccalilli

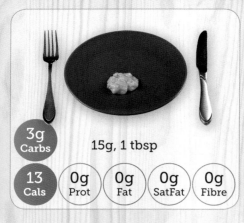

3g Carbs
15g, 1 tbsp

13 Cals | **0g** Prot | **0g** Fat | **0g** SatFat | **0g** Fibre

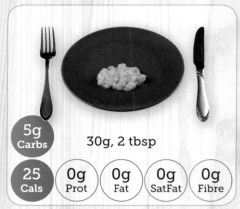

5g Carbs
30g, 2 tbsp

25 Cals | **0g** Prot | **0g** Fat | **0g** SatFat | **0g** Fibre

Pickle

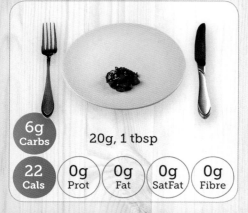

6g Carbs
20g, 1 tbsp

22 Cals | **0g** Prot | **0g** Fat | **0g** SatFat | **0g** Fibre

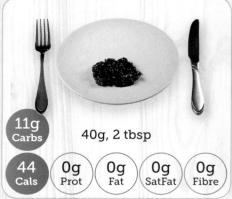

11g Carbs
40g, 2 tbsp

44 Cals | **0g** Prot | **0g** Fat | **0g** SatFat | **0g** Fibre

20cm Side Plate

Raita

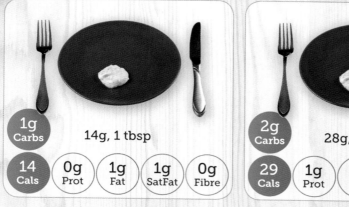

1g Carbs — 14g, 1 tbsp

14 Cals | **0g** Prot | **1g** Fat | **1g** SatFat | **0g** Fibre

2g Carbs — 28g, 2 tbsp

29 Cals | **1g** Prot | **2g** Fat | **1g** SatFat | **0g** Fibre

Salad Cream

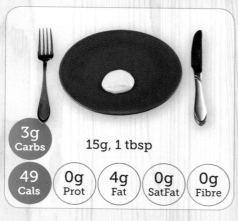
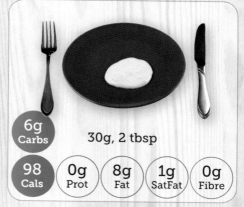

3g Carbs — 15g, 1 tbsp

49 Cals | **0g** Prot | **4g** Fat | **0g** SatFat | **0g** Fibre

6g Carbs — 30g, 2 tbsp

98 Cals | **0g** Prot | **8g** Fat | **1g** SatFat | **0g** Fibre

Soy Sauce

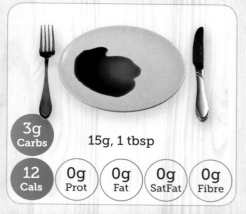
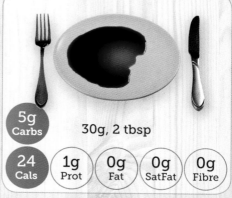

3g Carbs — 15g, 1 tbsp

12 Cals | **0g** Prot | **0g** Fat | **0g** SatFat | **0g** Fibre

5g Carbs — 30g, 2 tbsp

24 Cals | **1g** Prot | **0g** Fat | **0g** SatFat | **0g** Fibre

20cm Side Plate

Sweet Chilli Sauce

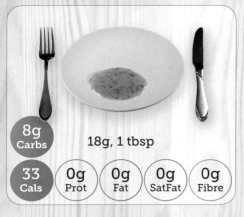

8g Carbs

18g, 1 tbsp

33 Cals | **0g** Prot | **0g** Fat | **0g** SatFat | **0g** Fibre

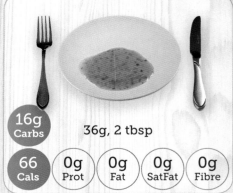

16g Carbs

36g, 2 tbsp

66 Cals | **0g** Prot | **0g** Fat | **0g** SatFat | **0g** Fibre

Sweet & Sour Sauce (takeaway)

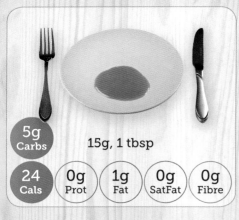

5g Carbs

15g, 1 tbsp

24 Cals | **0g** Prot | **1g** Fat | **0g** SatFat | **0g** Fibre

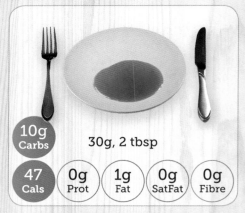

10g Carbs

30g, 2 tbsp

47 Cals | **0g** Prot | **1g** Fat | **0g** SatFat | **0g** Fibre

Tartare Sauce

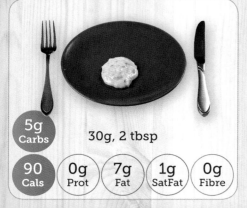

5g Carbs

30g, 2 tbsp

90 Cals | **0g** Prot | **7g** Fat | **1g** SatFat | **0g** Fibre

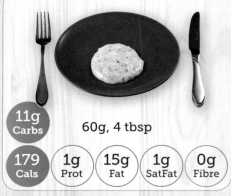

11g Carbs

60g, 4 tbsp

179 Cals | **1g** Prot | **15g** Fat | **1g** SatFat | **0g** Fibre

Thousand Island Dressing

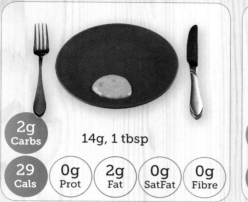

2g Carbs

14g, 1 tbsp

29 Cals | **0g** Prot | **2g** Fat | **0g** SatFat | **0g** Fibre

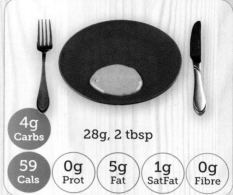

4g Carbs

28g, 2 tbsp

59 Cals | **0g** Prot | **5g** Fat | **1g** SatFat | **0g** Fibre

White Sauce (made with whole milk)

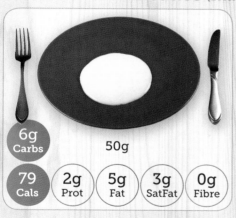

6g Carbs

50g

79 Cals | **2g** Prot | **5g** Fat | **3g** SatFat | **0g** Fibre

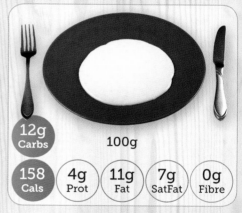

12g Carbs

100g

158 Cals | **4g** Prot | **11g** Fat | **7g** SatFat | **0g** Fibre

Worcestershire Sauce

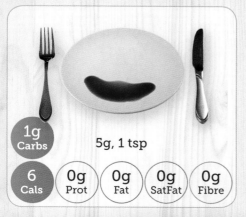

1g Carbs

5g, 1 tsp

6 Cals | **0g** Prot | **0g** Fat | **0g** SatFat | **0g** Fibre

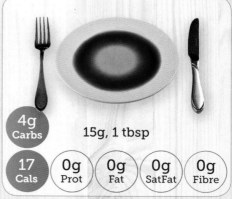

4g Carbs

15g, 1 tbsp

17 Cals | **0g** Prot | **0g** Fat | **0g** SatFat | **0g** Fibre

Ackee (tinned)

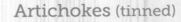

0g Carbs — 40g — **½** 5-a-day

60 Cals | **1g** Prot | **6g** Fat | **0g** SatFat | **1g** Fibre

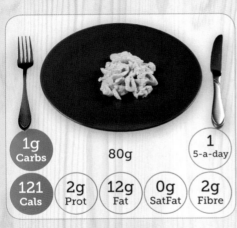

1g Carbs — 80g — **1** 5-a-day

121 Cals | **2g** Prot | **12g** Fat | **0g** SatFat | **2g** Fibre

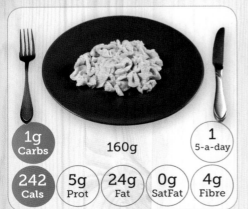

1g Carbs — 160g — **1** 5-a-day

242 Cals | **5g** Prot | **24g** Fat | **0g** SatFat | **4g** Fibre

Artichokes (tinned)

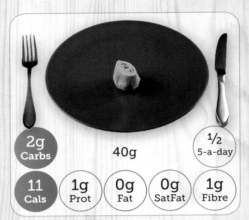

2g Carbs — 40g — **½** 5-a-day

11 Cals | **1g** Prot | **0g** Fat | **0g** SatFat | **1g** Fibre

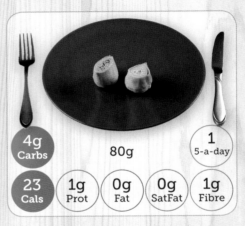

4g Carbs — 80g — **1** 5-a-day

23 Cals | **1g** Prot | **0g** Fat | **0g** SatFat | **1g** Fibre

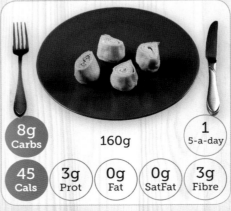

8g Carbs — 160g — **1** 5-a-day

45 Cals | **3g** Prot | **0g** Fat | **0g** SatFat | **3g** Fibre

Asparagus (boiled)

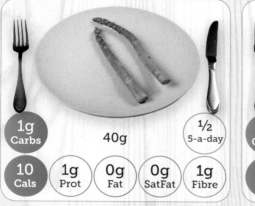

1g **Carbs**

40g

½ 5-a-day

10 **Cals** | 1g Prot | 0g Fat | 0g SatFat | 1g Fibre

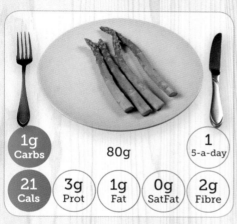

1g **Carbs**

80g

1 5-a-day

21 **Cals** | 3g Prot | 1g Fat | 0g SatFat | 2g Fibre

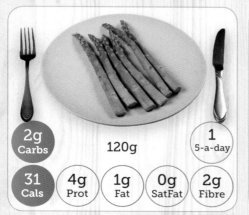

2g **Carbs**

120g

1 5-a-day

31 **Cals** | 4g Prot | 1g Fat | 0g SatFat | 2g Fibre

Aubergine (fried in oil)

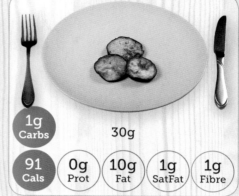

1g **Carbs**

30g

91 **Cals** | 0g Prot | 10g Fat | 1g SatFat | 1g Fibre

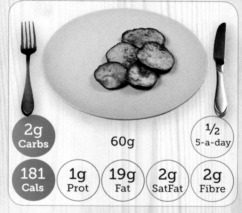

2g **Carbs**

60g

½ 5-a-day

181 **Cals** | 1g Prot | 19g Fat | 2g SatFat | 2g Fibre

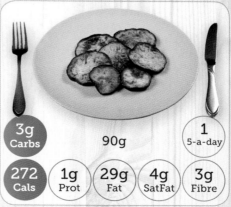

3g **Carbs**

90g

1 5-a-day

272 **Cals** | 1g Prot | 29g Fat | 4g SatFat | 3g Fibre

26cm Dinner Plate

Avocado

Baked Beans
(in tomato sauce)

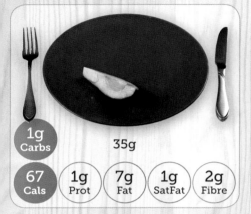

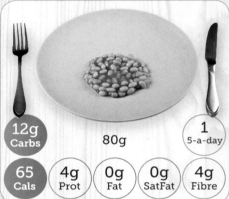

1g Carbs — 35g

67 Cals | **1g** Prot | **7g** Fat | **1g** SatFat | **2g** Fibre

12g Carbs — 80g — **1** 5-a-day

65 Cals | **4g** Prot | **0g** Fat | **0g** SatFat | **4g** Fibre

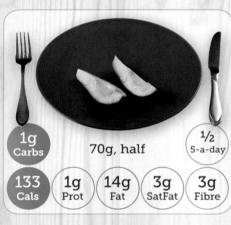

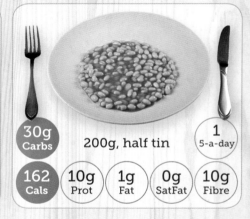

1g Carbs — 70g, half — **½** 5-a-day

133 Cals | **1g** Prot | **14g** Fat | **3g** SatFat | **3g** Fibre

30g Carbs — 200g, half tin — **1** 5-a-day

162 Cals | **10g** Prot | **1g** Fat | **0g** SatFat | **10g** Fibre

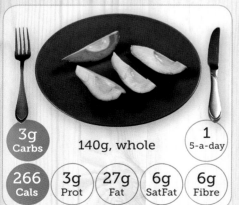

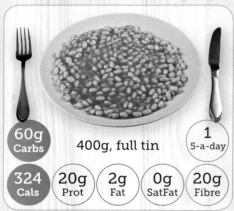

3g Carbs — 140g, whole — **1** 5-a-day

266 Cals | **3g** Prot | **27g** Fat | **6g** SatFat | **6g** Fibre

60g Carbs — 400g, full tin — **1** 5-a-day

324 Cals | **20g** Prot | **2g** Fat | **0g** SatFat | **20g** Fibre

Bamboo Shoots

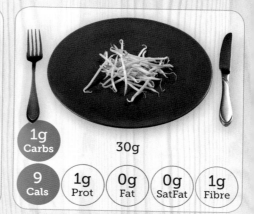

0g Carbs
30g
3 Cals | 0g Prot | 0g Fat | 0g SatFat | 1g Fibre

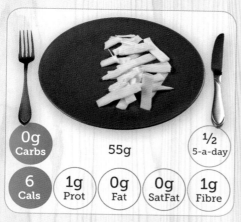

0g Carbs
55g
½ 5-a-day
6 Cals | 1g Prot | 0g Fat | 0g SatFat | 1g Fibre

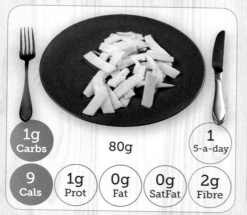

1g Carbs
80g
1 5-a-day
9 Cals | 1g Prot | 0g Fat | 0g SatFat | 2g Fibre

Bean Sprouts

1g Carbs
30g
9 Cals | 1g Prot | 0g Fat | 0g SatFat | 1g Fibre

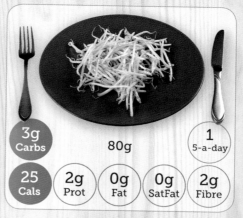

3g Carbs
80g
1 5-a-day
25 Cals | 2g Prot | 0g Fat | 0g SatFat | 2g Fibre

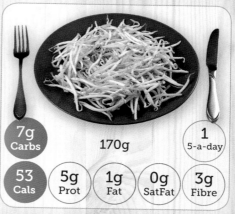

7g Carbs
170g
1 5-a-day
53 Cals | 5g Prot | 1g Fat | 0g SatFat | 3g Fibre

Beetroot (boiled)

Broad Beans (boiled)

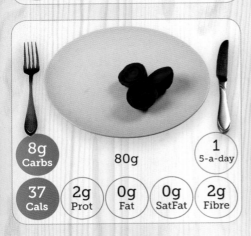

3g Carbs — 30g

14 Cals | **1g** Prot | **0g** Fat | **0g** SatFat | **1g** Fibre

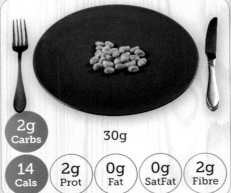

2g Carbs — 30g

14 Cals | **2g** Prot | **0g** Fat | **0g** SatFat | **2g** Fibre

8g Carbs — 80g — **1** 5-a-day

37 Cals | **2g** Prot | **0g** Fat | **0g** SatFat | **2g** Fibre

3g Carbs — 55g — **½** 5-a-day

26 Cals | **3g** Prot | **0g** Fat | **0g** SatFat | **4g** Fibre

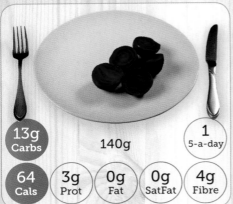

13g Carbs — 140g — **1** 5-a-day

64 Cals | **3g** Prot | **0g** Fat | **0g** SatFat | **4g** Fibre

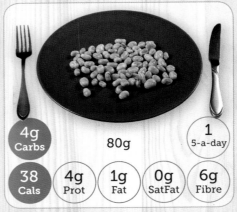

4g Carbs — 80g — **1** 5-a-day

38 Cals | **4g** Prot | **1g** Fat | **0g** SatFat | **6g** Fibre

Broccoli (boiled)

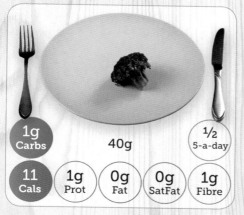

1g Carbs | 40g | ½ 5-a-day

11 Cals | 1g Prot | 0g Fat | 0g SatFat | 1g Fibre

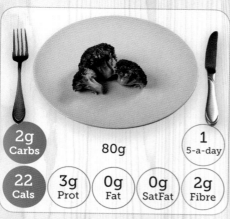

2g Carbs | 80g | 1 5-a-day

22 Cals | 3g Prot | 0g Fat | 0g SatFat | 2g Fibre

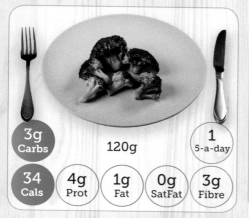

3g Carbs | 120g | 1 5-a-day

34 Cals | 4g Prot | 1g Fat | 0g SatFat | 3g Fibre

Brussels Sprouts (boiled)

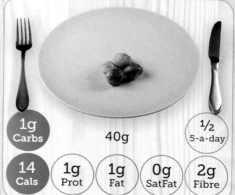

1g Carbs | 40g | ½ 5-a-day

14 Cals | 1g Prot | 1g Fat | 0g SatFat | 2g Fibre

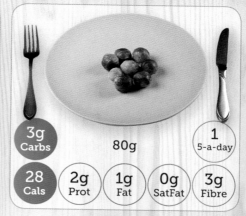

3g Carbs | 80g | 1 5-a-day

28 Cals | 2g Prot | 1g Fat | 0g SatFat | 3g Fibre

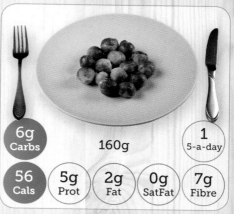

6g Carbs | 160g | 1 5-a-day

56 Cals | 5g Prot | 2g Fat | 0g SatFat | 7g Fibre

26cm Dinner Plate

Butter Beans

Butternut Squash (baked)

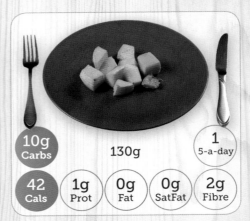

Butter Beans

5g Carbs — 40g — ½ 5-a-day
31 Cals | 2g Prot | 0g Fat | 0g SatFat | 2g Fibre

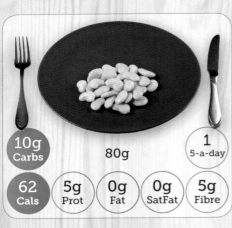

10g Carbs — 80g — 1 5-a-day
62 Cals | 5g Prot | 0g Fat | 0g SatFat | 5g Fibre

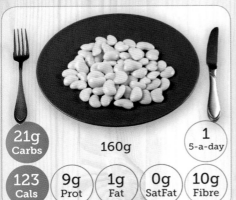

21g Carbs — 160g — 1 5-a-day
123 Cals | 9g Prot | 1g Fat | 0g SatFat | 10g Fibre

Butternut Squash (baked)

10g Carbs — 130g — 1 5-a-day
42 Cals | 1g Prot | 0g Fat | 0g SatFat | 2g Fibre

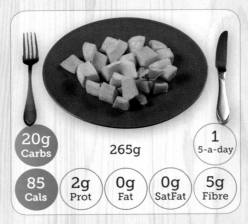

20g Carbs — 265g — 1 5-a-day
85 Cals | 2g Prot | 0g Fat | 0g SatFat | 5g Fibre

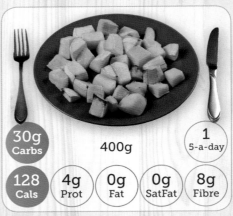

30g Carbs — 400g — 1 5-a-day
128 Cals | 4g Prot | 0g Fat | 0g SatFat | 8g Fibre

Cabbage (boiled)

Carrots (boiled)

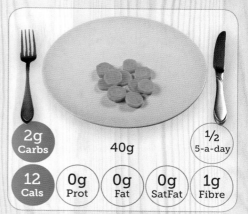

1g Carbs — 40g — ½ 5-a-day

7 Cals | **0g** Prot | **0g** Fat | **0g** SatFat | **1g** Fibre

2g Carbs — 40g — ½ 5-a-day

12 Cals | **0g** Prot | **0g** Fat | **0g** SatFat | **1g** Fibre

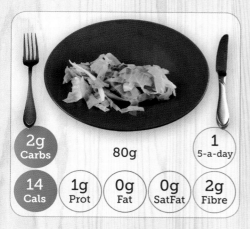

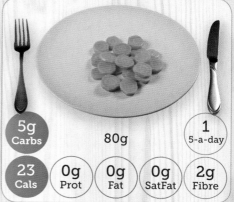

2g Carbs — 80g — 1 5-a-day

14 Cals | **1g** Prot | **0g** Fat | **0g** SatFat | **2g** Fibre

5g Carbs — 80g — 1 5-a-day

23 Cals | **0g** Prot | **0g** Fat | **0g** SatFat | **2g** Fibre

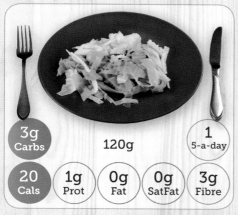

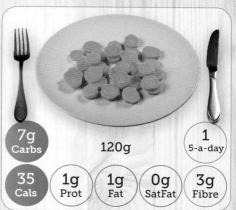

3g Carbs — 120g — 1 5-a-day

20 Cals | **1g** Prot | **0g** Fat | **0g** SatFat | **3g** Fibre

7g Carbs — 120g — 1 5-a-day

35 Cals | **1g** Prot | **1g** Fat | **0g** SatFat | **3g** Fibre

Cauliflower (boiled)

Celery

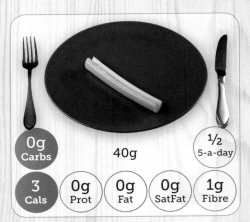

Cauliflower (boiled)

1g Carbs
40g
½ 5-a-day
12 Cals | 1g Prot | 0g Fat | 0g SatFat | 1g Fibre

0g Carbs
40g
½ 5-a-day
3 Cals | 0g Prot | 0g Fat | 0g SatFat | 1g Fibre

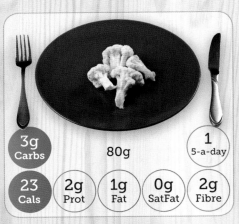

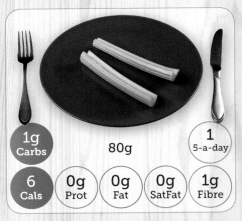

3g Carbs
80g
1 5-a-day
23 Cals | 2g Prot | 1g Fat | 0g SatFat | 2g Fibre

1g Carbs
80g
1 5-a-day
6 Cals | 0g Prot | 0g Fat | 0g SatFat | 1g Fibre

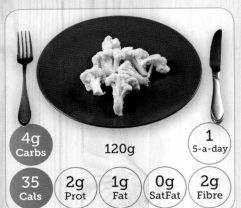

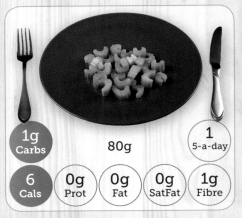

4g Carbs
120g
1 5-a-day
35 Cals | 2g Prot | 1g Fat | 0g SatFat | 2g Fibre

1g Carbs
80g
1 5-a-day
6 Cals | 0g Prot | 0g Fat | 0g SatFat | 1g Fibre

Cherry Tomatoes

Chickpeas (tinned)

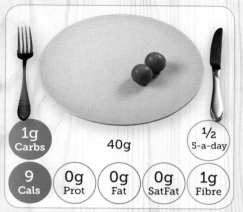

1g Carbs

40g

½ 5-a-day

9 Cals

0g Prot

0g Fat

0g SatFat

1g Fibre

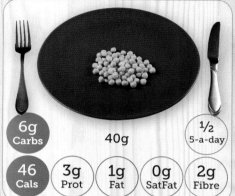

6g Carbs

40g

½ 5-a-day

46 Cals

3g Prot

1g Fat

0g SatFat

2g Fibre

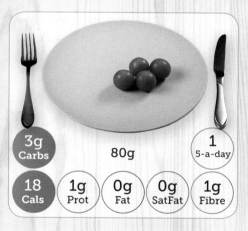

3g Carbs

80g

1 5-a-day

18 Cals

1g Prot

0g Fat

0g SatFat

1g Fibre

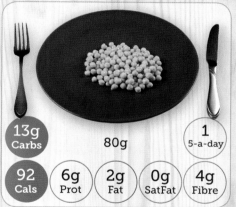

13g Carbs

80g

1 5-a-day

92 Cals

6g Prot

2g Fat

0g SatFat

4g Fibre

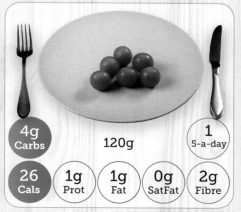

4g Carbs

120g

1 5-a-day

26 Cals

1g Prot

1g Fat

0g SatFat

2g Fibre

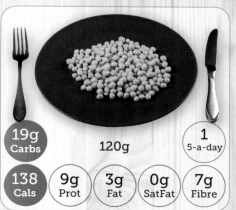

19g Carbs

120g

1 5-a-day

138 Cals

9g Prot

3g Fat

0g SatFat

7g Fibre

Courgette (boiled)

Cucumber

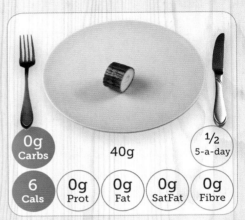

Courgette 40g:
- 1g Carbs
- 40g
- ½ 5-a-day
- 8 Cals
- 1g Prot
- 0g Fat
- 0g SatFat
- 1g Fibre

Cucumber 40g:
- 0g Carbs
- 40g
- ½ 5-a-day
- 6 Cals
- 0g Prot
- 0g Fat
- 0g SatFat
- 0g Fibre

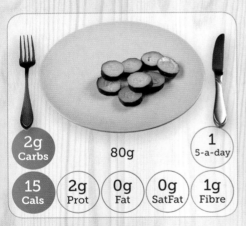
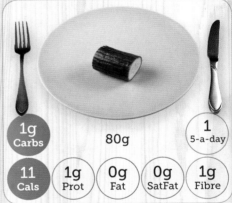

Courgette 80g:
- 2g Carbs
- 80g
- 1 5-a-day
- 15 Cals
- 2g Prot
- 0g Fat
- 0g SatFat
- 1g Fibre

Cucumber 80g:
- 1g Carbs
- 80g
- 1 5-a-day
- 11 Cals
- 1g Prot
- 0g Fat
- 0g SatFat
- 1g Fibre

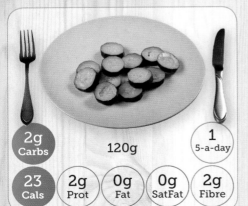
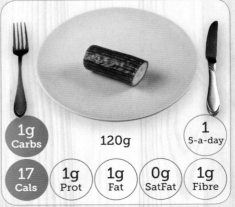

Courgette 120g:
- 2g Carbs
- 120g
- 1 5-a-day
- 23 Cals
- 2g Prot
- 0g Fat
- 0g SatFat
- 2g Fibre

Cucumber 120g:
- 1g Carbs
- 120g
- 1 5-a-day
- 17 Cals
- 1g Prot
- 1g Fat
- 0g SatFat
- 1g Fibre

Edamame Beans

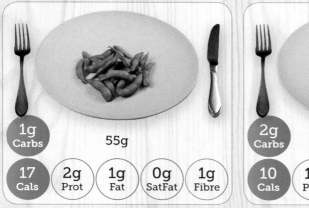

1g Carbs
55g
17 Cals | 2g Prot | 1g Fat | 0g SatFat | 1g Fibre

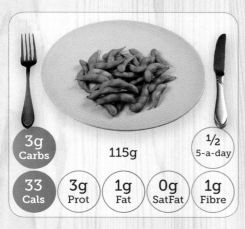

3g Carbs
115g
½ 5-a-day
33 Cals | 3g Prot | 1g Fat | 0g SatFat | 1g Fibre

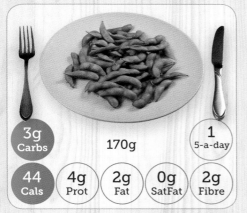

3g Carbs
170g
1 5-a-day
44 Cals | 4g Prot | 2g Fat | 0g SatFat | 2g Fibre

Green Beans (boiled)

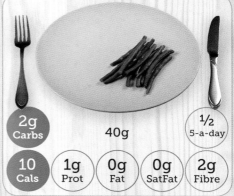

2g Carbs
40g
½ 5-a-day
10 Cals | 1g Prot | 0g Fat | 0g SatFat | 2g Fibre

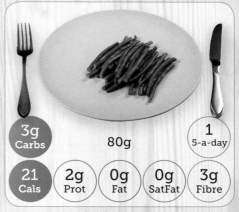

3g Carbs
80g
1 5-a-day
21 Cals | 2g Prot | 0g Fat | 0g SatFat | 3g Fibre

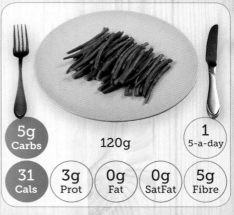

5g Carbs
120g
1 5-a-day
31 Cals | 3g Prot | 0g Fat | 0g SatFat | 5g Fibre

26cm Dinner Plate

Kidney Beans (tinned)

Leek (boiled)

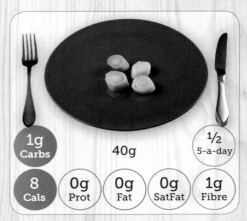

6g Carbs — 40g — ½ 5-a-day

37 Cals | **3g** Prot | **0g** Fat | **0g** SatFat | **3g** Fibre

1g Carbs — 40g — ½ 5-a-day

8 Cals | **0g** Prot | **0g** Fat | **0g** SatFat | **1g** Fibre

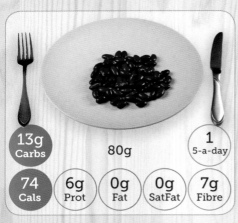
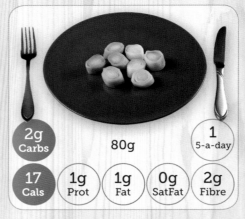

13g Carbs — 80g — 1 5-a-day

74 Cals | **6g** Prot | **0g** Fat | **0g** SatFat | **7g** Fibre

2g Carbs — 80g — 1 5-a-day

17 Cals | **1g** Prot | **1g** Fat | **0g** SatFat | **2g** Fibre

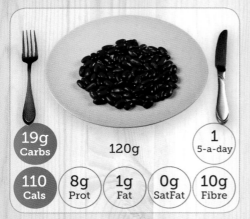
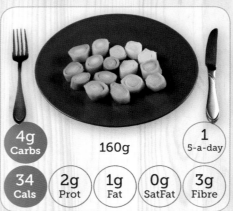

19g Carbs — 120g — 1 5-a-day

110 Cals | **8g** Prot | **1g** Fat | **0g** SatFat | **10g** Fibre

4g Carbs — 160g — 1 5-a-day

34 Cals | **2g** Prot | **1g** Fat | **0g** SatFat | **3g** Fibre

Lentils (tinned)

Lettuce

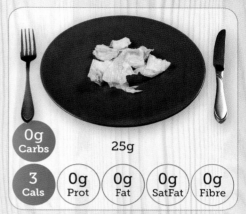

7g Carbs — 40g — ½ 5-a-day

41 Cals | **3g** Prot | **0g** Fat | **0g** SatFat | **1g** Fibre

0g Carbs — 25g

3 Cals | **0g** Prot | **0g** Fat | **0g** SatFat | **0g** Fibre

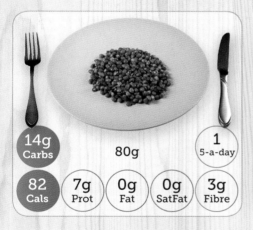
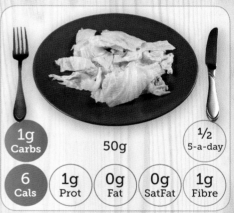

14g Carbs — 80g — 1 5-a-day

82 Cals | **7g** Prot | **0g** Fat | **0g** SatFat | **3g** Fibre

1g Carbs — 50g — ½ 5-a-day

6 Cals | **1g** Prot | **0g** Fat | **0g** SatFat | **1g** Fibre

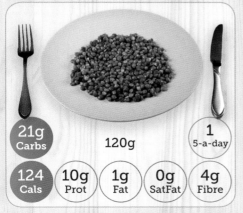
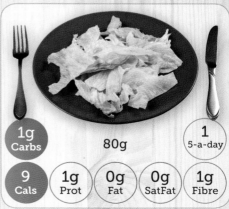

21g Carbs — 120g — 1 5-a-day

124 Cals | **10g** Prot | **1g** Fat | **0g** SatFat | **4g** Fibre

1g Carbs — 80g — 1 5-a-day

9 Cals | **1g** Prot | **0g** Fat | **0g** SatFat | **1g** Fibre

Mangetout (raw)   Mixed Salad Leaves

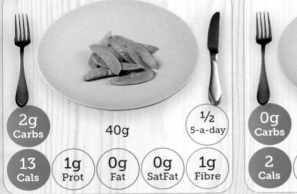

2g Carbs — 40g — ½ 5-a-day
13 Cals — 1g Prot — 0g Fat — 0g SatFat — 1g Fibre

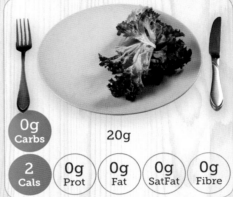

0g Carbs — 20g
2 Cals — 0g Prot — 0g Fat — 0g SatFat — 0g Fibre

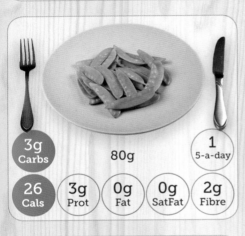

3g Carbs — 80g — 1 5-a-day
26 Cals — 3g Prot — 0g Fat — 0g SatFat — 2g Fibre

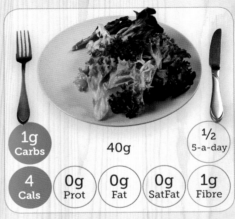

1g Carbs — 40g — ½ 5-a-day
4 Cals — 0g Prot — 0g Fat — 0g SatFat — 1g Fibre

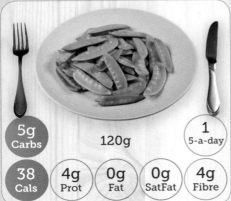

5g Carbs — 120g — 1 5-a-day
38 Cals — 4g Prot — 0g Fat — 0g SatFat — 4g Fibre

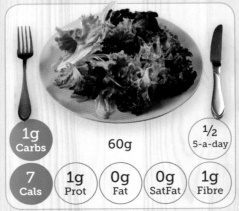

1g Carbs — 60g — ½ 5-a-day
7 Cals — 1g Prot — 0g Fat — 0g SatFat — 1g Fibre

Mushrooms (raw)

Mushrooms (fried in butter)

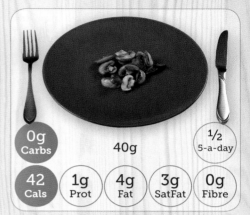

Mushrooms (raw) — 40g

0g Carbs | 40g | ½ 5-a-day
3 Cals | 0g Prot | 0g Fat | 0g SatFat | 0g Fibre

Mushrooms (fried in butter) — 40g

0g Carbs | 40g | ½ 5-a-day
42 Cals | 1g Prot | 4g Fat | 3g SatFat | 0g Fibre

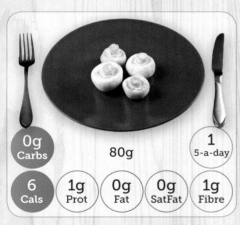

Mushrooms (raw) — 80g

0g Carbs | 80g | 1 5-a-day
6 Cals | 1g Prot | 0g Fat | 0g SatFat | 1g Fibre

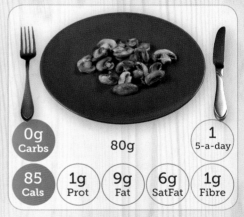

Mushrooms (fried in butter) — 80g

0g Carbs | 80g | 1 5-a-day
85 Cals | 1g Prot | 9g Fat | 6g SatFat | 1g Fibre

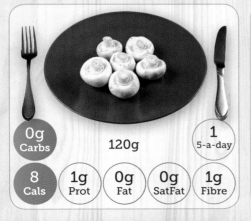

Mushrooms (raw) — 120g

0g Carbs | 120g | 1 5-a-day
8 Cals | 1g Prot | 0g Fat | 0g SatFat | 1g Fibre

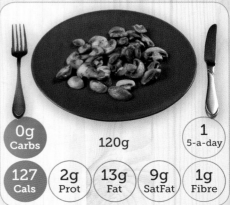

Mushrooms (fried in butter) — 120g

0g Carbs | 120g | 1 5-a-day
127 Cals | 2g Prot | 13g Fat | 9g SatFat | 1g Fibre

26cm Dinner Plate

Onions (raw)

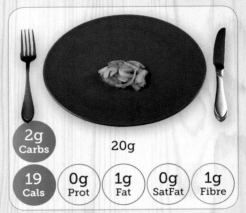

Onions (fried in oil)

Onions (raw) — 40g

3g Carbs · ½ 5-a-day · 14 Cals · 0g Prot · 0g Fat · 0g SatFat · 1g Fibre

Onions (fried in oil) — 20g

2g Carbs · 19 Cals · 0g Prot · 1g Fat · 0g SatFat · 1g Fibre

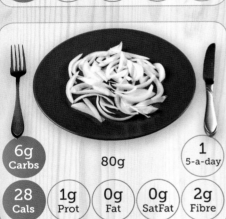

Onions (raw) — 80g

6g Carbs · 1 5-a-day · 28 Cals · 1g Prot · 0g Fat · 0g SatFat · 2g Fibre

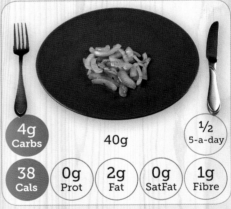

Onions (fried in oil) — 40g

4g Carbs · ½ 5-a-day · 38 Cals · 0g Prot · 2g Fat · 0g SatFat · 1g Fibre

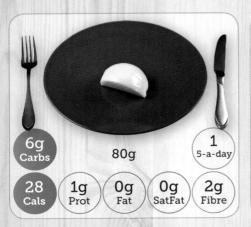

Onions (raw) — 80g

6g Carbs · 1 5-a-day · 28 Cals · 1g Prot · 0g Fat · 0g SatFat · 2g Fibre

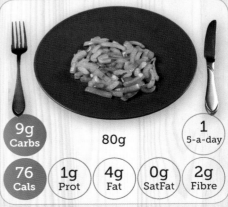

Onions (fried in oil) — 80g

9g Carbs · 1 5-a-day · 76 Cals · 1g Prot · 4g Fat · 0g SatFat · 2g Fibre

Okra (boiled)

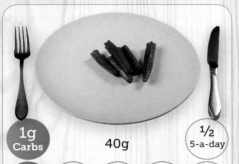

1g Carbs — 40g — ½ 5-a-day

11 Cals | 1g Prot | 0g Fat | 0g SatFat | 2g Fibre

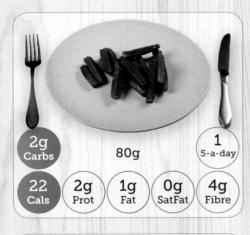

2g Carbs — 80g — 1 5-a-day

22 Cals | 2g Prot | 1g Fat | 0g SatFat | 4g Fibre

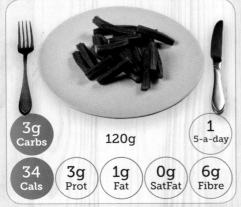

3g Carbs — 120g — 1 5-a-day

34 Cals | 3g Prot | 1g Fat | 0g SatFat | 6g Fibre

Pak Choi (boiled)

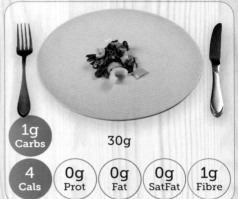

1g Carbs — 30g

4 Cals | 0g Prot | 0g Fat | 0g SatFat | 1g Fibre

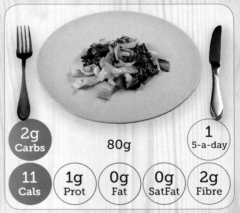

2g Carbs — 80g — 1 5-a-day

11 Cals | 1g Prot | 0g Fat | 0g SatFat | 2g Fibre

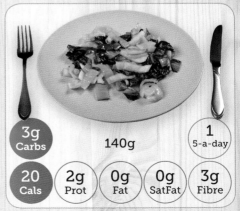

3g Carbs — 140g — 1 5-a-day

20 Cals | 2g Prot | 0g Fat | 0g SatFat | 3g Fibre

26cm Dinner Plate

Peas

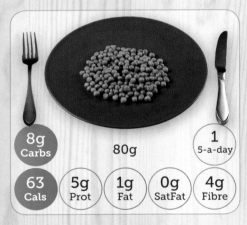

4g Carbs

40g

½ 5-a-day

32 Cals | 3g Prot | 1g Fat | 0g SatFat | 2g Fibre

Mushy Peas

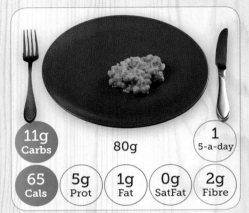

11g Carbs

80g

1 5-a-day

65 Cals | 5g Prot | 1g Fat | 0g SatFat | 2g Fibre

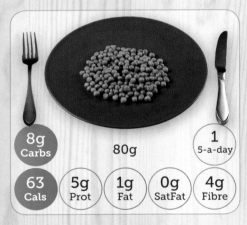

8g Carbs

80g

1 5-a-day

63 Cals | 5g Prot | 1g Fat | 0g SatFat | 4g Fibre

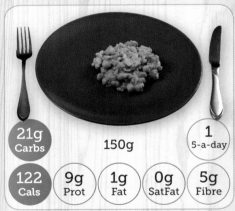

21g Carbs

150g

1 5-a-day

122 Cals | 9g Prot | 1g Fat | 0g SatFat | 5g Fibre

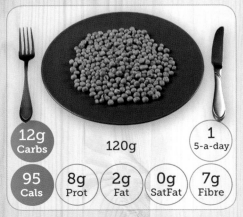

12g Carbs

120g

1 5-a-day

95 Cals | 8g Prot | 2g Fat | 0g SatFat | 7g Fibre

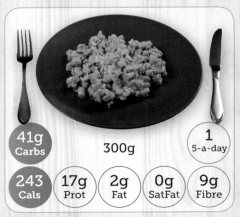

41g Carbs

300g

1 5-a-day

243 Cals | 17g Prot | 2g Fat | 0g SatFat | 9g Fibre

Parsnips (roasted)

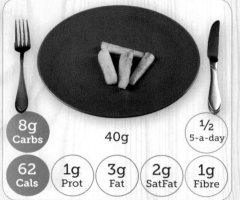

8g Carbs — 40g — ½ 5-a-day

62 Cals | 1g Prot | 3g Fat | 2g SatFat | 1g Fibre

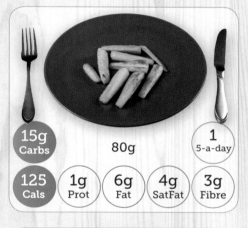

15g Carbs — 80g — 1 5-a-day

125 Cals | 1g Prot | 6g Fat | 4g SatFat | 3g Fibre

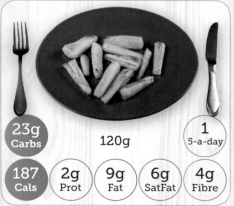

23g Carbs — 120g — 1 5-a-day

187 Cals | 2g Prot | 9g Fat | 6g SatFat | 4g Fibre

Peppers (raw)

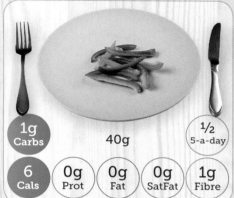

1g Carbs — 40g — ½ 5-a-day

6 Cals | 0g Prot | 0g Fat | 0g SatFat | 1g Fibre

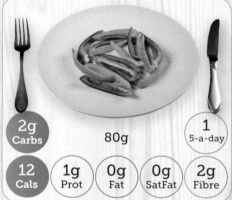

2g Carbs — 80g — 1 5-a-day

12 Cals | 1g Prot | 0g Fat | 0g SatFat | 2g Fibre

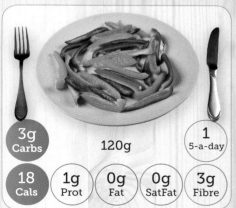

3g Carbs — 120g — 1 5-a-day

18 Cals | 1g Prot | 0g Fat | 0g SatFat | 3g Fibre

Plantain (boiled)

Plantain (fried)

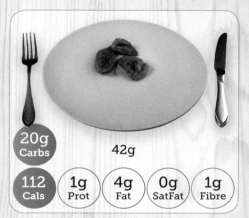

Plantain (boiled) — 40g

11g Carbs
45 Cals
0g Prot
0g Fat
0g SatFat
1g Fibre

Plantain (fried) — 42g

20g Carbs
112 Cals
1g Prot
4g Fat
0g SatFat
1g Fibre

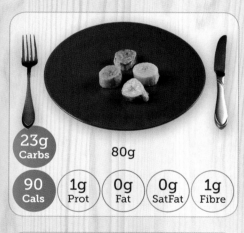

Plantain (boiled) — 80g

23g Carbs
90 Cals
1g Prot
0g Fat
0g SatFat
1g Fibre

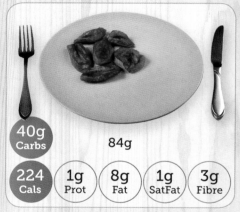

Plantain (fried) — 84g

40g Carbs
224 Cals
1g Prot
8g Fat
1g SatFat
3g Fibre

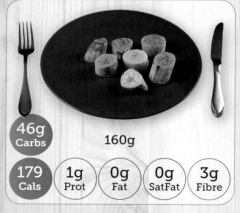

Plantain (boiled) — 160g

46g Carbs
179 Cals
1g Prot
0g Fat
0g SatFat
3g Fibre

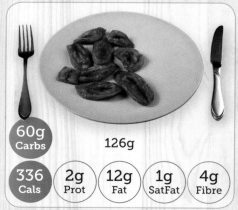

Plantain (fried) — 126g

60g Carbs
336 Cals
2g Prot
12g Fat
1g SatFat
4g Fibre

Radishes

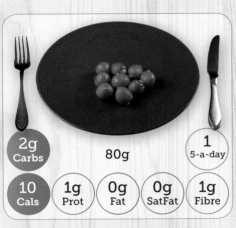

1g Carbs — 40g — ½ 5-a-day

5 Cals | 0g Prot | 0g Fat | 0g SatFat | 0g Fibre

2g Carbs — 80g — 1 5-a-day

10 Cals | 1g Prot | 0g Fat | 0g SatFat | 1g Fibre

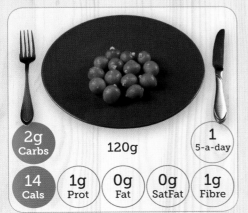

2g Carbs — 120g — 1 5-a-day

14 Cals | 1g Prot | 0g Fat | 0g SatFat | 1g Fibre

Rocket

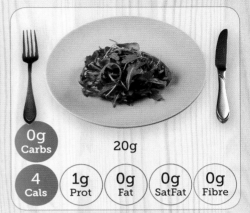

0g Carbs — 20g

4 Cals | 1g Prot | 0g Fat | 0g SatFat | 0g Fibre

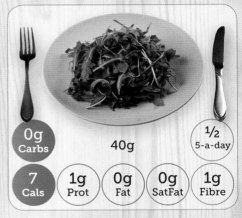

0g Carbs — 40g — ½ 5-a-day

7 Cals | 1g Prot | 0g Fat | 0g SatFat | 1g Fibre

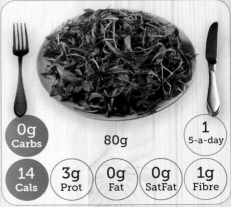

0g Carbs — 80g — 1 5-a-day

14 Cals | 3g Prot | 0g Fat | 0g SatFat | 1g Fibre

Spinach (boiled)

Spring Greens (boiled)

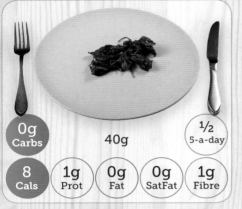

0g Carbs	40g	½ 5-a-day

8 Cals	1g Prot	0g Fat	0g SatFat	1g Fibre

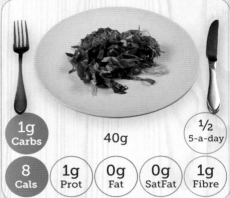

1g Carbs	40g	½ 5-a-day

8 Cals	1g Prot	0g Fat	0g SatFat	1g Fibre

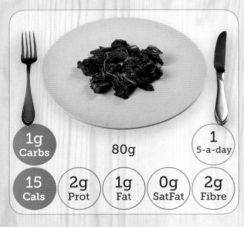

1g Carbs	80g	1 5-a-day

15 Cals	2g Prot	1g Fat	0g SatFat	2g Fibre

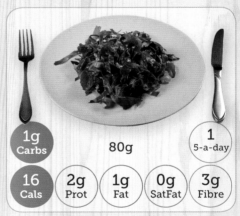

1g Carbs	80g	1 5-a-day

16 Cals	2g Prot	1g Fat	0g SatFat	3g Fibre

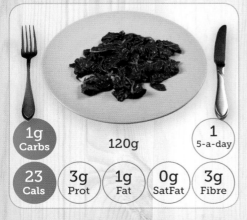

1g Carbs	120g	1 5-a-day

23 Cals	3g Prot	1g Fat	0g SatFat	3g Fibre

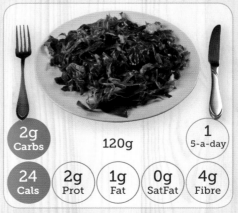

2g Carbs	120g	1 5-a-day

24 Cals	2g Prot	1g Fat	0g SatFat	4g Fibre

Sweetcorn

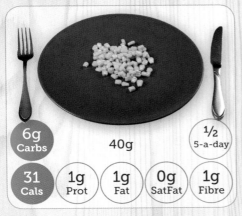

6g Carbs — 40g — ½ 5-a-day

31 Cals | 1g Prot | 1g Fat | 0g SatFat | 1g Fibre

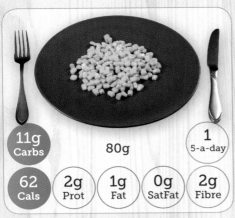

11g Carbs — 80g — 1 5-a-day

62 Cals | 2g Prot | 1g Fat | 0g SatFat | 2g Fibre

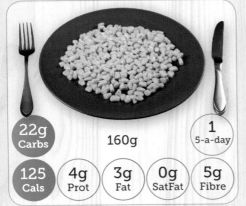

22g Carbs — 160g — 1 5-a-day

125 Cals | 4g Prot | 3g Fat | 0g SatFat | 5g Fibre

Corn on the Cob (boiled)

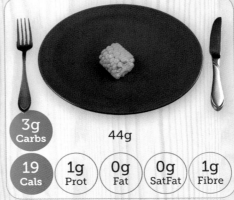

3g Carbs — 44g

19 Cals | 1g Prot | 0g Fat | 0g SatFat | 1g Fibre

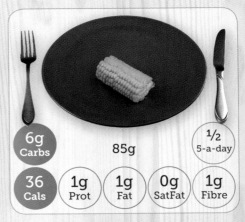

6g Carbs — 85g — ½ 5-a-day

36 Cals | 1g Prot | 1g Fat | 0g SatFat | 1g Fibre

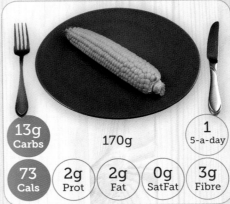

13g Carbs — 170g — 1 5-a-day

73 Cals | 2g Prot | 2g Fat | 0g SatFat | 3g Fibre

Sugar Snap Peas (boiled)

Tomato

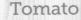

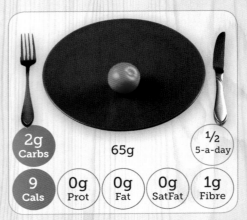

2g Carbs	40g	½ 5-a-day

13 Cals	1g Prot	0g Fat	0g SatFat	1g Fibre

2g Carbs	65g	½ 5-a-day

9 Cals	0g Prot	0g Fat	0g SatFat	1g Fibre

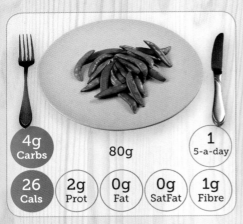

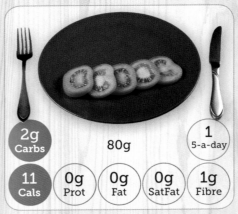

4g Carbs	80g	1 5-a-day

26 Cals	2g Prot	0g Fat	0g SatFat	1g Fibre

2g Carbs	80g	1 5-a-day

11 Cals	0g Prot	0g Fat	0g SatFat	1g Fibre

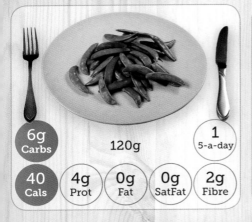

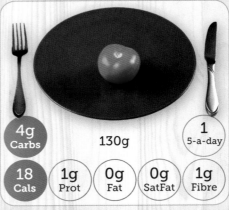

6g Carbs	120g	1 5-a-day

40 Cals	4g Prot	0g Fat	0g SatFat	2g Fibre

4g Carbs	130g	1 5-a-day

18 Cals	1g Prot	0g Fat	0g SatFat	1g Fibre

Turnip (boiled)

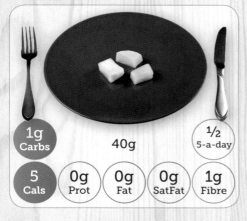

1g Carbs   40g   ½ 5-a-day

5 Cals | 0g Prot | 0g Fat | 0g SatFat | 1g Fibre

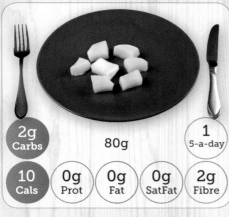

2g Carbs   80g   1 5-a-day

10 Cals | 0g Prot | 0g Fat | 0g SatFat | 2g Fibre

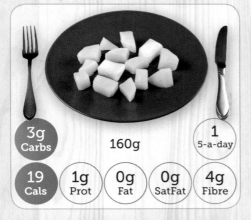

3g Carbs   160g   1 5-a-day

19 Cals | 1g Prot | 0g Fat | 0g SatFat | 4g Fibre

Watercress

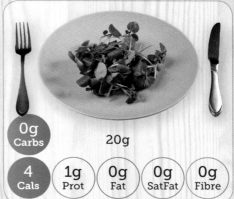

0g Carbs   20g

4 Cals | 1g Prot | 0g Fat | 0g SatFat | 0g Fibre

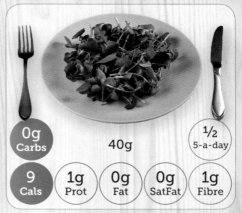

0g Carbs   40g   ½ 5-a-day

9 Cals | 1g Prot | 0g Fat | 0g SatFat | 1g Fibre

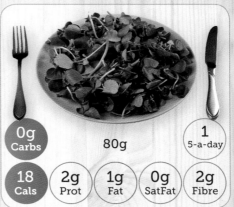

0g Carbs   80g   1 5-a-day

18 Cals | 2g Prot | 1g Fat | 0g SatFat | 2g Fibre

	Carbs	Cals	Prot	Fat	SatFat	Fibre
Beans & Pulses (per 100g weight)						
Aduki Beans (tinned)	23g	123	9g	0g	0g	7g
Black Eye Beans (tinned)	20g	116	9g	1g	0g	5g
Broad Beans (tinned)	13g	87	8g	1g	0g	7g
Chickpeas (tinned)	16g	115	7g	3g	0g	6g
Haricot Beans (tinned)	17g	95	7g	1g	0g	8g
Kidney Beans (tinned)	16g	92	7g	1g	0g	8g
Lentils (tinned)	17g	103	8g	1g	0g	3g
Lentils, Red Split (dried)	54g	315	24g	1g	0g	5g
Lentils, Green (dried)	50g	301	23g	2g	0g	10g
Lentils, Puy (dried)	58g	345	24g	2g	0g	20g
Mung Beans (dried)	46g	279	24g	1g	0g	10g
Pinto Beans (tinned)	24g	137	9g	1g	0g	6g
Soya Beans	5g	141	14g	7g	1g	8g
Vegetables RAW (per 100g weight)						
Artichokes (tinned)	5g	28	2g	0g	0g	2g
Asparagus	2g	25	3g	1g	0g	2g
Aubergine	2g	15	1g	0g	0g	3g
Beetroot	8g	36	2g	0g	0g	3g
Broccoli	3g	34	4g	1g	0g	4g
Brussels Sprouts	4g	42	4g	1g	0g	6g
Butternut Squash	8g	36	1g	0g	0g	2g
Cabbage, Green	4g	27	2g	0g	0g	4g
Cabbage, Red	4g	21	1g	0g	0g	3g
Carrots	8g	34	1g	0g	0g	4g
Cauliflower	4g	30	3g	0g	0g	2g
Celeriac	2g	18	1g	0g	0g	5g
Celery	1g	7	1g	0g	0g	1g
Courgette	2g	18	2g	0g	0g	1g
Cucumber	1g	14	1g	1g	0g	1g

	Carbs	Cals	Prot	Fat	SatFat	Fibre
Fennel	2g	2	1g	0g	0g	3g
Garlic	16g	98	8g	1g	0g	6g
Ginger	8g	44	2g	1g	0g	2g
Kale	1g	33	3g	2g	0g	4g
Leek	3g	22	2g	1g	0g	3g
Lettuce	1g	11	1g	0g	0g	2g
Lettuce, Lamb's	2g	14	1g	0g	0g	1g
Mangetout	4g	32	4g	0g	0g	3g
Marrow (flesh only)	2g	12	1g	0g	0g	1g
Mushrooms, Oyster	0g	8	2g	0g	0g	2g
Mushrooms, White	0g	7	1g	0g	0g	1g
Okra	3g	31	3g	1g	0g	5g
Onions	8g	35	1g	0g	0g	2g
Parsnip (peeled)	13g	64	2g	1g	0g	5g
Peas	11g	83	7g	2g	1g	5g
Pepper, Green	3g	15	1g	0g	0g	2g
Pepper, Red	4g	21	1g	0g	0g	2g
Plantain	29g	117	1g	0g	0g	2g
Pumpkin (flesh only)	2g	13	1g	0g	0g	1g
Radish Leaves	4g	33	4g	1g	0g	1g
Radishes	2g	12	1g	0g	0g	1g
Shallots	3g	20	2g	0g	0g	2g
Spinach	2g	25	3g	1g	0g	3g
Sugar Snap Peas	5g	34	3g	0g	0g	2g
Swede (flesh only)	5g	24	1g	0g	0g	3g
Sweetcorn	8g	60	3g	2g	0g	2g
Sweetcorn, On the Cob	5g	36	2g	1g	0g	1g
Tomato	3g	14	1g	0g	0g	1g
Tomato, Cherry	4g	22	1g	1g	0g	1g
Turnip (flesh only)	5g	23	1g	0g	0g	3g
Water Chestnuts	10g	46	1g	0g	0g	2g

26cm Dinner Plate

Quorn Chicken Pieces

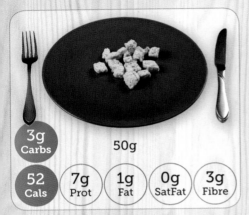

3g Carbs

50g

52 Cals | 7g Prot | 1g Fat | 0g SatFat | 3g Fibre

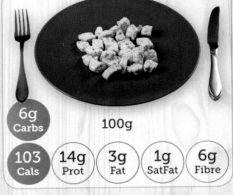

6g Carbs

100g

103 Cals | 14g Prot | 3g Fat | 1g SatFat | 6g Fibre

Quorn Burger (fried)

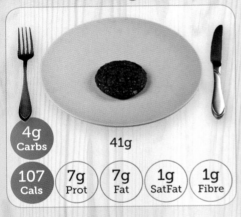

4g Carbs

41g

107 Cals | 7g Prot | 7g Fat | 1g SatFat | 1g Fibre

Quorn Burger (grilled)

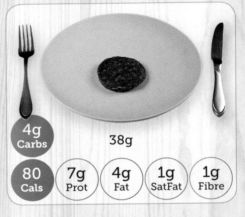

4g Carbs

38g

80 Cals | 7g Prot | 4g Fat | 1g SatFat | 1g Fibre

Quorn Sausage (fried)

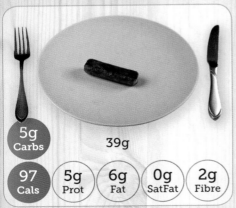

5g Carbs

39g

97 Cals | 5g Prot | 6g Fat | 0g SatFat | 2g Fibre

Quorn Sausage (grilled)

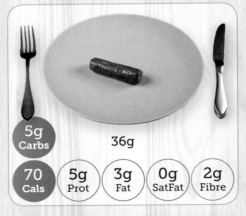

5g Carbs

36g

70 Cals | 5g Prot | 3g Fat | 0g SatFat | 2g Fibre

Tofu (fried)

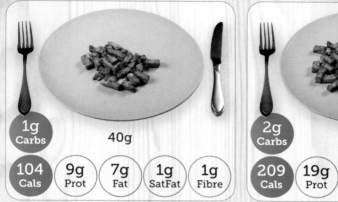

1g Carbs
40g

104 Cals | **9g** Prot | **7g** Fat | **1g** SatFat | **1g** Fibre

2g Carbs
80g

209 Cals | **19g** Prot | **14g** Fat | **2g** SatFat | **1g** Fibre

Veggie Burger (fried)

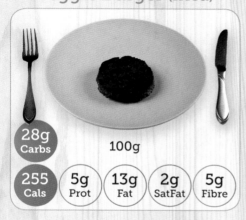

28g Carbs
100g

255 Cals | **5g** Prot | **13g** Fat | **2g** SatFat | **5g** Fibre

Veggie Burger (grilled)

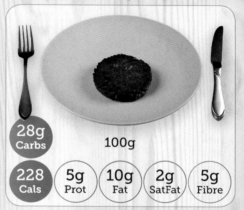

28g Carbs
100g

228 Cals | **5g** Prot | **10g** Fat | **2g** SatFat | **5g** Fibre

Veggie Sausage (fried)

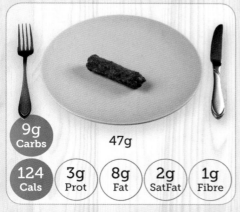

9g Carbs
47g

124 Cals | **3g** Prot | **8g** Fat | **2g** SatFat | **1g** Fibre

Veggie Sausage (grilled)

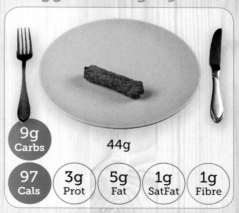

9g Carbs
44g

97 Cals | **3g** Prot | **5g** Fat | **1g** SatFat | **1g** Fibre

Fruit Yogurt

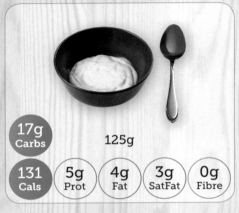

17g Carbs
125g

131 Cals | **5g** Prot | **4g** Fat | **3g** SatFat | **0g** Fibre

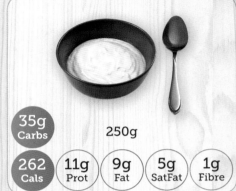

35g Carbs
250g

262 Cals | **11g** Prot | **9g** Fat | **5g** SatFat | **1g** Fibre

Fruit Yogurt (fat free)

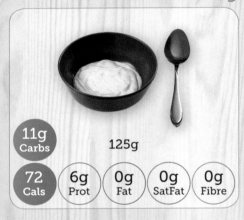

11g Carbs
125g

72 Cals | **6g** Prot | **0g** Fat | **0g** SatFat | **0g** Fibre

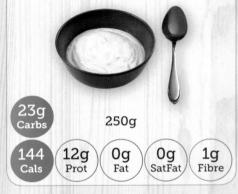

23g Carbs
250g

144 Cals | **12g** Prot | **0g** Fat | **0g** SatFat | **1g** Fibre

Fruit Yogurt Pot

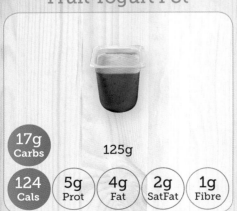

17g Carbs
125g

124 Cals | **5g** Prot | **4g** Fat | **2g** SatFat | **1g** Fibre

Fruit Yogurt Pot (fat free)

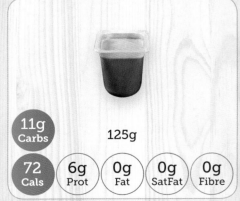

11g Carbs
125g

72 Cals | **6g** Prot | **0g** Fat | **0g** SatFat | **0g** Fibre

Greek Yogurt

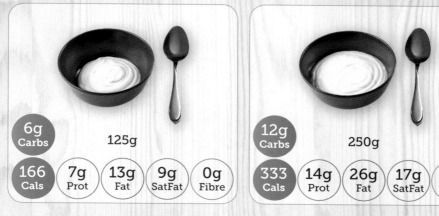

6g Carbs — 125g
166 Cals | **7g** Prot | **13g** Fat | **9g** SatFat | **0g** Fibre

12g Carbs — 250g
333 Cals | **14g** Prot | **26g** Fat | **17g** SatFat | **0g** Fibre

Greek Yogurt (low fat)

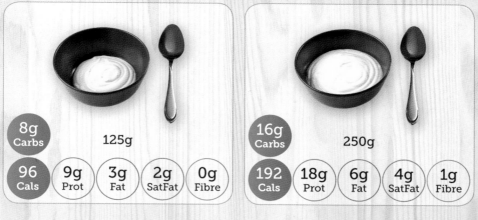

8g Carbs — 125g
96 Cals | **9g** Prot | **3g** Fat | **2g** SatFat | **0g** Fibre

16g Carbs — 250g
192 Cals | **18g** Prot | **6g** Fat | **4g** SatFat | **1g** Fibre

Soya Yogurt

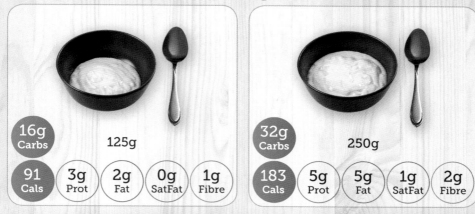

16g Carbs — 125g
91 Cals | **3g** Prot | **2g** Fat | **0g** SatFat | **1g** Fibre

32g Carbs — 250g
183 Cals | **5g** Prot | **5g** Fat | **1g** SatFat | **2g** Fibre

Natural Yogurt

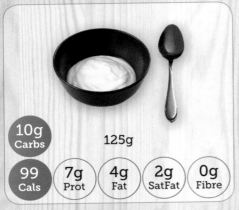

10g Carbs — 125g
99 Cals | **7g** Prot | **4g** Fat | **2g** SatFat | **0g** Fibre

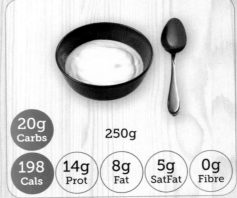

20g Carbs — 250g
198 Cals | **14g** Prot | **8g** Fat | **5g** SatFat | **0g** Fibre

Natural Yogurt (low fat)

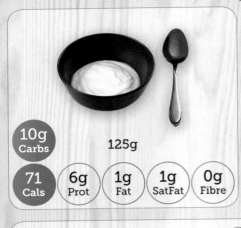

10g Carbs — 125g
71 Cals | **6g** Prot | **1g** Fat | **1g** SatFat | **0g** Fibre

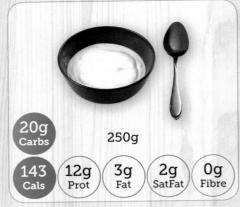

20g Carbs — 250g
143 Cals | **12g** Prot | **3g** Fat | **2g** SatFat | **0g** Fibre

Yogurt (per 100g weight)

	Carbs	Cals	Prot	Fat	SatFat	Fibre
Coconut	2g	55	4g	3g	1g	1g
Fruit	14g	105	4g	3g	2g	0g
Fruit (fat free)	9g	58	5g	0g	0g	0g
Greek	5g	133	6g	10g	7g	0g
Greek (low fat)	6g	77	7g	3g	2g	0g
Natural	8g	79	6g	3g	2g	0g
Natural (low fat)	8g	57	5g	1g	1g	0g
Soya	13g	73	2g	2g	0g	1g

Beef Burger (with cheese)

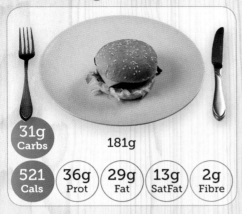

31g Carbs

181g

521 Cals | **36g** Prot | **29g** Fat | **13g** SatFat | **2g** Fibre

Chicken Burger

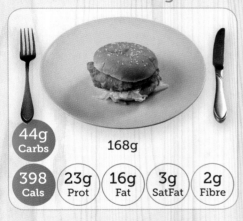

44g Carbs

168g

398 Cals | **23g** Prot | **16g** Fat | **3g** SatFat | **2g** Fibre

Veggie Burger

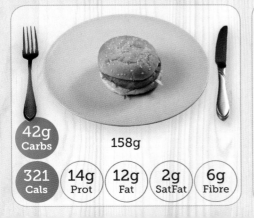

42g Carbs

158g

321 Cals | **14g** Prot | **12g** Fat | **2g** SatFat | **6g** Fibre

French Fries

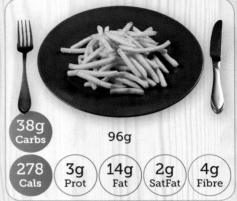

38g Carbs

96g

278 Cals | **3g** Prot | **14g** Fat | **2g** SatFat | **4g** Fibre

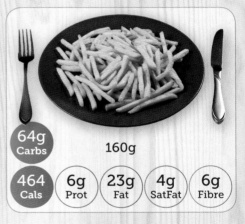

64g Carbs

160g

464 Cals | **6g** Prot | **23g** Fat | **4g** SatFat | **6g** Fibre

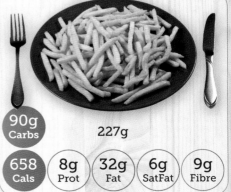

90g Carbs

227g

658 Cals | **8g** Prot | **32g** Fat | **6g** SatFat | **9g** Fibre

Chicken Nuggets

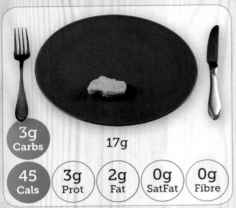

3g Carbs

17g

45 Cals | **3g** Prot | **2g** Fat | **0g** SatFat | **0g** Fibre

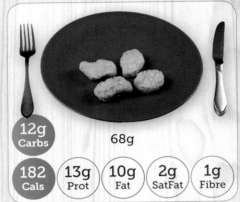

12g Carbs

68g

182 Cals | **13g** Prot | **10g** Fat | **2g** SatFat | **1g** Fibre

Fried Chicken (battered)

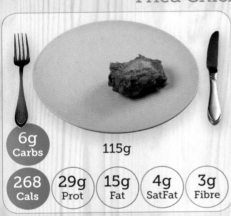

6g Carbs

115g

268 Cals | **29g** Prot | **15g** Fat | **4g** SatFat | **3g** Fibre

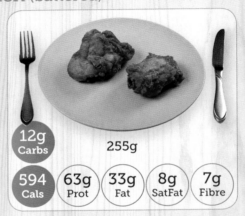

12g Carbs

255g

594 Cals | **63g** Prot | **33g** Fat | **8g** SatFat | **7g** Fibre

Hot Dog

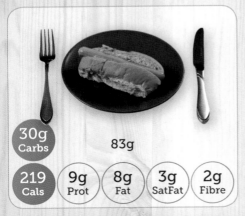

30g Carbs

83g

219 Cals | **9g** Prot | **8g** Fat | **3g** SatFat | **2g** Fibre

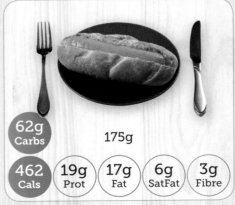

62g Carbs

175g

462 Cals | **19g** Prot | **17g** Fat | **6g** SatFat | **3g** Fibre

Doner Kebab

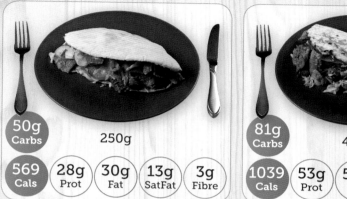

50g Carbs
250g
569 Cals | **28g** Prot | **30g** Fat | **13g** SatFat | **3g** Fibre

81g Carbs
415g
1039 Cals | **53g** Prot | **58g** Fat | **26g** SatFat | **5g** Fibre

Shish Kebab

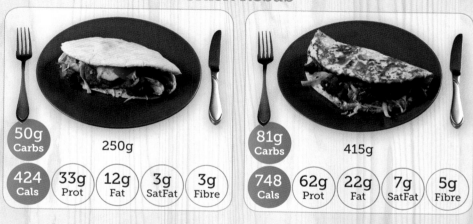

50g Carbs
250g
424 Cals | **33g** Prot | **12g** Fat | **3g** SatFat | **3g** Fibre

81g Carbs
415g
748 Cals | **62g** Prot | **22g** Fat | **7g** SatFat | **5g** Fibre

Falafel in Pitta

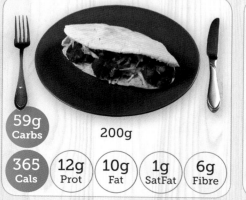
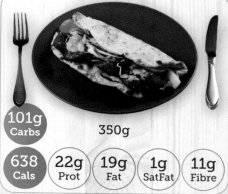

59g Carbs
200g
365 Cals | **12g** Prot | **10g** Fat | **1g** SatFat | **6g** Fibre

101g Carbs
350g
638 Cals | **22g** Prot | **19g** Fat | **1g** SatFat | **11g** Fibre

Fish

Chips

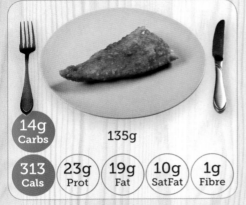

14g Carbs — 135g

313 Cals | **23g** Prot | **19g** Fat | **10g** SatFat | **1g** Fibre

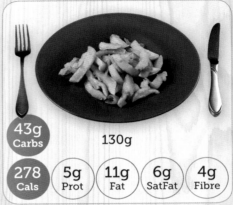

43g Carbs — 130g

278 Cals | **5g** Prot | **11g** Fat | **6g** SatFat | **4g** Fibre

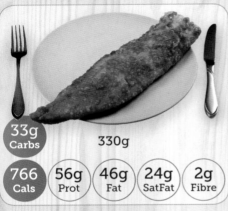

33g Carbs — 330g

766 Cals | **56g** Prot | **46g** Fat | **24g** SatFat | **2g** Fibre

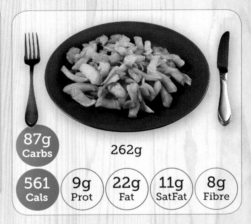

87g Carbs — 262g

561 Cals | **9g** Prot | **22g** Fat | **11g** SatFat | **8g** Fibre

Battered Sausage

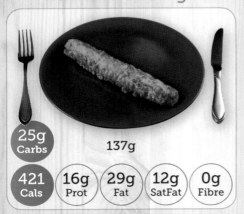

25g Carbs — 137g

421 Cals | **16g** Prot | **29g** Fat | **12g** SatFat | **0g** Fibre

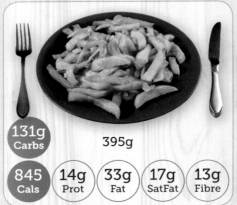

131g Carbs — 395g

845 Cals | **14g** Prot | **33g** Fat | **17g** SatFat | **13g** Fibre

Margherita Pizza (large, thin crust)

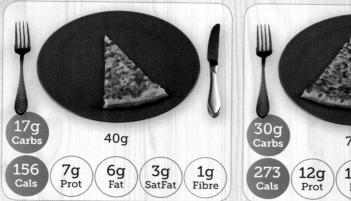

17g Carbs
40g

156 Cals | **7g** Prot | **6g** Fat | **3g** SatFat | **1g** Fibre

30g Carbs
70g

273 Cals | **12g** Prot | **11g** Fat | **5g** SatFat | **2g** Fibre

Pepperoni Pizza (large, thin crust)

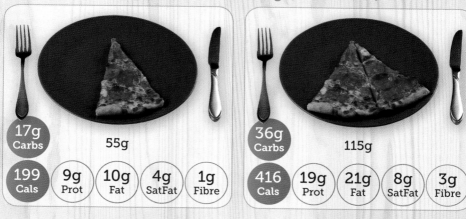

17g Carbs
55g

199 Cals | **9g** Prot | **10g** Fat | **4g** SatFat | **1g** Fibre

36g Carbs
115g

416 Cals | **19g** Prot | **21g** Fat | **8g** SatFat | **3g** Fibre

Vegetable Pizza (large, thin crust)

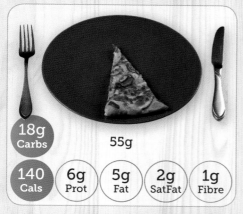
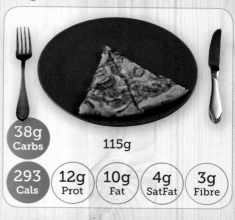

18g Carbs
55g

140 Cals | **6g** Prot | **5g** Fat | **2g** SatFat | **1g** Fibre

38g Carbs
115g

293 Cals | **12g** Prot | **10g** Fat | **4g** SatFat | **3g** Fibre

Margherita Pizza (large, deep pan)

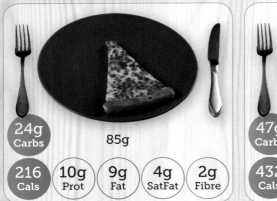

24g Carbs   85g

216 Cals | **10g** Prot | **9g** Fat | **4g** SatFat | **2g** Fibre

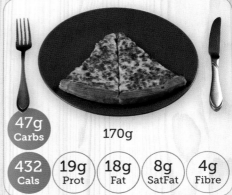

47g Carbs   170g

432 Cals | **19g** Prot | **18g** Fat | **8g** SatFat | **4g** Fibre

Pepperoni Pizza (large, deep pan)

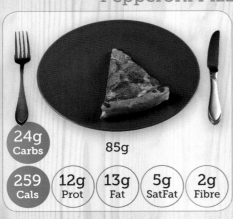

24g Carbs   85g

259 Cals | **12g** Prot | **13g** Fat | **5g** SatFat | **2g** Fibre

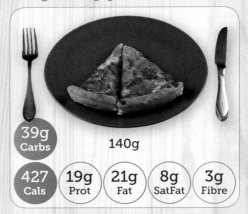

39g Carbs   140g

427 Cals | **19g** Prot | **21g** Fat | **8g** SatFat | **3g** Fibre

Vegetable Pizza (large, deep pan)

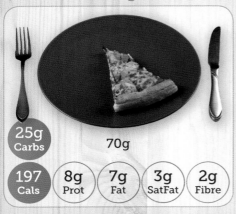

25g Carbs   70g

197 Cals | **8g** Prot | **7g** Fat | **3g** SatFat | **2g** Fibre

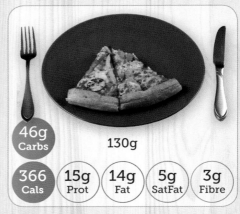

46g Carbs   130g

366 Cals | **15g** Prot | **14g** Fat | **5g** SatFat | **3g** Fibre

Margherita Pizza (large, stuffed crust)

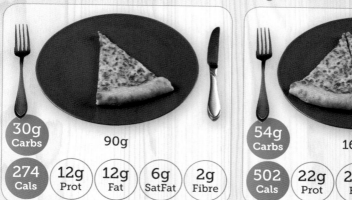

30g Carbs — 90g

274 Cals | **12g Prot** | **12g Fat** | **6g SatFat** | **2g Fibre**

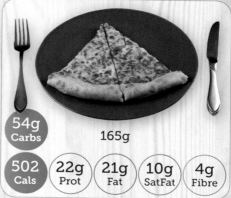

54g Carbs — 165g

502 Cals | **22g Prot** | **21g Fat** | **10g SatFat** | **4g Fibre**

Pepperoni Pizza (large, stuffed crust)

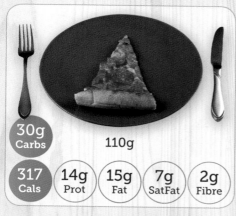

30g Carbs — 110g

317 Cals | **14g Prot** | **15g Fat** | **7g SatFat** | **2g Fibre**

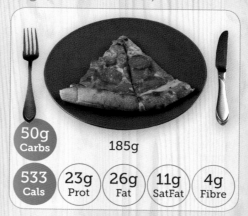

50g Carbs — 185g

533 Cals | **23g Prot** | **26g Fat** | **11g SatFat** | **4g Fibre**

Vegetable Pizza (large, stuffed crust)

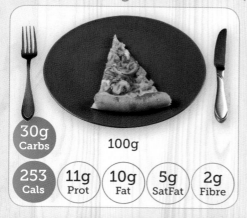

30g Carbs — 100g

253 Cals | **11g Prot** | **10g Fat** | **5g SatFat** | **2g Fibre**

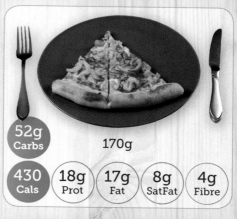

52g Carbs — 170g

430 Cals | **18g Prot** | **17g Fat** | **8g SatFat** | **4g Fibre**

26cm Dinner Plate / 22cm Large Bowl

Chicken Balls

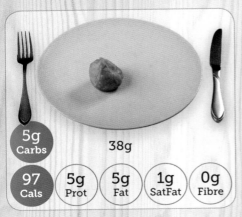

5g Carbs
38g

97 Cals | **5g** Prot | **5g** Fat | **1g** SatFat | **0g** Fibre

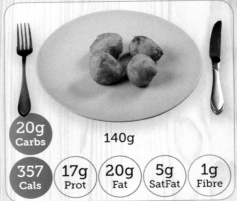

20g Carbs
140g

357 Cals | **17g** Prot | **20g** Fat | **5g** SatFat | **1g** Fibre

Duck Pancake

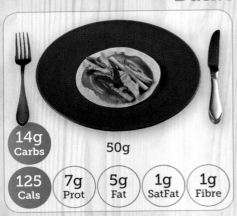

14g Carbs
50g

125 Cals | **7g** Prot | **5g** Fat | **1g** SatFat | **1g** Fibre

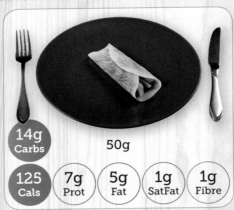

14g Carbs
50g

125 Cals | **7g** Prot | **5g** Fat | **1g** SatFat | **1g** Fibre

Prawn Crackers

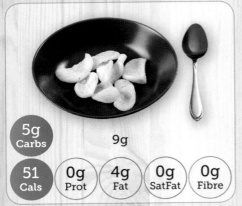

5g Carbs
9g

51 Cals | **0g** Prot | **4g** Fat | **0g** SatFat | **0g** Fibre

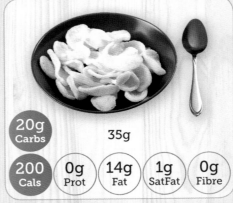

20g Carbs
35g

200 Cals | **0g** Prot | **14g** Fat | **1g** SatFat | **0g** Fibre

Prawn Toast

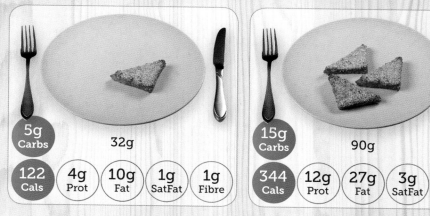

5g
Carbs

32g

122
Cals

4g
Prot

10g
Fat

1g
SatFat

1g
Fibre

15g
Carbs

90g

344
Cals

12g
Prot

27g
Fat

3g
SatFat

3g
Fibre

Spare Ribs

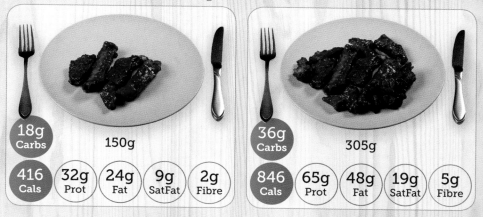

18g
Carbs

150g

416
Cals

32g
Prot

24g
Fat

9g
SatFat

2g
Fibre

36g
Carbs

305g

846
Cals

65g
Prot

48g
Fat

19g
SatFat

5g
Fibre

Spring Roll (meat)

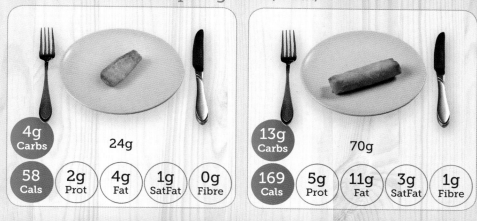

4g
Carbs

24g

58
Cals

2g
Prot

4g
Fat

1g
SatFat

0g
Fibre

13g
Carbs

70g

169
Cals

5g
Prot

11g
Fat

3g
SatFat

1g
Fibre

26cm Dinner Plate

Beef Chow Mein

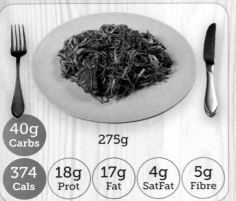

40g Carbs

275g

374 Cals | 18g Prot | 17g Fat | 4g SatFat | 5g Fibre

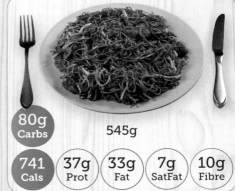

80g Carbs

545g

741 Cals | 37g Prot | 33g Fat | 7g SatFat | 10g Fibre

Beef in Black Bean Sauce

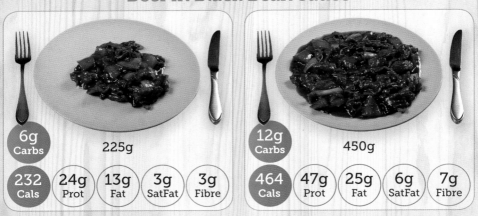

6g Carbs

225g

232 Cals | 24g Prot | 13g Fat | 3g SatFat | 3g Fibre

12g Carbs

450g

464 Cals | 47g Prot | 25g Fat | 6g SatFat | 7g Fibre

Chicken Curry

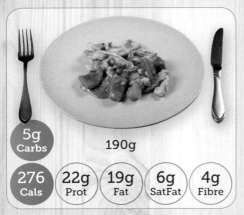

5g Carbs

190g

276 Cals | 22g Prot | 19g Fat | 6g SatFat | 4g Fibre

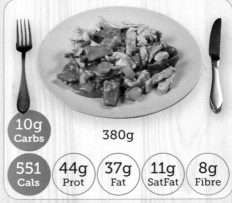

10g Carbs

380g

551 Cals | 44g Prot | 37g Fat | 11g SatFat | 8g Fibre

Crispy Shredded Beef

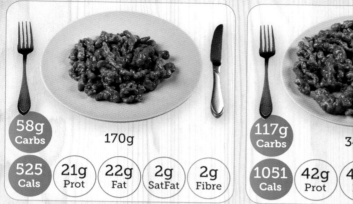

58g Carbs

170g

525 Cals | **21g** Prot | **22g** Fat | **2g** SatFat | **2g** Fibre

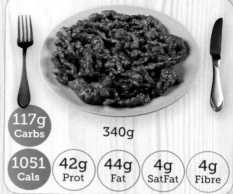

117g Carbs

340g

1051 Cals | **42g** Prot | **44g** Fat | **4g** SatFat | **4g** Fibre

Lemon Chicken

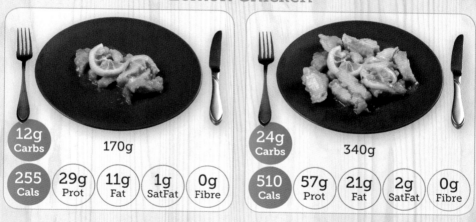

12g Carbs

170g

255 Cals | **29g** Prot | **11g** Fat | **1g** SatFat | **0g** Fibre

24g Carbs

340g

510 Cals | **57g** Prot | **21g** Fat | **2g** SatFat | **0g** Fibre

Roast Peking Duck

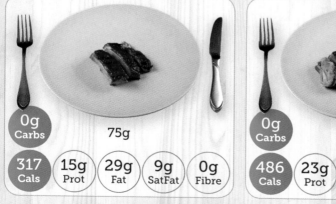

0g Carbs

75g

317 Cals | **15g** Prot | **29g** Fat | **9g** SatFat | **0g** Fibre

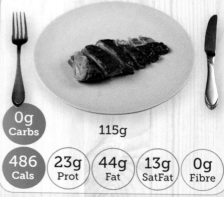

0g Carbs

115g

486 Cals | **23g** Prot | **44g** Fat | **13g** SatFat | **0g** Fibre

26cm Dinner Plate

Singapore Noodles

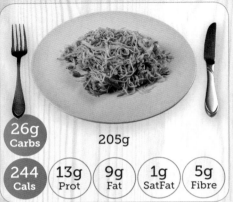

26g Carbs

205g

244 Cals | **13g** Prot | **9g** Fat | **1g** SatFat | **5g** Fibre

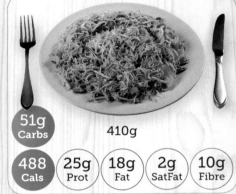

51g Carbs

410g

488 Cals | **25g** Prot | **18g** Fat | **2g** SatFat | **10g** Fibre

Sweet & Sour Pork

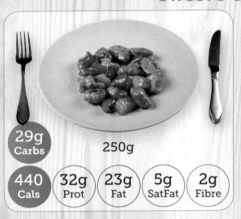

29g Carbs

250g

440 Cals | **32g** Prot | **23g** Fat | **5g** SatFat | **2g** Fibre

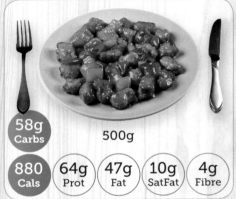

58g Carbs

500g

880 Cals | **64g** Prot | **47g** Fat | **10g** SatFat | **4g** Fibre

Szechuan Prawns

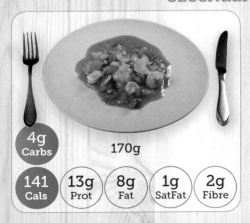

4g Carbs

170g

141 Cals | **13g** Prot | **8g** Fat | **1g** SatFat | **2g** Fibre

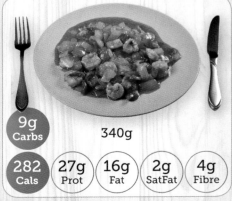

9g Carbs

340g

282 Cals | **27g** Prot | **16g** Fat | **2g** SatFat | **4g** Fibre

Miso Soup

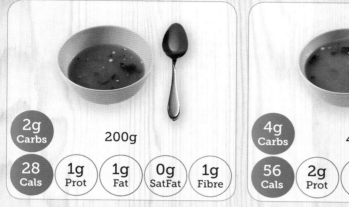

2g Carbs — 200g

28 Cals | **1g** Prot | **1g** Fat | **0g** SatFat | **1g** Fibre

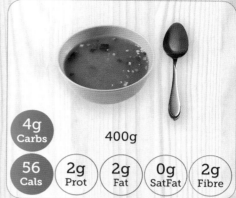

4g Carbs — 400g

56 Cals | **2g** Prot | **2g** Fat | **0g** SatFat | **2g** Fibre

Pork Gyoza

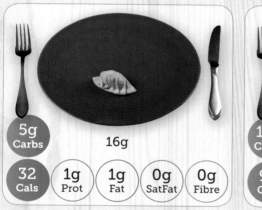

5g Carbs — 16g

32 Cals | **1g** Prot | **1g** Fat | **0g** SatFat | **0g** Fibre

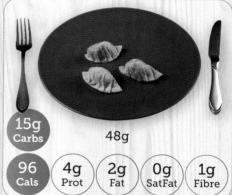

15g Carbs — 48g

96 Cals | **4g** Prot | **2g** Fat | **0g** SatFat | **1g** Fibre

Prawn Tempura

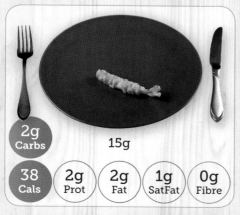

2g Carbs — 15g

38 Cals | **2g** Prot | **2g** Fat | **1g** SatFat | **0g** Fibre

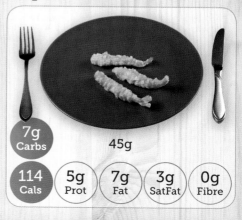

7g Carbs — 45g

114 Cals | **5g** Prot | **7g** Fat | **3g** SatFat | **0g** Fibre

26cm Dinner Plate

California Roll

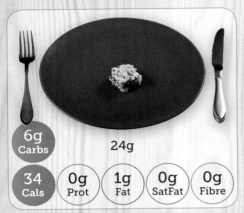

6g Carbs 24g

34 Cals | **0g** Prot | **1g** Fat | **0g** SatFat | **0g** Fibre

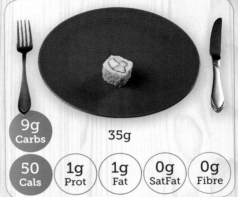

9g Carbs 35g

50 Cals | **1g** Prot | **1g** Fat | **0g** SatFat | **0g** Fibre

Prawn Maki

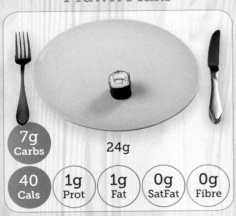

7g Carbs 24g

40 Cals | **1g** Prot | **1g** Fat | **0g** SatFat | **0g** Fibre

Prawn Nigiri

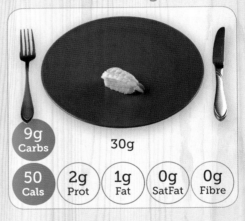

9g Carbs 30g

50 Cals | **2g** Prot | **1g** Fat | **0g** SatFat | **0g** Fibre

Salmon Nigiri

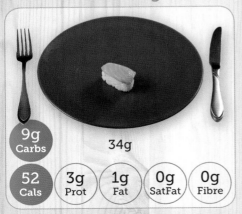

9g Carbs 34g

52 Cals | **3g** Prot | **1g** Fat | **0g** SatFat | **0g** Fibre

Tuna Nigiri

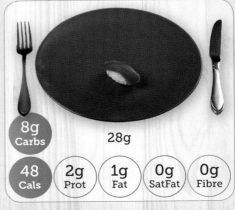

8g Carbs 28g

48 Cals | **2g** Prot | **1g** Fat | **0g** SatFat | **0g** Fibre

Mackerel Sashimi

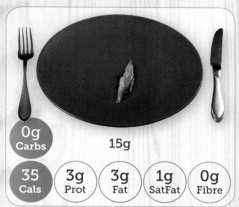

0g Carbs

15g

35 Cals | **3g** Prot | **3g** Fat | **1g** SatFat | **0g** Fibre

Salmon Sashimi

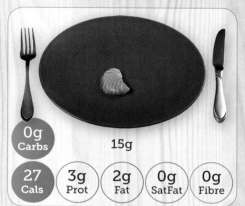

0g Carbs

15g

27 Cals | **3g** Prot | **2g** Fat | **0g** SatFat | **0g** Fibre

Tuna Sashimi

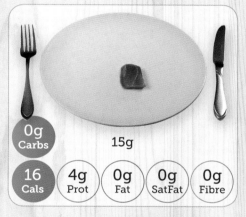

0g Carbs

15g

16 Cals | **4g** Prot | **0g** Fat | **0g** SatFat | **0g** Fibre

Rice Ball

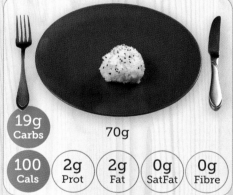

19g Carbs

70g

100 Cals | **2g** Prot | **2g** Fat | **0g** SatFat | **0g** Fibre

Chicken Teriyaki

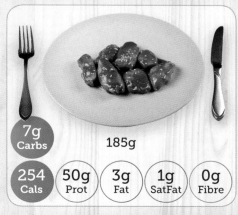

7g Carbs

185g

254 Cals | **50g** Prot | **3g** Fat | **1g** SatFat | **0g** Fibre

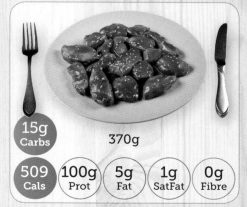

15g Carbs

370g

509 Cals | **100g** Prot | **5g** Fat | **1g** SatFat | **0g** Fibre

Onion Bhaji

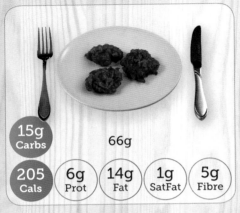

15g Carbs

66g

205 Cals | **6g** Prot | **14g** Fat | **1g** SatFat | **5g** Fibre

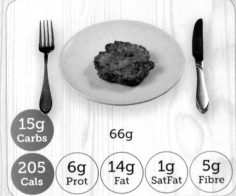

15g Carbs

66g

205 Cals | **6g** Prot | **14g** Fat | **1g** SatFat | **5g** Fibre

Lamb Samosa

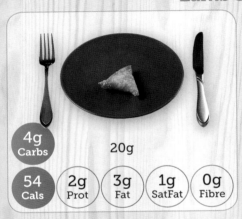

4g Carbs

20g

54 Cals | **2g** Prot | **3g** Fat | **1g** SatFat | **0g** Fibre

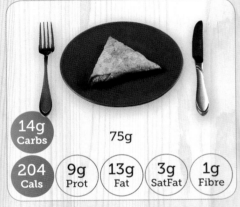

14g Carbs

75g

204 Cals | **9g** Prot | **13g** Fat | **3g** SatFat | **1g** Fibre

Vegetable Samosa

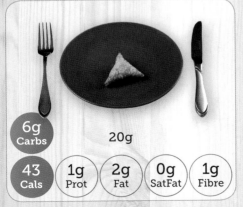

6g Carbs

20g

43 Cals | **1g** Prot | **2g** Fat | **0g** SatFat | **1g** Fibre

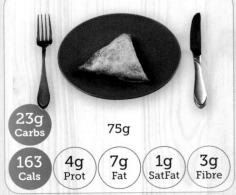

23g Carbs

75g

163 Cals | **4g** Prot | **7g** Fat | **1g** SatFat | **3g** Fibre

Vegetable Pakora

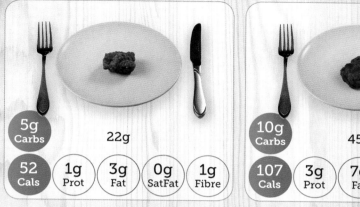
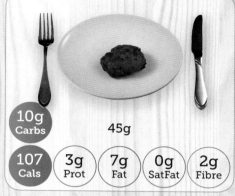

5g Carbs — 22g
52 Cals | **1g** Prot | **3g** Fat | **0g** SatFat | **1g** Fibre

10g Carbs — 45g
107 Cals | **3g** Prot | **7g** Fat | **0g** SatFat | **2g** Fibre

Bombay Potatoes

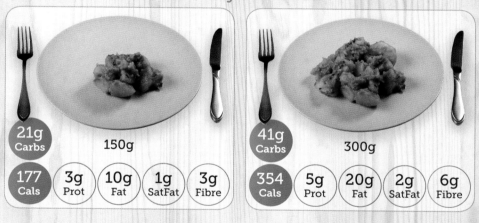

21g Carbs — 150g
177 Cals | **3g** Prot | **10g** Fat | **1g** SatFat | **3g** Fibre

41g Carbs — 300g
354 Cals | **5g** Prot | **20g** Fat | **2g** SatFat | **6g** Fibre

Sag Aloo Gobi

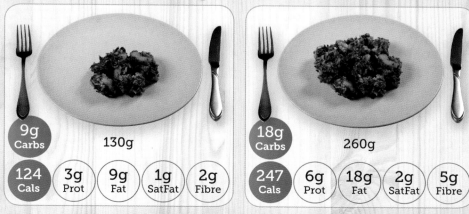

9g Carbs — 130g
124 Cals | **3g** Prot | **9g** Fat | **1g** SatFat | **2g** Fibre

18g Carbs — 260g
247 Cals | **6g** Prot | **18g** Fat | **2g** SatFat | **5g** Fibre

Chicken Korma

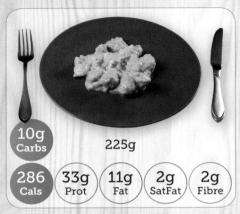

10g Carbs
225g

286 Cals | **33g** Prot | **11g** Fat | **2g** SatFat | **2g** Fibre

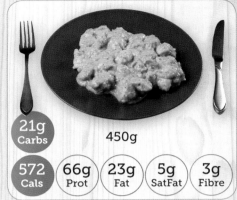

21g Carbs
450g

572 Cals | **66g** Prot | **23g** Fat | **5g** SatFat | **3g** Fibre

Chicken Tandoori

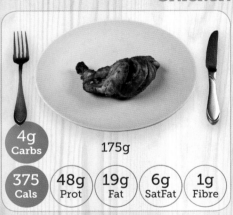

4g Carbs
175g

375 Cals | **48g** Prot | **19g** Fat | **6g** SatFat | **1g** Fibre

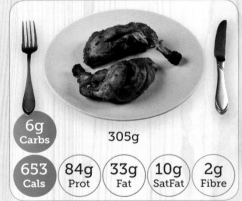

6g Carbs
305g

653 Cals | **84g** Prot | **33g** Fat | **10g** SatFat | **2g** Fibre

Chicken Tikka Masala

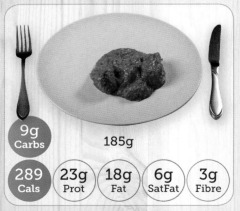

9g Carbs
185g

289 Cals | **23g** Prot | **18g** Fat | **6g** SatFat | **3g** Fibre

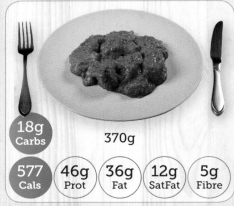

18g Carbs
370g

577 Cals | **46g** Prot | **36g** Fat | **12g** SatFat | **5g** Fibre

King Prawn Bhuna

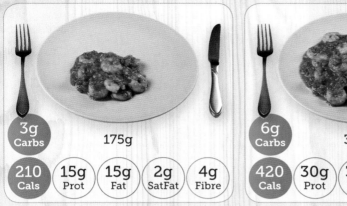

3g Carbs

175g

210 Cals | **15g** Prot | **15g** Fat | **2g** SatFat | **4g** Fibre

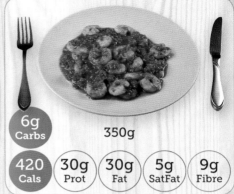

6g Carbs

350g

420 Cals | **30g** Prot | **30g** Fat | **5g** SatFat | **9g** Fibre

Lamb Biryani

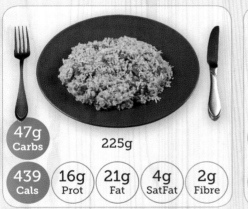

47g Carbs

225g

439 Cals | **16g** Prot | **21g** Fat | **4g** SatFat | **2g** Fibre

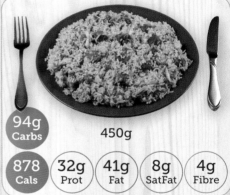

94g Carbs

450g

878 Cals | **32g** Prot | **41g** Fat | **8g** SatFat | **4g** Fibre

Lamb Rogan Josh

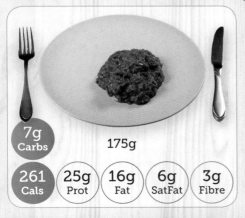

7g Carbs

175g

261 Cals | **25g** Prot | **16g** Fat | **6g** SatFat | **3g** Fibre

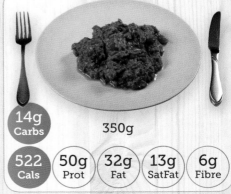

14g Carbs

350g

522 Cals | **50g** Prot | **32g** Fat | **13g** SatFat | **6g** Fibre

26cm Dinner Plate

Lentil Curry

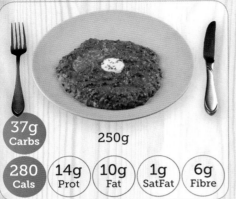

37g Carbs
250g
280 Cals | 14g Prot | 10g Fat | 1g SatFat | 6g Fibre

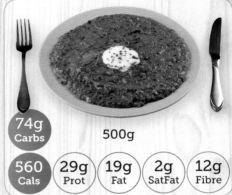

74g Carbs
500g
560 Cals | 29g Prot | 19g Fat | 2g SatFat | 12g Fibre

Vegetable Curry

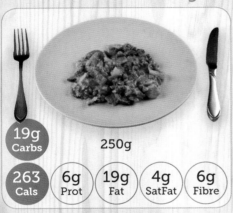

19g Carbs
250g
263 Cals | 6g Prot | 19g Fat | 4g SatFat | 6g Fibre

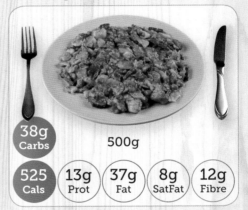

38g Carbs
500g
525 Cals | 13g Prot | 37g Fat | 8g SatFat | 12g Fibre

Beef Red Curry

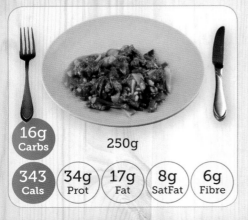

16g Carbs
250g
343 Cals | 34g Prot | 17g Fat | 8g SatFat | 6g Fibre

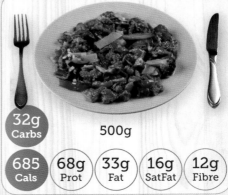

32g Carbs
500g
685 Cals | 68g Prot | 33g Fat | 16g SatFat | 12g Fibre

Chicken Green Curry

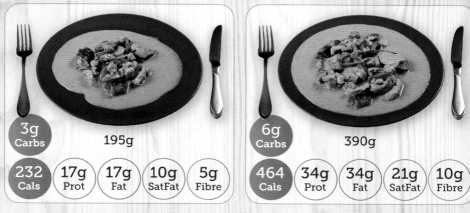

3g Carbs — 195g
232 Cals | **17g** Prot | **17g** Fat | **10g** SatFat | **5g** Fibre

6g Carbs — 390g
464 Cals | **34g** Prot | **34g** Fat | **21g** SatFat | **10g** Fibre

Beef Massaman Curry

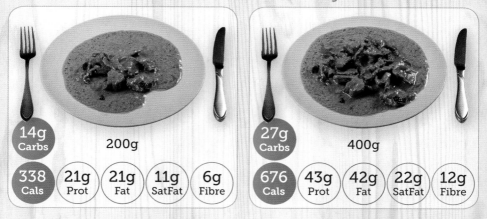

14g Carbs — 200g
338 Cals | **21g** Prot | **21g** Fat | **11g** SatFat | **6g** Fibre

27g Carbs — 400g
676 Cals | **43g** Prot | **42g** Fat | **22g** SatFat | **12g** Fibre

Prawn Pad Thai

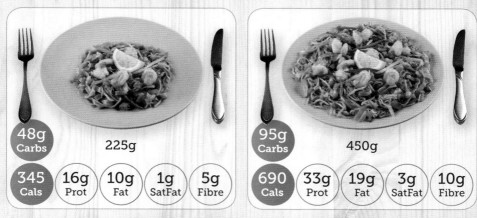

48g Carbs — 225g
345 Cals | **16g** Prot | **10g** Fat | **1g** SatFat | **5g** Fibre

95g Carbs — 450g
690 Cals | **33g** Prot | **19g** Fat | **3g** SatFat | **10g** Fibre

Chicken, Prawn & Pineapple Rice

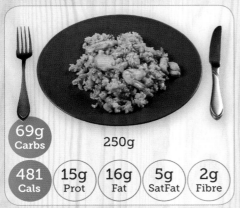

69g Carbs

250g

481 Cals | 15g Prot | 16g Fat | 5g SatFat | 2g Fibre

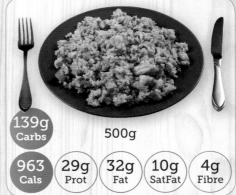

139g Carbs

500g

963 Cals | 29g Prot | 32g Fat | 10g SatFat | 4g Fibre

Chicken Satay

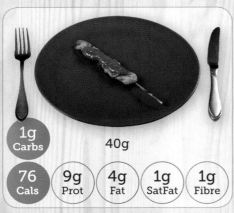

1g Carbs

40g

76 Cals | 9g Prot | 4g Fat | 1g SatFat | 1g Fibre

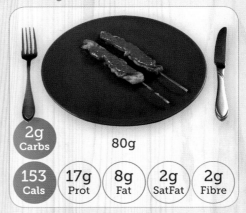

2g Carbs

80g

153 Cals | 17g Prot | 8g Fat | 2g SatFat | 2g Fibre

Tom Yum Soup (prawn)

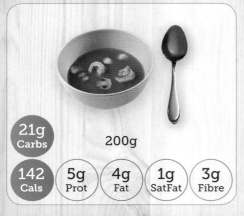

21g Carbs

200g

142 Cals | 5g Prot | 4g Fat | 1g SatFat | 3g Fibre

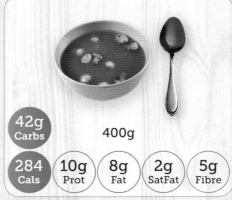

42g Carbs

400g

284 Cals | 10g Prot | 8g Fat | 2g SatFat | 5g Fibre

Nasi Goreng

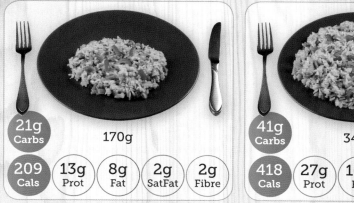

21g Carbs
170g
209 Cals · 13g Prot · 8g Fat · 2g SatFat · 2g Fibre

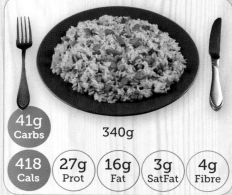

41g Carbs
340g
418 Cals · 27g Prot · 16g Fat · 3g SatFat · 4g Fibre

Paella

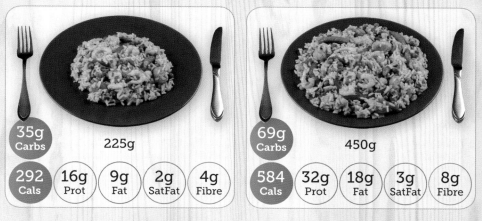

35g Carbs
225g
292 Cals · 16g Prot · 9g Fat · 2g SatFat · 4g Fibre

69g Carbs
450g
584 Cals · 32g Prot · 18g Fat · 3g SatFat · 8g Fibre

Nachos with Cheese

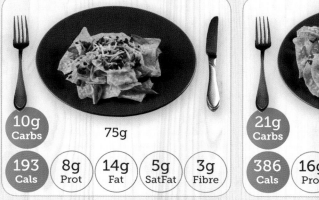

10g Carbs
75g
193 Cals · 8g Prot · 14g Fat · 5g SatFat · 3g Fibre

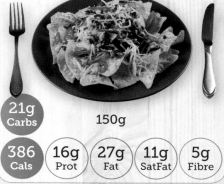

21g Carbs
150g
386 Cals · 16g Prot · 27g Fat · 11g SatFat · 5g Fibre

26cm Dinner Plate

Bean Burrito

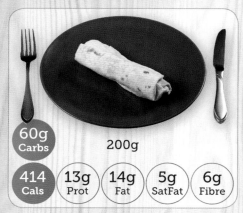

60g Carbs

200g

414 Cals | **13g** Prot | **14g** Fat | **5g** SatFat | **6g** Fibre

Bean Quesadilla

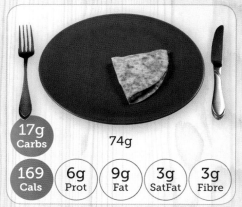

17g Carbs

74g

169 Cals | **6g** Prot | **9g** Fat | **3g** SatFat | **3g** Fibre

Beef Taco

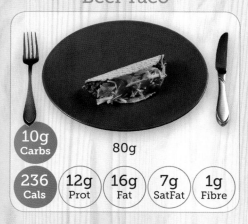

10g Carbs

80g

236 Cals | **12g** Prot | **16g** Fat | **7g** SatFat | **1g** Fibre

Chicken Burrito

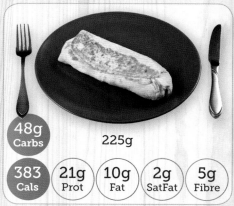

48g Carbs

225g

383 Cals | **21g** Prot | **10g** Fat | **2g** SatFat | **5g** Fibre

Chicken Enchilada

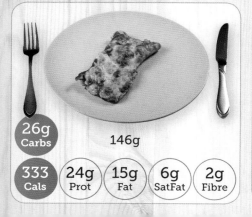

26g Carbs

146g

333 Cals | **24g** Prot | **15g** Fat | **6g** SatFat | **2g** Fibre

Chicken Fajita

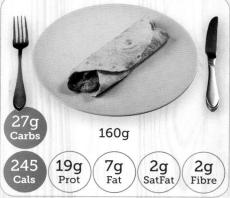

27g Carbs

160g

245 Cals | **19g** Prot | **7g** Fat | **2g** SatFat | **2g** Fibre

Burger King (per item)

	Carbs	Cals	Prot	Fat	SatFat	Fibre
Angus Classic	48g	580	31g	29g	9g	3g
Angus Smoked Bacon & Cheddar	49g	701	39g	38g	14g	3g
Big King	49g	587	29g	31g	11g	3g
Cheeseburger	33g	303	16g	12g	5g	2g
Chicken Burger	42g	392	11g	20g	4g	2g
Chicken Nuggets (6 pieces)	22g	318	17g	18g	5g	1g
Chicken Royale	49g	567	23g	31g	4g	3g
Double Whopper	46g	840	46g	52g	17g	3g
Fries (large)	52g	395	5g	18g	5g	4g
Fries (regular)	36g	277	4g	12g	4g	3g
Hamburger	32g	263	14g	9g	3g	2g
King Fish	44g	502	18g	28g	6g	3g
Whopper	46g	611	27g	35g	9g	3g
Whopper Junior	34g	335	14g	16g	4g	2g

Domino's Pizza (per medium slice, classic crust)

	Carbs	Cals	Prot	Fat	SatFat	Fibre
American Hot	20g	181	8g	8g	4g	1g
Cheese & Tomato	19g	144	6g	5g	3g	1g
Chicken Feast	20g	167	10g	8g	3g	1g
Deluxe	20g	180	8g	8g	4g	1g
Extravaganza	20g	199	10g	9g	5g	2g
Farmhouse	20g	156	8g	5g	3g	1g
Hawaiian	20g	158	8g	5g	3g	1g
Hot & Spicy	20g	152	7g	5g	3g	1g
Meat Lovers	19g	192	9g	9g	4g	1g
Meateor	23g	214	9g	10g	4g	1g
Tuna Delight	20g	161	8g	5g	3g	1g
Veg-A-Roma	21g	161	6g	6g	2g	1g
Vegetarian Supreme	20g	151	6g	5g	3g	1g
Vegi Volcano	20g	167	8g	6g	3g	1g

EAT (per item)

	Carbs	Cals	Prot	Fat	SatFat	Fibre
Apple & Berry Bircher Muesli	45g	379	15g	16g	1g	8g
Beef & Ale Pie	59g	553	22g	28g	15g	4g
Beef Ragu Soup (big)	21g	283	21g	11g	4g	4g
Cheddar Ploughmans Sandwich	68g	638	27g	30g	15g	4g
Chicken & Vegetable Soup (big)	19g	172	19g	2g	0g	3g
Chicken & Mushroom Pie	57g	685	28g	38g	21g	4g
Chicken & Bacon Caesar Sandwich	52g	543	29g	25g	5g	4g
Chicken Pho Broth Pot	50g	330	25g	2g	0g	3g
Ham & Free Range Egg Bloomer	48g	573	32g	29g	8g	5g
Hoi Sin Duck Gyoza Broth Pot	70g	398	18g	4g	1g	5g
Hot & Sour Chicken Soup (big)	16g	140	15g	2g	0g	2g
Hot Smoked Salmon & Potato Salad	16g	334	15g	22g	4g	3g
Roasted Butternut Squash & Feta Pie	41g	630	18g	44g	24g	4g
Sesame Shiitake Mushroom Broth	37g	338	16g	11g	2g	5g

KFC (per item)

	Carbs	Cals	Prot	Fat	SatFat	Fibre
Chicken Breast	6g	260	33g	12g	2g	-
Chicken Drumstick	7g	170	32g	10g	2g	-
Chicken Thigh	7g	285	22g	21g	5g	-
Chicken Wing	5g	185	17g	11g	2g	-
Coleslaw (regular)	8g	145	1g	12g	1g	-
Fillet Burger	47g	440	29g	15g	2g	-
Fillet Tower Burger	65g	620	32g	26g	5g	-
Fries (regular)	42g	310	4g	15g	2g	-
Fries (large)	61g	450	6g	21g	3g	-
Hot Wings	4g	85	5g	6g	1g	-
Kids Burger	31g	260	17g	7g	1g	-
Popcorn Chicken (regular)	15g	285	21g	16g	3g	-
Zinger Burger	48g	450	26g	18g	3g	-
Zinger Tower Burger	63g	620	29g	29g	6g	-

McDonald's (per item)

	Carbs	Cals	Prot	Fat	SatFat	Fibre
Bacon & Egg McMuffin	27g	348	21g	17g	6g	2g
Big Mac	43g	508	26g	25g	10g	4g
Cheeseburger	31g	301	16g	12g	6g	2g
Chicken McNuggets (6 pieces)	18g	259	16g	13g	2g	1g
Chocolate Milkshake (regular)	66g	380	10g	8g	5g	2g
Fillet 'o' Fish	36g	329	15g	13g	3g	3g
Fries (large)	55g	444	4g	22g	2g	5g
Fries (regular)	42g	337	3g	17g	2g	4g
Hamburger	30g	250	13g	8g	3g	2g
McChicken Sandwich	43g	388	17g	16g	2g	3g
Quarter Pounder with Cheese	37g	518	31g	27g	13g	3g
Sausage & Egg McMuffin	27g	430	26g	24g	9g	2g
Smarties McFlurry	48g	322	6g	12g	8g	1g
Strawberry Milkshake	68g	379	9g	8g	5g	1g

Nando's (per item)

	Carbs	Cals	Prot	Fat	SatFat	Fibre
½ Chicken	4g	644	92g	29g	7g	0g
¼ Chicken (breast)	4g	330	58g	9g	2g	0g
5 Chicken Wings	0g	336	36g	21g	5g	1g
Butterfly Burger	42g	568	64g	15g	3g	5g
Chicken Butterfly	0g	331	57g	11g	2g	1g
Chicken Thighs	1g	582	71g	33g	7g	2g
Chips (regular)	79g	546	8g	21g	1g	8g
Grilled Chicken Burger	42g	388	35g	8g	1g	4g
Grilled Chicken Wrap	59g	586	37g	22g	3g	3g
Mushroom & Halloumi Burger	59g	670	21g	38g	11g	5g
Mushroom & Halloumi Wrap	60g	784	22g	50g	13g	4g
Veggie Burger	65g	463	18g	14g	2g	6g
Veggie Pitta	64g	447	18g	12g	1g	5g
Whole Chicken	8g	1266	183g	56g	14g	0g

	Carbs	Cals	Prot	Fat	SatFat	Fibre
Pizza Express (per item)						
American	91g	804	39g	33g	14g	6g
Calzone Classico	100g	953	47g	43g	15g	8g
Dough Balls	42g	347	8g	17g	10g	3g
Fiorentina	93g	830	44g	33g	13g	7g
Four Seasons	92g	679	30g	23g	7g	7g
Garlic Bread	42g	239	8g	5g	3g	3g
La Reine	92g	740	39g	26g	11g	7g
Lasagna Classica	45g	623	38g	33g	16g	0g
Margherita	91g	683	33g	23g	10g	6g
Melanzane Parmigiana	26g	607	22g	45g	16g	8g
Niçoise Salad	45g	532	38g	23g	4g	4g
Giardiniera	96g	906	35g	44g	12g	10g
Pollo Pesto	86g	1136	43g	68g	29g	4g
Sloppy Giuseppe	98g	952	53g	39g	18g	8g
Pret (per item)						
Avocado & Herb Salad Wrap	39g	499	12g	31g	6g	-
Bacon & Egg Breakfast Roll	28g	459	24g	27g	10g	-
Brie, Tomato & Basil Baguette	54g	430	16g	16g	8g	3g
Chicken Avocado Sandwich	45g	482	25g	22g	4g	7g
Chicken Caesar & Bacon Baguette	62g	622	32g	26g	5g	4g
Chicken, Broccoli & Brown Rice Soup	14g	126	11g	3g	1g	2g
Free-Range Egg Mayo Sandwich	51g	367	19g	11g	1g	3g
Hoisin Duck Salad Wrap	48g	451	22g	17g	3g	-
Miso Soup	4g	32	2g	1g	0g	0g
Tuna Mayo & Cucumber Baguette	57g	539	24g	23g	2g	3g
Humous Salad Wrap	42g	430	11g	22g	3g	5g
Roasted Pumpkin Soup	18g	152	6g	5g	1g	-
Tuscan Bean Soup	21g	156	6g	5g	1g	-
Wild Crayfish & Rocket Sandwich	44g	394	22g	14g	1g	3g

Subway (per 6 inch sub, Italian bread)

	Carbs	Cals	Prot	Fat	SatFat	Fibre
Bacon, Egg and Cheese	45g	498	28g	22g	9g	3g
Beef	39g	274	22g	3g	1g	3g
Chicken & Bacon Ranch Melt	42g	494	37g	19g	8g	3g
Chicken Breast	40g	295	26g	3g	1g	3g
Club	40g	302	28g	3g	1g	3g
Italian B.M.T.	40g	387	20g	17g	7g	3g
Meatball Marinara	50g	426	23g	15g	7g	6g
Spicy Italian	39g	463	20g	25g	11g	3g
Steak and Cheese	42g	335	24g	8g	4g	3g
Subway Melt	40g	350	27g	9g	4g	3g
Tuna	40g	347	19g	12g	2g	3g
Turkey Breast	39g	260	27g	2g	1g	3g
Veggie Delite	37g	302	9g	2g	1g	6g
Veggie Patty	45g	364	20g	10g	3g	7g

Wagamama (per item)

	Carbs	Cals	Prot	Fat	SatFat	Fibre
Beef Massaman Curry	160g	1338	57g	52g	13g	7g
Chicken and Prawn Pad-Thai	73g	723	35g	30g	5g	9g
Chicken Katsu Curry	126g	1147	47g	50g	12g	5g
Chicken Raisukaree	152g	1371	42g	64g	25g	8g
Chicken Ramen	62g	513	41g	11g	2g	3g
Chilli Sirloin Steak Ramen	79g	665	68g	7g	2g	8g
Ginger Chicken Udon	79g	751	39g	29g	5g	10g
Seafood Ramen	71g	821	68g	28g	5g	5g
Surendra's Curry with Tilapia	157g	1352	39g	61g	13g	8g
Teriyaki Lamb	53g	890	54g	51g	11g	4g
Teriyaki Salmon Soba	68g	803	45g	38g	4g	6g
Yaki Soba	62g	700	35g	33g	4g	6g
Yaki Udon	79g	705	34g	26g	4g	10g
Yasai Ramen	53g	558	22g	28g	4g	5g

Index

■ = Gluten Free   ■ = per 100g

A

Ackee 278
Aduki Beans 304
Advocaat 112
Alcohol 109–113
Ale 109
All Bran 50, 61
Almond Milk 195, 198
Almonds 201
Alpen Bar 255
Apple 118, 131
    Chutney 267
    Danish 70
    (dried) 132, 135
    Juice 99
    Pie 84
    & Rhubarb Crumble 84
    Strudel 85
Apricots 117, 131
    (dried) 132, 135
Arrabbiata 156
Artichokes 278, 304
Asparagus 279, 304
Aubergine 279, 304
Avocado 280

B

Bacon 174, 193–194
Bagel 41
Baguette 43
Baked Beans 145, 280
    on Toast 144
    & Sausages 171
Baked Potato. *See* Jacket Potato
Bakery 70–75
Bakewell Tart 67
Baking Ingredients 76
Baklava 67
Bamboo Shoots 281
Banana 119, 131
    Bread 43
    Chips 133
Banoffee Pie 85

Bap 40
Barley 243
Basmati Rice 233, 243
Battenburg 71
Battered
    Fish 183
    Sausage 314
BBQ
    Chicken Wings 180
    Ribs 172
    Sauce 267
Bean
    Burrito 334
    Quesadilla 334
    Sprouts 281
Beans 304
    Aduki 304
    Baked 145, 280
    Black Eye 304
    Broad 282, 304
    Butter 284
    Edamame 289
    Green 289
    Haricot 304
    Kidney 290, 304
    Mung 304
    on Toast 144
    Pinto 304
    Soya 304
Béarnaise Sauce 267
Beef 176–178, 192
    Burger 177, 311
    Chow Mein 320
    Corned 177
    Crispy Shredded 321
    in Black Bean Sauce 320
    Massaman Curry 331
    Mince 192
    Patty 152
    Red Curry 330
    Roast 177
    Sausage 192
    Slice 176
    Steak 178, 192
    Stew 146
    Taco 334
    Wafer-thin 176
Beer 109
Beetroot 282, 304
Belgian Bun 75

Bhaji 326
Bhuna 329
Biryani 329
Biscuits 32–35, 141
Black
    Bean Sauce with Beef 320
    Eye Beans 304
    Forest Gateau 86
    Pudding 172
Blackberries 118, 131
BLT 244
Blueberries 120, 131
Blueberry Muffin 73
Blue Stilton. *See* Stilton
Boiled Egg 114
Bok Choy. *See* Pak Choy
Bolognese 164
Bombay
    Mix 247
    Potatoes 327
Bourbon Cream 32
Braising Steak 192
Brandy 113
Bran Flakes 50, 61
Brazil Nuts 201
Bread 38–48, 138–140
    & Butter Pudding 86
Breaded Fish 183
Breadstick 36, 140
Breakfast 49–66
    Tart 66
Brie 77
Brioche 49
Broad Beans 282, 304
Broccoli 283, 304
    & Stilton Soup 257
Brownie 87
Brown Sauce 268
Brussels
    Pâté 172
    Sprouts 283, 304
Buckwheat 243
Bulgur Wheat 240, 243
Burger 177
    Beef 311
    Bun 42
    Chicken 311
    Veggie 307, 311
Burger King 335

Burrito 334
Butter 260
    Beans 284
Butternut Squash 284, 304

C

Cabbage 285, 304
Caesar
    Dressing 268
    Salad 161
Cakes 69–71
Calamari 191
California Roll 324
Camembert 77
Cappuccino 105
Carbonara 165
Caribbean Dumplings 152
Carrot Cake 67
Carrots 285, 304
Cashews 201
Cashew Stir-fry 165
Cassava 232
    Chips 230, 232
Caster Sugar 76
Cauliflower 286, 304
Celeriac 304
Celery 286, 304
Cereal 50–58, 61, 136
    Bar 255
Champagne 112
Chapati 48
Cheddar 77–78
    Cracker 36
Cheese 77–83
    Macaroni 156
    Nachos 333
    Omelette 115
    & Pickle Sandwich 244
    Sandwich Grilled 245
    Scone 75
    Slice 82
    Straw 36
Cheesecake 87
Cherries 120, 131
Cherry Tomatoes 287

■ = Gluten Free   ■ = per 100g

Chicken 180–182, 193
  & Bacon Pie 158
  Balls 318
  Breast 181
  Burger 311
  Burrito 334
  Caesar Salad 161
  Curry 148, 320
  Drumsticks 180
  Enchilada 334
  Fajita 334
  Fried 312
  Goujon 145, **172**
  Green Curry 331
  Jerk 153
  Kiev 182
  Korma 328
  Lemon 321
  Noodle Soup 257
  Nuggets 312
  Pizza 159
  & Prawn Rice 332
  Roast 181
  Salad Sandwich 244
  Satay 332
  Stir-fry 166
  Tandoori 328
  Teriyaki 325
  Tikka Masala 328
  Wafer-thin 175
  Wings 180
Chickpea Flour 76
Chickpeas 287, 304
Chilli
  con Carne 147
  Sauce 268
Chinese Takeaway 318–322
Chips. *See also* **French Fries**
  Deep Fried 221, 232
  Oven 222, 232
  Takeaway 314
Choc Ice 92
Chocolate 251–254
  Brownie 87
  Bunny 254
  Cake 67
  Chip Cookie 32, 141
  Chip Twist 70
  Digestive 32, 141
  Éclair 71

Honeycomb Balls 253
Ice Cream 90
Individual 253
Mint 253
Mousse 88
Muffin 73
& Nut Cone 92
Nut Spread 263
Oat Biscuit 32
Orange 254
Ring Doughnut 72
Sandwich Biscuit 32
Snaps 51, 61
Torte 88
with Hazelnuts 252
Chorizo 175
Choux Pastry 76
Chow Mein 320
Christmas Pudding 89
Chutney. *See also* **Pickle**
  Apple 267
  Mango 271
Ciabatta 42
Cider 110
Cinnamon Swirl 70
Clementine 121, 131
Clotted Cream 199
Cocoa Powder 76
Coconut
  Desiccated 76
  Milk 195, 198
  Yogurt 310
Cod 189, 194
Coffee 105, 107–108
  & Walnut Cake 68
Cola 102
  Bottles 256
Coleslaw 167
Coley 194
Confectionery 250–254, 256
Cooked Breakfast 63
Cookie 32, 141
Cordial. *See* **Squash**
Corn
  Flake Cake 71
  Flakes 51, 61
  on the Cob 301, 305
Corned Beef 177
  Hash 146
Cornflour 76

Cornish Pasty 170
Cornmeal Porridge 59, 61
Coronation Chicken Sandwich 245
Cottage Cheese 79
Courgette 288, 304
Couscous 241, 243
Crab
    Meat 191
    Sticks. *See* Seafood Sticks
Crackers 36–37
Cranberries 121, 131
    (dried) 133, 135
Cranberry
    Juice 99
    Sauce 269
Cream 199–200
    Cheese 79
    Cracker 36
Crème
    Brûlée 92
    Fraîche 200
Crispbread 36, 140
Crisps 247
Crispy Shredded Beef 321
Croissant 49
Croquette 229, 232
Croutons 42
Crumble 84
Crumpet 41
Crunchy Clusters 61
Crusty Roll 40
Cucumber 288, 304
Cup Cake 71
Curry
    Beef Massaman 331
    Beef Red 330
    Chicken 148, 320
    Chicken Green 331
    Chicken Korma 328
    Chicken Tikka Masala 328
    Goat & Potato 153
    King Prawn Bhuna 329
    Lamb Rogan Josh 329
    Lentil 149, 330
    Vegetable 150, 330
Custard 89
    Cream 33
    Powder 76
    Slice 71
    Tart 71

D

Danish Pastries 70
Dark Chocolate 251
Dates (dried) 133, 135
Dauphinoise Potatoes 223, 232
Demerara Sugar 76
Desiccated Coconut 76
Desserts 84–98
Dextrose Tablets 256
Diet Cola 102
Digestive 33, 141
    Chocolate 32, 141
    Savoury 37
Domino's Pizza 335
Doner Kebab 313
Double Cream 199
Doughnuts 72–73
Dried Fruit 132–135, 135
    & Nuts 202
Duck 193
    Pancake 318
    Roast Peking 321
Dumplings 146
    Caribbean 152

E

Easter Egg 254
EAT 336
Eba 230, 232
Edam 79
Edamame Beans 289
Egg 76
    Fried Rice 236, 243
    Mayo Sandwich 245
    Noodles 217, 220
    White 76
    Yolk 76
Eggs 114–116
    Benedict 116
    Florentine 116
Eggy Bread 66
Enchilada 334
English
    Muffin 41
    Mustard 273
Espresso 108

■ = Gluten Free   ■ = per 100g

F

Fajita 334
Falafel in Pitta 313
Fennel 305
Feta 80
Fibre Flakes 136
Fig Roll 33
Figs 121, 131
   (dried) 134, 135
Filo Pastry 76
Finger Roll 42
Fish
   Battered 183, 314
   Breaded 183
   Cake 184
   & Chip Takeaway 314
   Fingers 145, **184**
   Fried 153
   Goujon 184
   Pie 151
   Stew 152
   Takeaway 314
Flapjack 74
Flaxseeds 205
Flour 76
Focaccia 43
French Fries 311
Fresh Cream Doughnut 73
Fried
   Bread 66
   Chicken 312
   Egg 114
   Fish 153
Fries 311. *See also* **Chips**
Frittata 160
Frosted Flakes 52, 61
Fruit 117–130, 131
   Cake 68
   Cocktail 122, 131
   (dried) 132–135, 135
   & Fibre 52, 61
   Scone 75
   Trellis 70
   Yogurt 308, 310
Fudge 250
Fufu 231, 232
   Flour 76

G

Game 192
Gammon 173
Gari 230, 232
   Flour 76
Garlic 305
   Bread 44
Ghee 261
Gherkins 167
Gin 113
Ginger 305
   Biscuit 33
   Cake 68
   Stem 76
Gingerbread Man 33
Glazed Ring Doughnut 72
Gluten Free 136–143
Gnocchi 223, 232
Goat & Potato Curry 153
Goat's
   Cheese 80
   Milk 195
Goose 193
Gooseberries 131
Goujon
   Chicken 145, **172**
   Fish 184
Grains 240–242, 243
Granola 53, 61
Granulated Sugar 76
Grapefruit 122, 131
   Juice 99
Grapenuts 61
Grapes 122, 131
Gravy 269
Greek
   Salad 161
   Yogurt 309, 310
Green Beans 289
Grilled Cheese Sandwich 245
Guacamole 269
Gyoza 323

H

Haddock 189, 194
Haggis 171
Halloumi 80

Ham
  Salad Sandwich 246
  Slice 176
  Wafer-thin 176
Haricot Beans 304
Hash Brown 229, 232
Hazelnuts 202
Hemp Milk 195
Hollandaise Sauce 270
Honey 263
  Nut Flakes 53, 61
  Puffed Wheat 54, 61
Horseradish Sauce 270
Hot
  Chocolate 106
  Cross Bun 75
  Dog 312
  Malt Drink 108
Houmous 270

I

Iceberg Lettuce 305
Ice Cream 90
  Cone 92
  Lolly 92
Iced
  Bun 75
  Ring 33
  Tea 104
Icing Sugar 76
Indian Takeaway 326–330
Irish Cream 112

J

Jacket Potato 224, 232
Jaffa Cake 34
Jam 263
  Doughnut 72
  Ring 34
Jamaican Beef Patty 152
Japanese Takeaway 323–325
Jelly 93
  Babies 256
  Beans 256
Jerk Chicken 153
Jollof Rice 152, 236, 243
Juice 99–100

K

Kale 305
Kebab 313
Ketchup 271
KFC 336
Kidney Beans 290, 304
Kiev 182
King Prawn Bhuna 329
King Prawns 185
Kipper 194
  Breakfast 63
Kiwi 123, 131
Korma 328

L

Lager 109
Lamb 179, 192–193
  Biryani 329
  Chop 179, 192–193
  Mince 192–193
  Roast 179
  Rogan Josh 329
  Samosa 326
  Steak 179
Lard 261
Lasagne 154
Latte 107
Leek 290, 305
Lemon
  Chicken 321
  Curd 264
  Meringue Pie 94
  Sorbet 91
Lemonade 103, 104
Lentil Curry 149, 330
Lentils 291, 304
Lettuce 291, 305
Licorice Allsorts 256
Lime Pickle 271
Linseeds 205
Lucozade Energy 103

M

Macadamia Nuts 202
Macaroni 206
  Cheese 156
Mackerel 188, 194
  Sashimi 325

■ = Gluten Free   ■ = per 100g

Maki Prawn 324
Malt
    Drink 104
    Hot Drink 108
    Loaf 69
Malted Milk 34
Malted Wheats 54, 61
Mangetout 292, 305
Mango 123, 131
    Chutney 271
Maple Syrup 264
Margarine 260
Margherita Pizza 315–317
Marmalade 264
Marmite 265
Marrow 305
Marshmallows 250
Marzipan 76
Mashed
    Potato 162, 225, 232
    Sweet Potato 227, 232
Massaman Curry 331
Mayonnaise 272
McDonald's 337
Meal Accompaniments 167
Melon 124, 130, 131
Meringue
    Nest 74
    Pie 94
Mexican
    Rice 237, 243
    Takeaway 334
Milk 195–198, 198
    Almond 195, 198
    Coconut 195, 198
    Goat's 195
    Hemp 195
    in bowl 58
    Oat 195
    Rice 195
    Soya 198, 198
Milk Chocolate 251
    Biscuit Bar 34
    Finger 34
    Wafer 34
Milkshake 198
Mince
    Beef 192
    Lamb 192–193
    Pie 74
    Pork 193–194

Mini Eggs 254
Mint Sauce 272
Miso Soup 323
Mixed Salad Leaves 292
Mousse 88
Mozzarella 81
Muesli 55, 61, 137
    Spelt 61
Muffin 73
Multigrain Hoops 56, 61
Mung Beans 304
Muscovado Sugar 76
Mushroom
    Risotto 155
    Soup 258
Mushrooms 293, 305
Mushy Peas 296
Mussels 194
Mustard 273

N

Naan Bread 47, 140
Nachos with Cheese 333
Nakd Bar 255
Nando's 337
Nasi Goreng 333
Natural Yogurt 310, 310
Nectarine 126, 131
New Potatoes 224, 232
Nice Biscuit 35
Nigiri 324
Noodles 217–218, 220
    Singapore 322
Noodle Soup 257
Nuts 201–204

O

Oat
    Flakes 61
    Milk 195
Oat Biscuit 35, 61
    Breakfast 58
    Chocolate 32
Oatcake 37
Oatmeal 76
Oats 61
Oil 262
Okra 295, 305
Olive Oil 262
    Spread 261

Olives 167
Omelette 115
Onion
    Bhaji 326
    Rings 168
    Soup 259
Onions 294, 305
    Pickled 168
Orange 124, 131
    Juice 100
Oven Chips 145, 222, 232
Oyster Mushrooms 305

P

Pad Thai with Prawns 331
Paella 333
Pain au
    Chocolat 49
    Raisins 70
Pak Choy 295
Pakora 327
Palm Oil 262
Pancake 64–65
    Duck 318
    Scotch 66
Pancetta 175
Panini 42
Panna Cotta 92
Papaya 125, 131
Paratha 48
Parma Ham 175
Parmesan 81
Parsley Sauce 273
Parsnips 297, 305
Partridge 192
Pasta 142–143, 206–216,
        219–220, 220
    Bake 157
    Bows 207
    Shapes 219
    Shells 208
    Twists 142, 209
Pastry 76
Pasty 170
Pâté 172
Peaches 126, 131
Peanut Butter 265
Peanuts 203
Pearl Barley 243
Pearled Spelt 243

Pears 127, 131
Peas 145, 296, 305
    Mushy 296
    Sugar Snap 302, 305
Pecan Plait 70
Pecans 203
Peking Duck 321
Penne 142, 210
    Arrabbiata 156
Pepperoni Pizza 159, 315–317
Peppers 297, 305
Persimmon 127, 131
Pesto 274
Pheasant 192
Piccalilli 274
Pickle 274
Pickled Onions 168
Pie
    Apple 84
    Banoffee 85
    Chicken & Bacon 158
    Fish 151
    Lemon Meringue 94
    Pork 170
    Shepherd's 163
    Steak 158
    Top Crust 158
Pilau Rice 237, 243
Pineapple 128, 131
    (dried) 134
    Juice 100
Pine Nuts 203
Pink Wafer 35
Pinto Beans 304
Pistachios 204
Pitta Bread 46, 140
Pizza 315–317
    Base 140
    Margherita 315-317
    Oven 159
    Pepperoni 315-317
    Vegetable 315-317
Pizza Express 338
Plaice 189
Plantain 298, 305
Plum 128, 131
Poached Egg 114
Polenta 242, 243
Pollock 194
Pomegranate 125, 131

■ = Gluten Free   ■ = per 100g

Popcorn 248
Poppadom 47
Poppy Seeded Roll 41
Pork 172–176, 193–194
    Belly 193–194
    Chop 173, 193–194
    Gyoza 323
    Mince 193–194
    Pie 170
    Roast 173
    Steak 193–194
    Sweet & Sour 322
Porridge 60, 61, 137
    Cornmeal 59, 61
Port 112
Potato
    Croquette 229, 232
    Jacket/Baked 224, 232
    Rosti 229, 232
    Salad 228, 232
    Slices 226, 232
    Smiles 145, 229, 232
    Waffle 229, 232
Potatoes 221–229, 232
    Bombay 327
Poultry 193
Prawn
    Bhuna 329
    Crackers 318
    Mayo Sandwich 246
    Pad Thai 331
    Soup 332
    Sushi 324
    Szechuan 322
    Tempura 323
    Toast 319
Prawns 185, 194
PRET 338
Pretzels 249
Processed Cheese Slice 82
Profiteroles 94
Prosciutto 175
Prunes 134, 135
Puffed Cracker 37
Puff Pastry 76
Pulses 304
Pumpernickel 44
Pumpkin 305
    Seeds 205
Puri 48
Puy Lentils 304

Q
Quesadilla 334
Quiche Lorraine 160
Quinoa 240, 243
Quorn 306

R
Rabbit 192
Rack of Lamb 192–193
Radishes 299, 305
Radish Leaves 305
Raisin Bites 56, 61
Raisin Bread 44
Raisins 135, 135
Raita 275
Rapeseed Oil 262
Raspberries 129, 131
Raspberry Sorbet 91
Ravioli
    Fresh 211
    Tinned 219
Red Leicester 83
Red Wine 111
Rhubarb 129, 131
    & Apple Crumble 84
Ribs 172
    Spare 319
Rice 233–239, 243
    Ball 325
    Basmati 233, 243
    Brown 149, 234, 243
    Cake 37, 140
    Chicken & Prawn 332
    Easy Cook 243
    Egg Fried 236, 243
    Jollof 152, 236, 243
    Long Grain 235, 243
    Mexican 237, 243
    Milk 195
    Noodles 218, 220
    & Peas 153, 238, 243
    Pilau 237, 243
    Pudding 95
    Snaps 57, 61
    Special Fried 238, 243
    Sticky White 239, 243
    White 147–148, 150, 235, 243
    Wholegrain 234, 243
    Wild 239, 243

Rich Tea 35
Ricotta 82
Risotto 155
Roast
    Beef 177
    Chicken 181
    Lamb 179
    Peking Duck 321
    Pork 173
    Potatoes 226, 232
    Turkey 182
Rocket 299
Rogan Josh 329
Roll 139
    Crusty 40
    Finger 42
    Poppy Seeded 41
Roti 48
Roulade 95
Rum 113
Rump Steak 178, 192
Rye
    Bread 45
    Flour 76

S

Sag Aloo Gobi 327
Salad
    Chicken Caesar 161
    Cream 275
    Greek 161
    Leaves 292
    Potato 228, 232
    Tuna Niçoise 161
Salami 175
Salmon 194
    Frittata 160
    Nigiri 324
    Sashimi 325
    Smoked 188
    Steak 190
    Tinned 186
Saltfish 188
Samosa 326
Sandwiches 244–246
Sardines 187, 194
Sashimi 325
Satay Chicken 332
Satsuma 129
Sauces 267–277

Sausage 174, 194
    Battered 314
    Beef 192
    & Mash 162
    Pork 170
    Veggie 307
    & Yorkshire Pudding 166
Sausages & Beans 171
Savoury
    Biscuit 141
    Digestive 37
Scallops 189, 194
Scampi 184
Scotch Egg 116
Scotch Pancake 66
Scrambled Eggs 114
    with Tomato & Halloumi 63
Sea Bream 194
Seafood 183–191, 194
    Sticks 191
Seeds 205
Self-Raising Flour 76
Sesame Oil 262
Shallots 305
Shepherd's Pie 163
Sherry 112
Shish Kebab 313
Shortbread Finger 35
Shortcake 35
Shortcrust Pastry 76
Singapore Noodles 322
Single Cream 199
Sirloin Steak 178, 192
Sliced Bread 38–39, 138–140
Smoked
    Mackerel 188
    Salmon 188
Smoothie 101
Snacks 247–249, 255
Sorbet 91
Soup 257–259
    Miso 323
    Tom Yum 332
Sourdough 45
Soured Cream 200
Soya
    Beans 304
    Milk 198, 198
    Nuts 204
    Yogurt 309, 310

■ = Gluten Free   ■ = per 100g

Soy Sauce 275
Spaghetti 143, 212–213, 220
  Bolognese 164
  Carbonara 165
  Hoops 220
  Tinned 219
Spare Ribs 319
Special
  Flakes 57, 61, 136
  Fried Rice 238, 243
Spelt
  Bread 45
  Muesli 61
  Pearled 243
Spinach 300, 305
Spirits 113
Spotted Dick 96
Spreadable Cheese 82
Spreads 260–265
Spring
  Greens 300
  Roll 319
Squash 101
  Butternut 284, 304
Squid Rings. *See* Calamari
Squirty Cheese 82
Steak
  Beef 192
  & Kidney Pudding 158
  Lamb 179
  Pie 158
  Pork 193–194
  & Potato Pie 158
  Rump 178, 192
  Sirloin 178, 192
Stem Ginger 76
Stewing Steak 192
Sticky
  Toffee Pudding 96
  White Rice 239, 243
Stilton 83
  & Broccoli Soup 257
Stir-fry 165–166
Stout 109
Strawberries 130, 131
Strawberry
  Delight 97
  Tartlet 92
Streaky Bacon 174, 193–194
Strudel 85

Stuffing 169
Subway 339
Sugar 76, 108, 266
  Ring Doughnut 72
Sugar Snap Peas 302, 305
Sultanas 135, 135
Summer Pudding 97
Sun-dried Tomatoes 168
Sunflower Seeds 205
Sushi 324
Swede 305
Sweet
  Biscuit 141
  Chilli Sauce 276
  Liqueur 113
  Potato 227, 232
  Potato Mash 227, 232
  & Sour Pork 322
  & Sour Sauce 276
  White Wine 111
Sweetcorn 301, 305
Sweetener 266
Sweets 256
Swiss Roll 69
Szechuan Prawns 322

T

Taco
  Beef 334
  Shell 46
Tagliatelle 143, 214
Tandoori Chicken 328
Tart 66
Tartare Sauce 276
Tartlet 92
Tea 108
  Biscuit 141
  Cake 41
  Iced 104
Tempura Prawn 323
Teriyaki Chicken 325
Thai Takeaway 330–333
Thousand Island Dressing 277
Tikka Masala Chicken 328
Tiramisu 98
Toad in the Hole 166
Toast 62
  Beans on 144
  Prawn 319
  Toppings 263–265

■ = Gluten Free   ■ = per 100g

Tofu (fried) 307
Tomato 302, 305
   Cherry 287, 305
   Juice 100
   Soup 259
   Sun-dried 168
Tom Yum Soup 332
Top Crust Pie 158
Torte 88
Tortellini 215
Tortilla 47
   Chips 249
Trifle 98
Trout 190, 194
Tubers 230–231, 232
Tuna
   Mayo Sandwich 246
   Niçoise Salad 161
   Nigiri 324
   Sashimi 325
   Steak 190, 194
   Tinned 186
Turkey 193
   Breast 182
   Roast 182
   Slice 176
   Wafer-thin 176
Turkish Flatbread 46
Turnip 303, 305

V

Vanilla Ice Cream 90
Vegetable
   Curry 330
   Oil 262
   Pakora 327
   Pizza 315–317
   & Potato Curry 150
   Samosa 326
   Soup 258
Vegetables 278–303, 304–305
Vegetarian Alternatives 306–307
Veggie
   Burger 307, 311
   Lasagne 154
   Sausage 307
Venison 192
Vermicelli 216, 220
Vermouth 112

Victoria Sponge 69
Vodka 113

W

Wafer 34, 35
Wafer-thin
   Beef 176
   Chicken 175
   Ham 176
   Turkey 176
Waffle 66
   Potato 229, 232
Wagamama 339
Walnut & Coffee Cake 68
Walnuts 204
Water
   Biscuit 37
   Chestnuts 305
Watercress 303
Watermelon 130, 131
Wedges 228, 232
Wensleydale with Cranberries 83
Wheat
   Biscuit 58, 61
   Pillow 58, 61
Whipped Cream 200
Whisky 113
White
   Chocolate 252
   Sauce 277
   Wine 111
Wholegrain Cracker 37
Wild Rice 239, 243
Wine 111
   Gums 256
WKD 110
Worcestershire Sauce 277

Y

Yam 231, 232
Yogurt 308–310, 310
   Coconut 310
   Fruit 308, 310
   Greek 309, 310
   Natural 310, 310
   Soya 309, 310
Yorkshire Pudding 169
Yum Yum 73

About the Authors

Chris Cheyette BSc (Hons) MSc RD
Diabetes Specialist Dietitian

Chris is a Diabetes Specialist Dietitian within the NHS, working with people with type 1, type 2 and gestational diabetes. Chris has spearheaded a number of projects over the years, many with the aim of improving diabetes educational resources. These include an educational DVD for young people with diabetes, which earned him the 2007 British Dietetic Association Elizabeth Washington Award. Chris has also published a number of journal articles on weight management and diabetes. He regularly undertakes local and national presentations to healthcare professionals, has done TV & newspaper interviews, and has participated as a guest expert in online discussions.

Yello Balolia BA (Hons)
Creative Entrepreneur

Having achieved a first class honours degree in Photography, Canada-born, Blackpool-bred and now London-based Yello used his entrepreneurial and creative skills to found Chello Publishing Limited with Chris Cheyette, to publish Carbs & Cals (**www.carbsandcals.com**), the bestselling and multi-award-winning book and app for diabetes and weight management. He has also undertaken a series of creative projects including The Cure for Normal: a YouTube channel inspiring people to look at the world differently (**www.curefornormal.com**), Magical: a 3-day music & arts festival (**www.magicalfestival.co.uk**), and private art commissions (**www.yellobalolia.com**).

Awards

BDA 2019 Elizabeth Washington
Award for Educational Work

Best Dietary Management Initiative at the Quality in Care Awards 2014

New Product of the Year in the Complete Nutrition Awards 2012

BDA 2011 Dame Barbara Clayton
Award for Innovation & Excellence

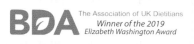

BDA — The Association of UK Dietitians — Winner of the 2019 Elizabeth Washington Award

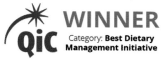

QiC — WINNER — Category: **Best Dietary Management Initiative** — Quality in Care Programme 2014

BDA — The Association of UK Dietitians — Winner of the 2011 Dame Barbara Clayton Award

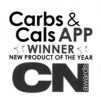

Carbs & Cals APP — WINNER — NEW PRODUCT OF THE YEAR — CN awards

Carbs & Cals